Massage Yourself

Self-massage of muscles, tendons and ligaments

First Edition

Rowland Benjamin D.O.

Copyright © 2022
First Edition September 2022

Published by R Benjamin
Western Australia

Massage Yourself (Print version)

ISBN 978-0-9581119-2-8

Preface

I am an osteopath and several years ago I was treating a patient with a rotator cuff tear following a sporting injury. He was a mine worker who only came home once a month and so was unable to attend my clinic for regular treatment. I had given him the appropriate exercises to stretch and strengthen key tissues, but he really needed more treatment - specifically transverse friction for 30 seconds every two or three days. This was usually something I did as part of a broader treatment. But as the mine worker was out of town for a month, I knew this was not going to happen. So, I showed him where to position his arm to expose the rotator cuff tendon, where to locate it and how to treat it himself. The patient recovered quickly, there was no pain and over that month his cuff tear had repaired. This approach proved useful for other patients who needed to come in for short sessions but were unavailable or inconvenienced by having to come in for such a short treatment. So began my teaching of self-massage to my patients and the journey that was to become this book.

'Massage Yourself' was written for several reasons. It defines my method of massage as one based on anatomy and logic, provides a comprehensive list of self-massage techniques covering the muscles, tendons and ligament of the body, empowers people with the skills to help their body function better and to treat specific soft tissues problems and helps them develop greater awareness of their own bodies and name its different parts.

I strive to bring a creative angle into my work and about three years ago I decided it would be fun to turn my massage techniques on myself. I thought it would be interesting to take the rules or principles of the techniques that I use on my patients and apply them to techniques on my own body. By being both the giver and receiver of the massage, I challenged the idea that massage was only something that was passively received by you or done to you. I wanted to combine my knowledge of anatomy and massage and create a system of self-massage that would be useful, add something new to the large repository of existing scientific knowledge and push a few boundaries.

I have been studying, teaching and writing books about massage for many years, as well as using it to treat patients, and the knowledge that I have acquired has helped me write this book. The material that I have accumulated from writing my earlier books has been useful for the creation of this book and the material from this book will be useful for my next book, entitled 'Treat Yourself' as well as for hand-outs for my patients. Self-massage is a useful tool and the material from this book should result in quicker and better outcomes in my clinic.

When I started work on this book, I focused on developing and testing the techniques on myself. I knew anatomy and the principles of massage, and I did not want to just follow another authors' publication and duplicate what had already been written. It had to be worked out by me on myself first-hand. The questions I asked myself as I attempted to work out each technique was what posture do I adopt for greatest safety and efficiency? what is the best way to reach the soft tissue - do I push with my hand or massage tool or use my body weight? and how do I move the limb or body part of the tissue that is being massaged?

After working out the mechanics of the technique I began writing out a list of step by step bullet points in a Word document on my computer. When this was done I played the 'Read Aloud' function in the Review section of Word and followed the instructions. Listening to what I had written, and doing the technique in real time, helped me modify the text so that it flowed and was clearer for the reader.

After refining the text, I started taking photographs of myself doing the techniques, trying different angles and lighting to show what I was doing. Although the selfies were useful experiments, the quality of the photographs was poor and so I employed Simon Harrington, who had a good camera, better lighting and an eye for taking a great photograph.

The graphic design involved adjusting the contrast and effects on the photographs and resizing them, creating the muscle diagrams, and creating line drawings from the photographs and then laying out the images among the text.

Self-massage can complement treatment by helping to fix problems or remove the need for treatment by preventing health problems developing. Self-massage can reduce treatment time and improve the health and efficiency of your muscles, tendons and ligaments without the need for expensive equipment, and once learned, can be used safely at home. Self-massage is suitable for the sedentary person or athlete, the layperson or professional.

Massage Yourself is comprehensive and concise. It contains a list of safe and effective massage techniques, and it focuses on specific areas of the body and targets specific muscles and muscle groups without unnecessary repetition. It covers two main types of technique: kneading and friction, and explains which soft tissues are being massaged and where they are located, which part of your hand or massage tool is best to use and it explains how to do the massage technique.

Massage Yourself is clear, easy to read, user friendly and contains hundreds of photographs and line drawings showing massage techniques for every part of the body, as well as anatomy illustrations explaining which muscles are being massaged. The bullet points take you through the techniques step-by-step.

Self-massage works well with manual therapies and medicine in general. The techniques can be used prescriptively for a wide range of problems encountered by the therapist. It is especially useful when lots of short sessions of treatment are needed but are inconvenient for the patient. A patient can be working on his or her problem between treatments. Working from home can be so much easier and time saving.

The book is useful for anyone who works with their own body including manual workers, musicians, dancers, yoga students, personal trainers, sports coaches, athletes and sports people. It is also useful for anyone who works on other people's bodies including masseurs, osteopaths, physiotherapists, chiropractors, manual therapists, yoga teachers, naturopaths, medical doctors, exercise physiologists, Pilates and aerobics teachers.

Massage Yourself is divided into introduction, techniques and appendix. The introduction defines some of the key terms, goals and concepts around self-massage, explains how massage works and how it can be used. It discusses the difference between massage and self-massage and the pros and cons of self-massage. It looks at the dozen or so places on the hand from where contact and pressure is applied to the soft tissues and the three massage tools recommended in this book: the two rubber balls in a net, the tightly rolled-up towel and the wadi, and indications and contraindication for their use. It explains the purpose of the techniques and the differences between them.

The introduction also looks at other types of massage, as well as anatomy, ergonomics, the working environment, palpation (the art and skill of feeling soft tissues), props, the ideal routine, side effects and as well it provides tips on how to do self-massage, especially for first time users. It lists medical conditions requiring caution and looks at how gravity, lifestyle, genetics and the curvatures of the spine affect posture.

The technique section is divided into part A jaw and spine, part B upper limb and part C lower limb and contains the massage techniques, including the starting positions (standing, sitting on a chair, laying on your back or kneeling on the floor) and the actions needed for the execution of the technique. This main section works through the soft tissues of the body in the following order: jaw, suboccipital, cervical and thoracic spine, ribs, lumbar and sacroiliac spine, shoulder, arm, elbow, forearm, wrist, hand, hip, thigh, knee, leg, ankle and foot.

The appendix contains a glossary of anatomical terms used in this book. I have used words that everyone can understand, but in a technical book like this some words will inevitably fall outside the domain of common usage. When these words needed to be explained they were added to the list in the appendix. Also in the appendix is a list of muscles and their actions. Each joint is listed, followed by its of movement and the muscles that produce that movement.

I am confident Massage Yourself will be of great benefit to all serious users and I hope you enjoy doing the techniques and exploring the muscles, tendons and ligaments of your body.

Biography

The author, Rowland Benjamin has worked as an Osteopath for thirty-seven years and in the health and massage field of massage for over forty years. In the late 1970s he established yoga schools in Australia and the U.K and worked with yoga and massage for several years before training as an Osteopath at the N.S.W. College of Natural Therapies and the Pacific College of Osteopathic medicine, Sydney, Australia. He set up his first Osteopathic practice in July 1985 in Sydney, Australia. In 1987 he moved to Liverpool, UK and worked for a year there and used the time for postgraduate studies at The British School of Osteopathy.

Rowland started working as a lecturer in 1987 teaching 'Natural medicine' for Liverpool City Council and 'Natural living' at Burton Manor College, Cheshire, U.K. Since then, he has lectured in Alternative medicine, Natural living, Soft tissue technique, Surface anatomy, Transverse friction, Deep tissue massage, Contemporary health issues, Life skills, Hydrotherapy and Advanced massage at various colleges in Perth, Western Australia.

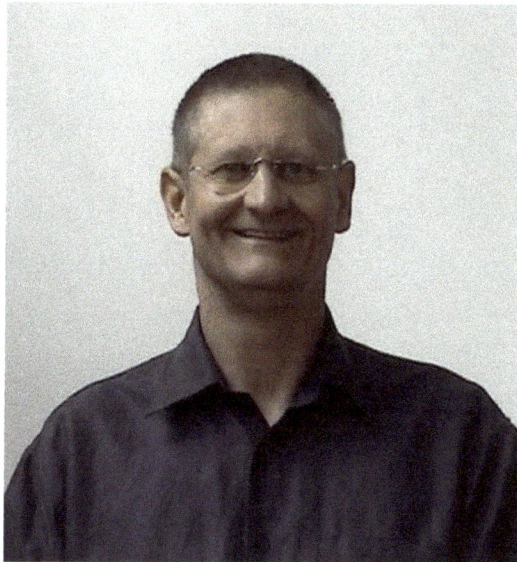

During his career as an Osteopath Rowland has worked in Australia and the UK in private practice and as a locum. His first book 'Myofaction - Myofascial Manipulation' was published in 2002 and has sold widely. In 2015 he published 'Safe Stretch' that looked at individual differences and took them into account when prescribing the right stretches. www.safe-stretch.info. Rowland also authors environmental books that use cartoons and the written word to explain and generate greater awareness about the issues www.ecofreakocartoons.com

The author has travelled extensively throughout Australia, New Zealand, Asia, the Middle East, Europe, Africa, North America, Central America and South America. He has worked as an environmental activist and lobbyist for over forty years and currently runs Information for Action www.informaction.org.

In the 1990s he engaged in a musical career for a few years, writing and performing his song in Australia and the UK. Since 2010 he has been working on the construction of a Permaculture based orchard and nature area in Bridgetown, Western Australia where he resides and practices osteopathy. Progress at Bridgetown Hillside Garden can be viewed at www.bhg.org.au. He continues to practice evidence based and anatomy based manual therapy using self-help systems such as stretching and self-massage to empower his patients.

Acknowledgments

I would like to thank Simon Harrington for his photography, Mike Eales for keeping my computers running, Leo Wai Kwan Lee for help setting up the Massage Yourself website www.massage-yourself.com, Tim Wilson for his pastel drawing on the header of the website, Doreen Mackman for proofreading my book and my partner Nirada, for her feedback and help with taking photographs.

Contents

List of Techniques

x

Introduction to Massage Yourself

Theory and Practice

Massage is a form of manual therapy or physical therapy. It is the practice of manipulating the soft tissues: muscles, tendons, ligaments and fascia, and the fluids of the body with an applicator, usually your hand or hands, another part of your body or a massage tool. This book is concerned with self-treatment, self-help and personal empowerment and describes a remedial massage system where you massage yourself.

In general, the goals of massage are to:

- reduce pain
- restore function when there is dysfunction
- optimise muscle flexibility and joint range of movement
- improve posture and treat the effects of postural fatigue
- increase resilience so that you can cope better with physical and mental stress
- enhance health, vitality and wellbeing

The self-massage techniques described in this book can be used proactively to build better structural integrity in muscles, tendons and ligaments and help prevent musculoskeletal problems developing, and they can be used in response to illness and dysfunction to treat musculoskeletal problems. The musculoskeletal system includes your bones, cartilage, ligaments, tendons and muscles. Tissues are made from cells with a similar structure and an extracellular matrix. Soft tissues are tissues that are not hardened by the processes of ossification or calcification such as bones and teeth. They connect, support, or surround other structures and organs of the body and include muscles, tendons, ligaments, fascia, nerves, fibrous tissues, fat, blood vessels, and synovial membranes.

All the techniques in this book can be used by the layperson and there is no need to be under anyone's supervision if you are doing the self-massage techniques proactively. But when there is a health problem that needs self-massage, it is important to get an assessment and have an accurate diagnosis of the condition from a qualified health professional. It is difficult to examine oneself, especially your own spine, and it is important to know whether the tissues involved with your problem are tendons, ligaments or muscles or something else. This is not a self-diagnosis book. People without medical training should be under the supervision of a tertiary trained health professional, a physical therapist such as an osteopath if they want to treat themselves with the techniques described in this book. The therapist should be able to give you the name of your condition and the soft tissues you need to massage, show you where they are and teach you how to massage them.

The word 'massage' is used in the title of this book 'Massage Yourself' because it keeps the title concise. There are dozens of kinds of massage, but the type described in this book is remedial massage or soft tissue manipulation. 'Massage Yourself' could have been entitled 'Self-directed Soft Tissue Manipulation' or 'Manipulate Your Own Soft Tissues' but 'Massage Yourself' is more succinct. The full title of this book is 'Massage Yourself - Self-massage of muscles, tendons and ligaments' because of the wide range of soft tissues being covered.

There are advantages and disadvantages to massaging yourself. One advantage of self-massage is that it gives you independence and allows you to choose when and where you do the massaging. It gives you control over the amount of force to use and how long to hold the pressure. And because you can feel the tissue that you are massaging, this feedback allows you to move your applicator to exactly the right place, and often the place that hurts the most is the source of the problem. Another advantage is it gives you time to relax the muscle before removing the applicator pressure and moving on to another area. With self-massage you can back-off if the muscle is going into spasm or too painful or increase the pressure if it is easy to let go of the muscle tension. Your ability to relax effectively depends on the technique, how well you relax, and your skill level. You are likely to get better at letting go of the muscle the more you do the self-massage techniques.

A disadvantage of self-massage is that a masseur will usually be able to generate greater force on the tissue than you can when working on yourself because they have the mechanical advantage of their body weight. Also, a masseur will usually have greater technical and palpation skills than you and may have years of experience.

Applicators

An applicator is a part of your hand or another part of your body or a massage tool. Here are the applicators, listed in order from the most used applicator to the least used: 1. The tip of your thumb 2. One fingertip, usually the tip of your index finger 3. The tips of your index, middle and ring fingers together 4. The tip or outside of your thumb, in opposition with and the tips of one or two fingers using a grasping, push-pull action 5. The outside of your thumb 6. The pad of your thumb 7. The flat area that forms your knuckles when your fist is clenched - it includes most of your finger joints and half of the back of your fingers 8. One knuckle or a row of knuckles of your clenched fist 9. The pad of muscles at the base of your thumb (thenar eminence) 10. The heel of your hand. 11. Your pisiform bone

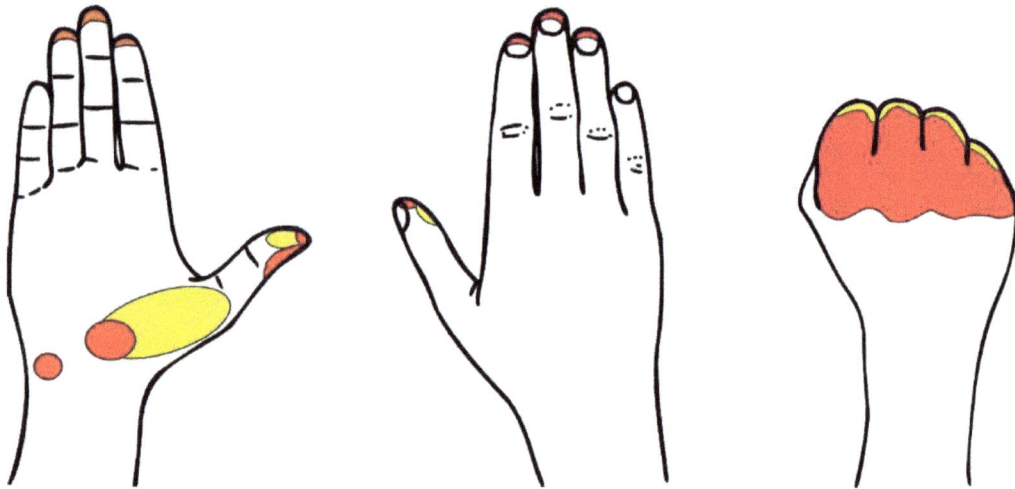

Massage tools are used to increase leverage and apply force on a muscle, tendon or ligament. They come in many different shapes and sizes to either transmit a broad force over a wide area of muscle or focus a narrow force over a small area of muscle, ligament or tendon. The three main massage tools used in this book are two rubber balls in a net, a tightly rolled-up towel and the wadi, two wheels linked by a narrow neck, and made from wood.

There are several important contraindications for massage tool use. Do not do any of the techniques involving lying on your back over a massage tool if you are overweight, have any spinal pathology such as osteoporosis, osteoarthritis, an increased kyphosis or an inflexible spine. Do not lie over a massage tool if it is uncomfortable. Sensitive bones at the back of the thoracic spine and rib cage may be irritated and painful if the massage tool is too hard. The rolled-up towel techniques should be done without the rolled-up towel if you have an increased kyphosis or any of the conditions listed above. If you have a rigid and flexed spine, then instead of using a massage tool under your back you may need a small pillow under your head to stop it dropping back into hyperextension. If the flexibility of your spine improves you may be able to reduce the height of the pillow.

The two rubber balls in a net are for kneading or inhibition and produce a moderate force over a broad area of muscle. One ball can function as a handle for the other ball or both balls can be used together on the muscle. The balls are made from medium density rubber or synthetic plastic material for optimum comfort and firmness. The net is a small bag, usually made from fishing net material but you could use a sock or stocking.

The tightly rolled-up towel is for inhibition and produces a mild to moderate force over a broad area of muscle. A threadbare towel or thin cotton T-towel is ironed flat and then carefully rolled into a dense cylindrical massage tool about 20 cm long and 4 cm in diameter. The rolled-up towel is mainly used on the spinal muscles but can be used on the shoulders or hips. It should be firm but comfortable to lie on.

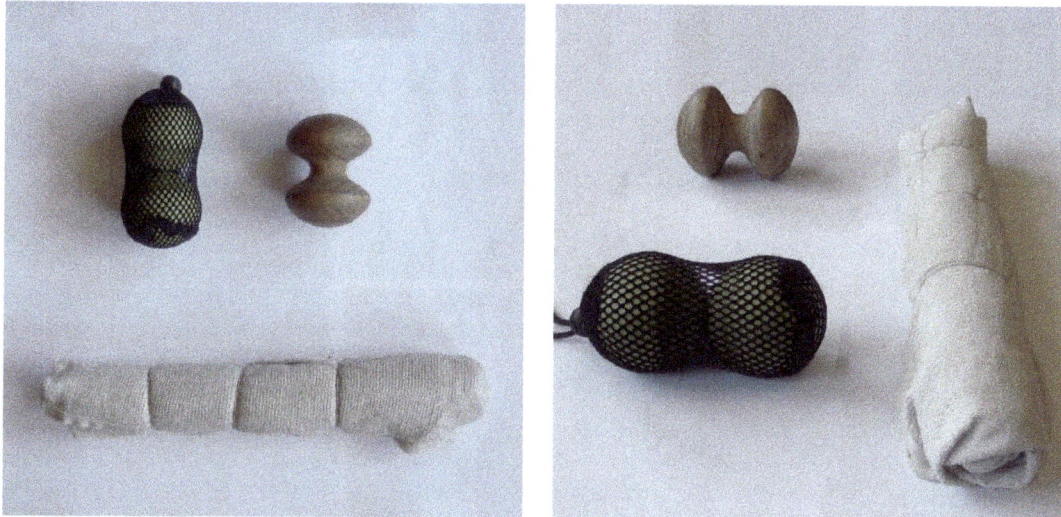

The wadi
The wadi consists of two slightly pointed wheels or half balls joined by a narrow neck. This massage tool is made from wood but could be made of a synthetic rubber or plastic compound. It is the firmest of the massage tools so it can easily push hard into the muscle. One wheel can function as a handle for the other wheel, or both wheels can be used together on the muscle.

Techniques used in this book

Kneading - also known as Cross Fibre Kneading

During kneading the applicator applies a mild to moderate force and a slow rhythmical pressure across muscle fibres. Muscle fibres are muscle cells, and a muscle is made up of many fibres, which vary in length, and can extend the entire length of a long muscle. The amount of force that needs to be used by the applicator depends on the thickness of the muscle, overlying fascia and skin, and whether the muscle is deep and situated under other muscles. During kneading you should try to relax the target muscle and overlying muscles.

Kneading involves the simultaneous combination of transverse, longitudinal and torsional forces acting on a muscle. These forces are the primary mechanism responsible for lengthening muscle fibres and decreasing muscle tension. Most tension is taken up with the transverse force, but effective kneading takes up tension with all forces. The more tension taken up by one, the less there is available for another, so it is important not to go too hard with one so there is no freedom left in the muscle for the others. The proportion of each also depends on the size, shape and depth of the muscle being kneaded. Focused breathing can also be used during kneading to induce relaxation. The applicator moves five to ten millimetres across the muscle - depending on the applicator, the size and depth of the muscle and the elasticity of the muscle and the skin.

Kneading involves:

1. compression and transverse forces - moving perpendicular to the muscle fibres. This cross-fibre action is analogous to bending the string on a bow or guitar string.

2. rotation, twisting or torsional forces - usually the combined action of the fingertips and thumb. This rotatory action of the hand is analogous to kneading dough or putty.

3. longitudinal forces - stretching the muscle by moving the two ends apart. This longitudinal action is analogous to pulling on either ends of an elastic strap.

Kneading increases cellular exchange for the nourishment, oxygenation and removal of waste from the muscle fibres.

4. Applying a force across a muscle will result in the movement of fluids within and around the muscle. This is analogous to squeezing a wet sponge.

Kneading is a mechanism for removing undesirable fibrous tissue that has accumulated between muscle fibres.

5. Applying a force across a muscle may also result in the dislodgement of loose fibrous tissue, such as scar tissue, wedged between muscle fibres. This mechanical action is analogous to unravelling fibres of a ball of wool that have become stuck together.

The goals of kneading are to:

- increase the length of muscle fibres
- decrease muscle tension and hence reduce stress
- increase blood and lymph for nourishment and oxygenation of muscle fibres
- remove waste that builds up within a muscle fibre as a result of energy use
- remove fibrous and scar tissue that may accumulate between muscle fibres
- reduce involuntary muscle contractions or spasms
- increase muscle strength, stamina and efficiency

The applicator can be:

- the tip, pad or outside of your thumb
- a row of fingertips
- one or all the knuckles of your clenched fist
- the pad at the base of your thumb
- the heel of your hand
- two balls in a net or a wadi

The kneading cycle

The graph below is an approximate representation of how applicator pressure and breathing change with time during the kneading and inhibition cycles. The exact detail of each cycle will vary according to the size and elasticity of the muscle being kneaded and the level of muscle irritability. In this hypothetical scenario the kneading cycle runs over a period of eight seconds, with the inhalation phase as two seconds and the exhalation phase as six seconds. The dark line represents the pressure that can be exerted with the transverse, longitudinal and torsion forces. The light line represents the breathing.

Synchronised breathing is mainly used when you are lying on your back over an applicator during an inhibition technique but can be used during kneading. Focused breathing helps relax muscles and is a useful timekeeper for the kneading cycle. During kneading or inhibition do not go to full inhalation. About 80% inhalation is optimal because this is comfortable and will facilitate the greatest relaxation.

With applicator contact on the muscle at 0 seconds (a) inhale over a period of approximately 2 seconds. During the first 0.5 seconds of kneading take up the skin slack and allow the muscle to get use to the initial pressure of the applicator (a to b). Irritable muscles can take several seconds to settle after the initial applicator contact so half a second may not be enough. For the next 1.5 seconds increase the applicator pressure with compression (b to c).

At the point of 80% inhalation (x) there is about 50% applicator force on the muscle. Begin exhalation and increase the applicator pressure by increasing the transverse force and introducing the longitudinal force. At about four seconds introduce torsion (d to e). At about five seconds combine the compressional, transverse, longitudinal and torsional forces. The applicator force is now about 80%. Continue holding the combined forces for about 2.5 seconds more (e to f). At about 7.5 seconds, which is just before full exhalation, reduce the applicator pressure and withdraw the applicator contact (f to g).

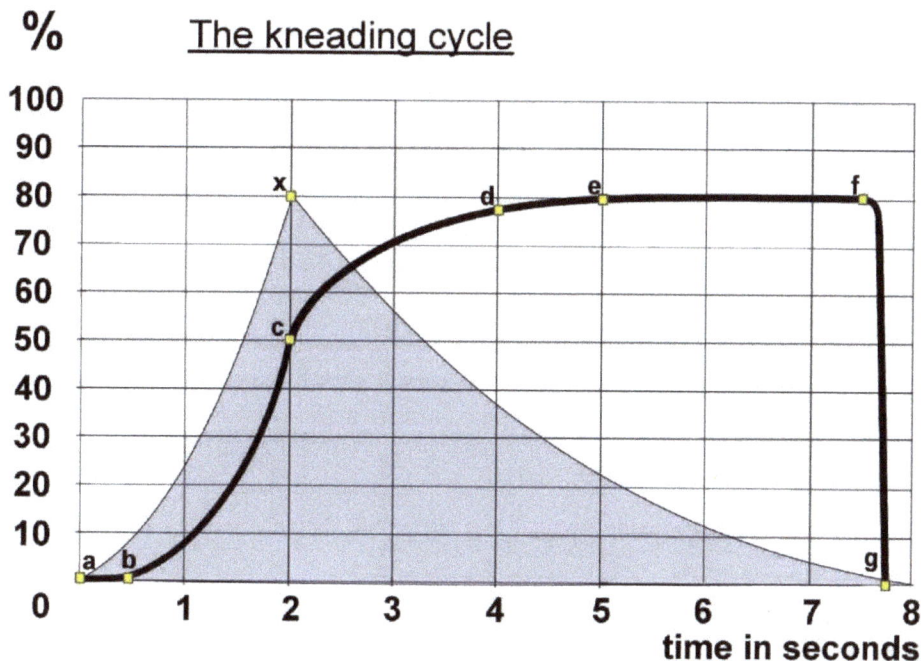

Inhibition

Inhibition uses firm sustained pressure over a small to medium area of muscle and may involve mindful relaxation and respiratory cooperation. Inhibition is especially useful for relaxing muscle spasms. The pressure should be increased slowly and released slowly. Many of the techniques for the shoulders, hips, ribs and spine involve inhibition. They require lying over a ball, wadi or tightly rolled-up towel and consciously relaxing as the muscle is being compressed.

The muscle being massaged lies between the applicator and a bone. Inhibition involves pushing the applicator into the muscle and compressing it against the bone. Inhibition is a modified type of kneading because in both techniques the applicator pushes transversely or at right angles to the muscle fibres. The difference between kneading and inhibition is that kneading uses transverse pressure across the muscle and bone whereas inhibition uses transverse pressure into the muscle and bone. The amount of compression depends on how deep the tissue is.

Recognising the level of muscle irritability is important if the right amount of pressure is to be applied during kneading or inhibition. Too much pressure on a highly irritable muscle may be counterproductive because it may cause the muscle to contract. Sense the tissue reactivity against the pressure of your applicator and respond appropriately by increasing or decreasing your pressure according to the feedback from the muscle.

Focused breathing can be used with any kneading technique but is mainly used with inhibition. Breathe by inhaling slowly through the nose and then exhaling slowly through the nose or mouth. Do not force the breathing - it should be natural. The abdomen and diaphragm should remain relaxed. Feel for a release of tension in the muscles during exhalation. Increase your applicator pressure during exhalation and release the applicator pressure just before the start of inhalation and reposition the applicator during inhalation for the start of the next phase of kneading.

The goals of inhibition are to:

- increase the length of muscle fibres
- decrease muscle tension
- reduce involuntary muscle contractions or spasms
- increase blood and lymph for nourishment and oxygenation of muscle fibres
- remove waste that builds up within a muscle fibre

The applicator can be:

- a wadi or similar blunt pointy object
- two rubber balls in a net
- a tightly rolled-up towel

Stretching

Stretching is the slow, rhythmical, purposeful, gradual increase in longitudinal force to separate the ends of muscles, ligaments or fascia. Stretching is a technique to lengthen short tissues and relax muscles. It can be used alone or as part of the kneading technique.

Stretching of muscle should be slow enough to minimise the impact of the stretch reflex - an involuntary muscle contraction. Fascia is tougher than muscle and requires a slow and strong longitudinal stretching force with a medium to heavy transverse pressure. For information on stretching please consult my book 'Safe Stretch.'

Friction - also known as Transverse Friction

During friction, the applicator applies quick back and forth movements with a moderate to firm force across a small area of a ligament, joint capsule, tendon or fibrous muscle. Friction can also be used across tendons and their sheaths and for breaking down adhesions between muscles, fascia, ligaments, tendons and bones. Friction is used for chronic conditions and in general is not used for acute conditions where tissues are inflamed and painful.

The applicator moves a short distance - between one and five millimetres depending on the elasticity of the skin. The applicator and the skin should move as one.

Friction is perpendicular to the direction of the fibres. Work across the ligament, tendon or tendon sheath to dislodge loosely attached fibrous tissue. The fibrous material is then moved into the circulation and to the liver for reuse or removal from the body. Work systematically and cover all the injured area. Apply sufficient pressure to go deep enough but keep your muscles relaxed. When working on a tendon sheath keep the tendon taught.

Friction is usually only applied over the tissue for 30 seconds to 2 minutes twice a week, until the condition improves. Rest and strapping may be indicated for the first 48 hours after injury. Ice packs may be applied to the area after using friction to reduce pain and inflammation. Apply the ice pack for 15 to 20 minutes.

Collagen is part of the natural structure of muscles, tendons and ligaments. After injury, the collagen and other structural proteins tend to get laid down randomly within the tissue, making it weaker, less elastic and vulnerable to further injury. Friction and kneading can help realign the collagen fibres after injury, so the tissue is stronger and more pliable. They are particularly effective when combined with targeted stretching and strengthening exercises.

The goals of friction are to:

- remove unwanted fibrous scar tissue between ligament, tendon and muscle fibres
- remove the fibrous inner lining of synovial sheaths causing tenosynovitis
- increase the nourishment and oxygenation of ligament, tendon or muscle fibres
- assist in the removal of waste from ligament, tendon or muscle fibres

The applicator can be:

- the tip of your thumb or a finger
- one of the knuckles of your clenched fist
- a wadi or blunt pointy object.

Other considerations

All the techniques in this book are based on human anatomy of the body and a basic knowledge of anatomy is helpful for using this book, particularly for identifying the tissues that are the source of your pain. But if you do not know any anatomy then anatomical descriptions and images of the region are provided at the beginning of each technique or group of techniques. Although pain can be referred from another part of the body, referred pain is the exception rather than the rule and most pain usually originates at the site of the dysfunction. If you know the name of the tissue that is painful, then you are usually part of the way to diagnosing the problem.

The book explains how to massage yourself with the minimum effort and the greatest efficiency. Body positions are chosen that are the most practical and involve the least effort. Many of the technique use gravity and the weight of the body to do the work. Pushing is easier and favoured over pulling and the thumb is stronger and favoured over the fingers.

There are many types of massage, but Swedish massage is arguably the most common form in the Western world. It uses a range of techniques including kneading, friction, effleurage, tapotement and passive stretching. Tapotement involves rapid and repeated striking of the body with the side of the hands to tone the muscles. Effleurage involves long massage strokes towards the heart to promote relaxation and facilitate better circulation. Passive stretching involves moving the ends of a muscle apart while it is relaxed.

Swedish massage uses massage oil to facilitate movement across the skin with a part of the hand or forearm. Although there are some benefits to using oil, such as greater fluidity of movement, which can help the masseur find unwanted fibrous changes within muscles, the techniques described in this book do not use oil because the disadvantages far outweigh the advantages. Effective kneading and friction require firm anchoring of thumb or fingers on a bone or muscle and good thumb or finger contact with the tissue you are massaging. This is not possible if there is excess oil on the skin because you keep sliding off.

It is difficult to focus your pressure on a small area of muscle, tendon or ligament and maintain firm contact with these tissues if your skin is too oily and slippery. The skin produces its own natural oils and there is usually enough oil and ample elasticity in the skin to allow movement across the tissue and avoid unwanted friction. The applicator and skin should move together across the tissues, and they should move just far enough, so they do not cause painful friction.

The only exceptions to not using oil may be if the skin is extremely dry or there is too much body hair over a particular area. Once oil is applied to the skin it is difficult to remove so it is better not to use it or to only use a small amount on a small area and to use it at the end of the massage when most of the kneading and friction techniques have been done.

Props used in self-massaging

Techniques done standing can usually be done seated in a chair and techniques that are done seated in a chair can usually be done standing. When lying on the floor lie on a high-density foam mat for greater comfort. If you do not have access to a mat, then a carpet will do. In certain techniques a wall is useful for keeping the spine or body straight and vertical, for support and as a reference point.

Daily considerations

Self-massage is ideally done on an empty stomach but can be done after a light meal. The duration of the self-massage can be for few minutes, once or twice a day, to one hour a day. It can be done daily or weekly. And if you can't adopt a regular routine because you are busy or unstructured, then do it when you can.

It is a good idea to take a day off from self-massaging once a week to give the muscles a rest from the routine. Do something else or rest completely. Rest allows your muscles to relax and rejuvenate. Too much massage can be counterproductive and a problem for some people, particularly massaging the same area. It can over-stimulate or irritate muscles that need to be left alone, and instead of relaxing the muscles it can make them tighter.

Self-massage for the first time

If this is your first attempt at self-massage then go lightly until you build up your skills. Practice coordinating the movement of your applicator with the movement of the muscle or part being massaged. Focus on your posture, moving your body efficiently and executing the technique correctly. Develop fluidity of movement. Breathing is useful as a timekeeper for the kneading process and helping relax the muscle you are working on, but only focus on the breathing after you have mastered the technique.

Normal flexibility is required to do the self-massage techniques effectively and so if you have a joint restriction or muscle shortness then you may have problems with some of the techniques. Wear clothing that allows easy movement and access to the muscle you are massaging, such as a t-shirt, short pants or a bathing costume. Remove distractions that will interfere with your concentration.

There may be some muscle soreness after the first time doing self-massage. Delayed onset muscle soreness may be caused by microscopic tearing of the muscle fibres and inflammation. If this occurs, then use lighter pressure. Start slowly and build up. There are great benefits from self-massage but everyone is different. For the first few days notice how your body responds to the massage and if there are no problems then proceed.

Throughout this book the text, photographs and diagrams consistently refer to the right side of your body, so it is necessary to transpose the information to the left side. Massage each limb and each side of your body and compare them. If one side is tighter, then focus on this side. Alternate between left and right sides and keep repeating this with greater emphasis on the tighter side. Doing the self-massage a second or even a third time is preferable to doing it once but if you are time constrained then doing it once is fine.

Even with a mirror it is not easy to see the back of our body but certain clues at the front of our body suggest what might be happening at the back. Round shoulders suggest an increased thoracic kyphosis, a high shoulder suggests a scoliosis with the convexity on the side of the high shoulder and a chin forward posture suggest a dowager hump.

To really know the structures at the back of your body you need a photograph of your back and then you need a manual therapist to interpret the photograph, and give you feedback about where key muscles are located. Get them to draw a diagram showing the shape of your spine or press on the different muscles or areas of your back and give you feedback about where they are located on the photograph. With continued feedback you will get to know the muscles and areas of your back that are not visible.

Another option is to get an X-ray taken of your back. Static plain film anteroposterior spinal X-rays taken standing and erect are particularly useful for learning where bony landmarks are located. Ask your therapist to press on the various bones and give you feedback about where the bones are on the X-ray.

Medical conditions requiring caution

If you are elderly, have an underlying health condition, are recovering from illness or if there is anything that is likely to cause problems with self-massage then consult your doctor or qualified health professional before starting self-massage. Mild pain may be helped with self-massage but if the pain is extreme or ongoing or if you do not know what is causing the pain then get a diagnosis. Self-massage may make it worse.

Some health issues may prevent you from physically doing some of the techniques in this book. For example osteoarthritis and other forms of joint stiffness can prevent you moving freely. People who bruise easily or feel sore after a regular massage should go lighter with self-massage. If the bruising and soreness continues then get health advice. When the number of platelets in the blood are low this can cause bleeding problems and self-massage may be unwise. Other contraindications include fractures, burns, wounds, cancer, deep vein thrombosis, severe osteoporosis and medication that causes blood-thinning.

Do not use self-massage immediately after an injury involving localised swelling and high levels of pain. Apply ice packs intermittently and rest the area for 24 hours or longer depending on the severity of the injury. After the acute phase has settled use light self-massage and gradually increase the intensity over a few days or weeks. Self-massage is best for chronic injuries or intermittent problems that are in remission.

Palpation

Palpation is the art and skill of feeling and recognising the different tissues of the body, identifying gross abnormal changes in these tissues, and recognising the difference between healthy and unhealthy tissues. This takes time and practice, but palpation is an important part of self-massage.

One of the most basic changes that can be felt in muscle is hypertonicity, which is when a muscle becomes tense and short. Muscles contract, and hypertonicity occurs when a muscle contracts too hard or too often. This is usually in response to overuse, overloading, pain, psychological stress, or as a compensation for a problem in another part of the body. Hypertonicity is usually a temporary change that is relatively easy to correct with light kneading, inhibition or stretching. But if the hypertonicity is stubborn then stronger and more persistent kneading may be required.

Prolonged use or overuse, overloading or stress can result in fibrosis, which is when a muscle becomes hard and fibrous due to fibrous infiltration into and around the muscle cells. In the spine, the muscles take on a feeling of ropiness with long hard bands of fibrous connective tissue replacing the relatively soft muscles. In other parts of the body the fibrous changes take on a feeling of lumpiness with round or oval shaped masses developing in the muscle. Friction and strong kneading are usually required when there is fibrosis.

Injury to a muscle, tendon or ligament usually results in the formation of scar tissue. When there is a minor injury the scar tissue may not be directly palpable. Minor injuries often result in tiny tears in the tissue and the only identifiable sign of the scar tissue is the presence of pain at the site of the tear. When there is a major injury, the scar may be felt as a lump within the soft tissue. Scar tissue should be removed with a combination of friction, kneading and passive stretching.

Muscles that are hypertonic, fibrous or scarred will offer greater resistance to kneading and passive stretching compared with normal muscles. Fibrous or scared muscles will be less elastic and have a firmer feel than hypertonic muscles because they involve structural changes, and these will require stronger massage.

Other changes that can be palpated in and around tissues include swelling, which is felt as bogginess, hypertrophy or muscle growth, which can be felt as a thick pad of muscle and atrophy or muscle wasting, which can be felt as the absence or diminution of muscle mass compared with the same muscle on the other side of the body.

Posture

Posture is concerned with the carriage of the body. Good posture depends on strong ligament support around the joints and optimal muscle tone and balance between the left and right sides of the body and the front and back. The genes we inherit from our parents play a major role in determining our posture. Genes affect the size and shape of our bones, joints and muscles, the laxity of our ligaments and the curves of our spine. People with genes for a good structure tend to develop less problems and people with genes for poor structure must work harder to keep a good posture by adopting good sitting habits and doing the right exercises.

Spinal curves

A good spinal posture is one with moderate curves - a modest thoracic kyphosis and lumbar and cervical lordosis, and minimal or absent scoliosis. A poor spinal posture is one with exaggerated, reduced or reversed curves - an increased or decreased lordosis or kyphosis, or a reversed lordosis or kyphosis or an extreme scoliosis.

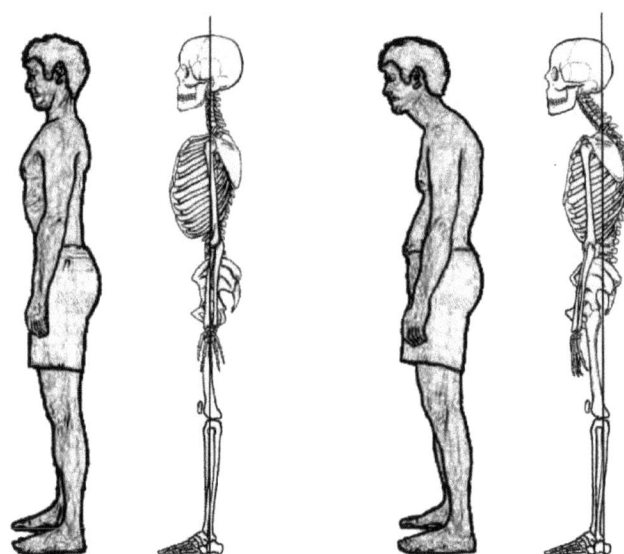

Normal posture   **Slouched posture**

Moderate spinal curves are good because the body is closer to its centre of gravity and so the back and shoulder muscles do not need to work so hard. They only need to contract lightly and intermittently and have periods of rest. Increased spinal curves are bad because the apex of each curve is further from the body's centre of gravity and some muscles must work harder. Working strongly and continuously can eventually result in muscle fatigue. Reduced spinal curves are bad because curves act like springs absorbing shock during activity and a straight spine suffers from greater wear on the intervertebral discs and joints.

Postural fatigue

Prolonged sitting or standing, especially in the presence of a poor posture, can lead to structural changes in muscles, affecting muscle tone, power and elasticity. Some muscles become shorter, and some become longer. With the slouched forward posture, muscles attached to the back of the rib cage, thoracic spine and shoulders must work harder against the continuous action of gravity taking the body forwards and downwards. Overworked muscles fatigue and eventually become fibrous and less efficient at contracting. The erector spinae, trapezius, levator scapulae and rhomboid muscles lengthen and become more fibrous whereas the suboccipital and upper posterior cervical muscles, anterior scalene, pectoralis major and minor, iliopsoas, hamstrings and calf muscle become shorter.

Gravity

The influence gravity has on our body is significant and is frequently underrated. Over our lifetime gravity causes our intervertebral discs to get thinner and we get shorter and less flexible in our spine. We also lose flexibility in the rest of the body as our muscles, ligaments and fasciae become distended. This distension causes the position of our organs to change and our circulation to be compromised. The loss of elasticity in our muscles and ligaments is also aggravated by demineralisation in our bones and the loss of cartilage in our joints.

Techniques

Part A The jaw, spine and rib cage

THE JAW

Massaging the jaw muscles, **temporalis** and **masseter** can be useful for overuse syndromes, anxiety disorders such as bruxism (the habitual grinding of the teeth), tension headaches, the relief of stress, and some dental problems, for example malocclusion (when the teeth do not meet properly). It may also be beneficial for singers and musicians who play a wind instrument.

1.1a Kneading temporalis using your fingertips

- Stand, sit on a chair, lay on your back or kneel on the floor.
- Lift your left arm and grasp the dome of your skull on top of your head.
- Lift your right arm and place your fingertips on the side of your head just above and behind your right ear.
- The temporalis muscle is very thin and hard to distinguish but can be felt under your fingertips by repeatedly clenching and relaxing your jaw.

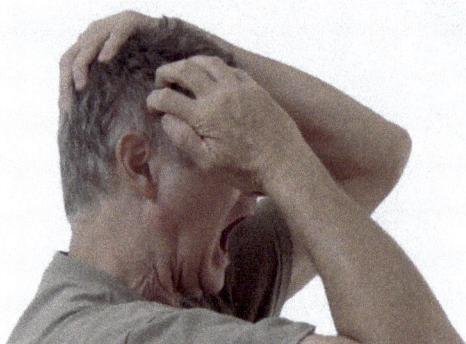

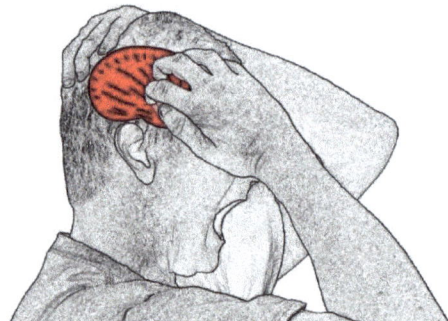

- Open your mouth a little bit to put a mild stretch on temporalis.
- Slide your fingertips forwards and across the side of your head as you open your jaw to the fully opened position.
- Follow a semicircular arc parallel with the top of your ear.

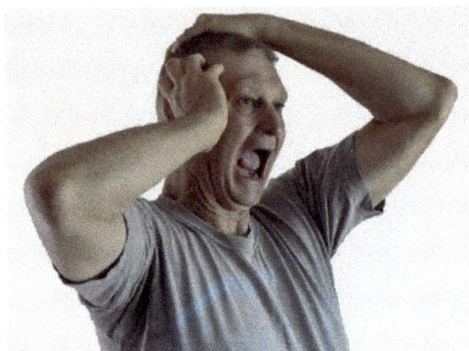

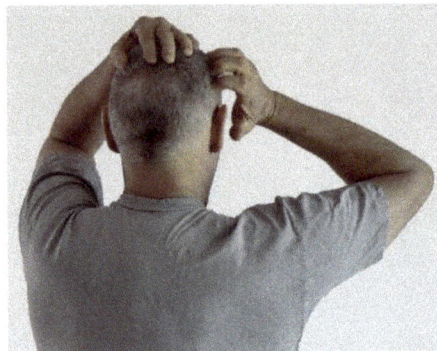

- Repeat the movement from back to front along parallel strips across the temple until you reach edge of the eye socket but do not press hard on the eye socket.

Temporalis arises from the temporal bone on the side of the skull, just above and in front of the ear, and from the under-surface of a layer of fascia covering the muscle. The fibres from this thin fan-shaped muscle converge on a tendon which passes under a bony arch and attaches on the top and front of the mandible.

The muscle acts at the temporomandibular joint (TMJ) to close the jaw during biting, chewing and speech.

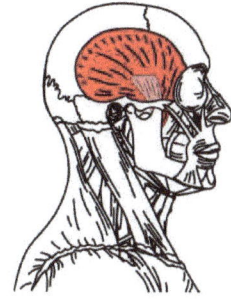

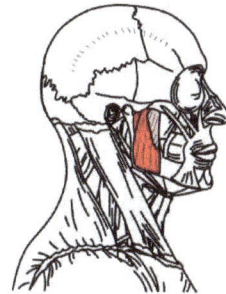

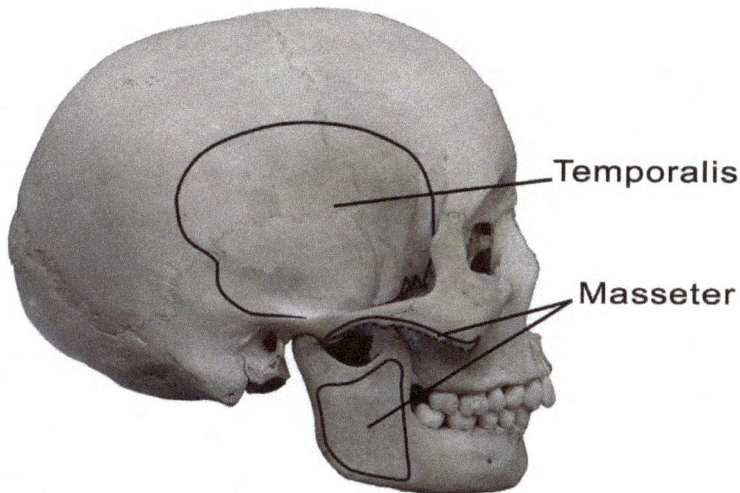

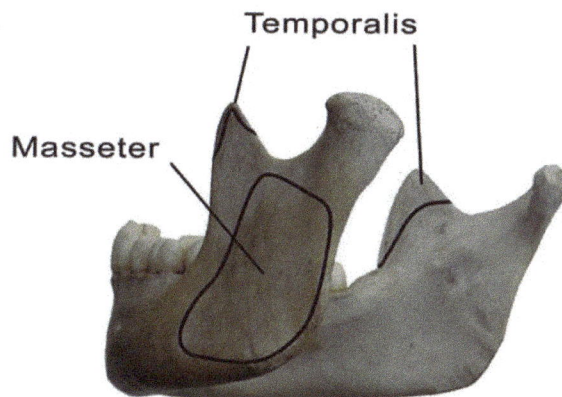

Masseter arises on the bony arch running across the side of the face above the jaw and attaches on the side of the flat rectangular area of bone at the back of the mandible. The rectangular muscle has three layers and is covered by fascia which make the muscle difficult to palpate unless it is contracted.

The muscle acts at the temporomandibular joint (TMJ) to close the jaw during biting, chewing and speech.

The skull and mandible

1.1b Kneading masseter using the tip of your thumb

- Stand, sit on a chair, lay on your back or kneel on the floor.
- Lift your left arm and grasp the dome of your skull on top of your head.
- Lift your right arm and place the tip of your thumb on the side of your jaw just below your ear.

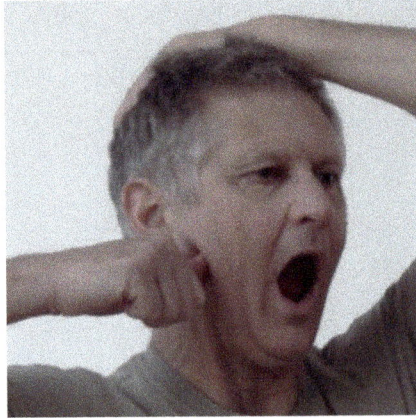

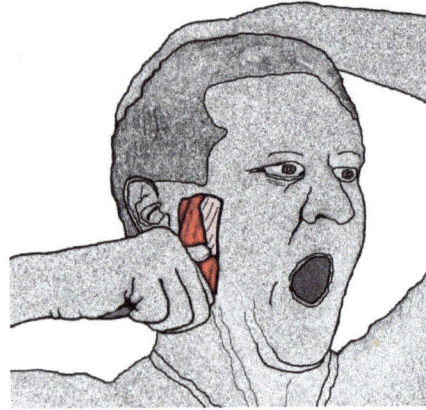

- Open your mouth a little bit to put a mild stretch on masseter.
- Slide the tip of your thumb forwards and across the muscle as you open your jaw to the fully opened position.

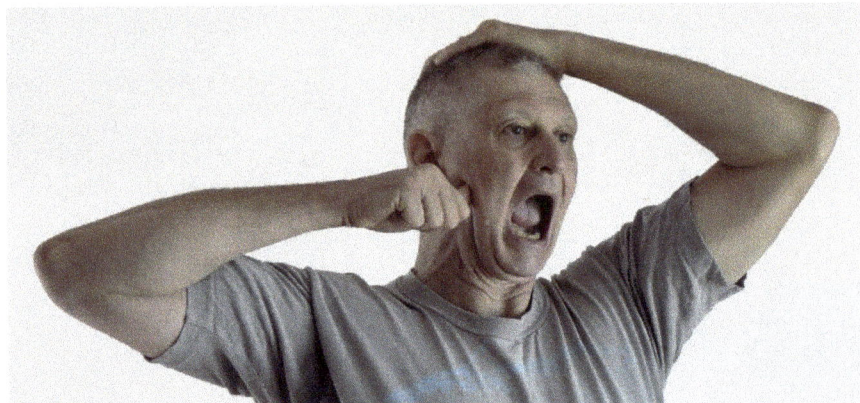

- Follow a line parallel with the bony arch running across the side of your head and work down the mandible until you reach the bottom.
- The muscle has three layers and is covered by thick fascia and so is quite hard but systematically cover the whole rectangular area of bone.

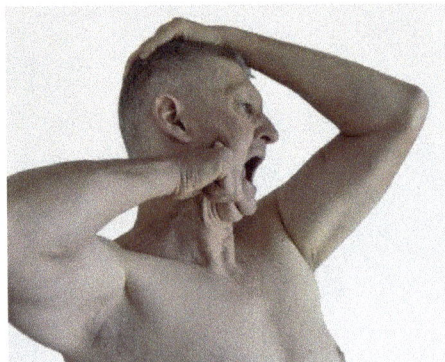

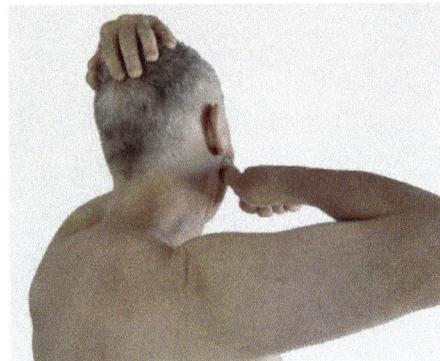

THE SUBOCCIPITAL SPINE

Massaging the suboccipital muscles can help tension headaches, neck pain, muscle spasms, whiplash injuries for example from a motor vehicle accident and conditions linked with poor posture especially the chin forward posture (anterior occiput). It may benefit people who work on computers or mobile phones.

The suboccipital spine consists of the occiput, which forms the base of the skull, the first two vertebrae of the spine, the atlas and axis, and the muscles.

The suboccipital muscles are a group of small muscles located at the top of the neck and back of the head, deep under the base of the skull and trapezius. They produce head rotation, sidebending and backwards tilt.

1. **Rectus capitis posterior minor** runs from the bottom of the occiput to the back of the arch of the atlas.

2. **Rectus capitis posterior major** runs from the bottom of the occiput to the spinous process of the axis.

3. **Obliquus capitis inferior** runs from the transverse process of the atlas to the spinous process of the axis.

4. **Obliquus capitis superior** runs from the bottom of the occiput to back of the transverse process of the atlas.

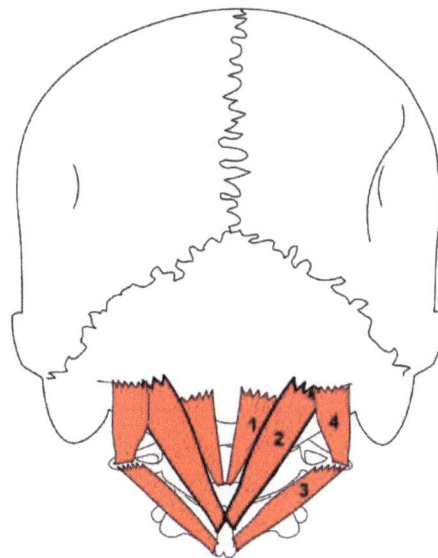

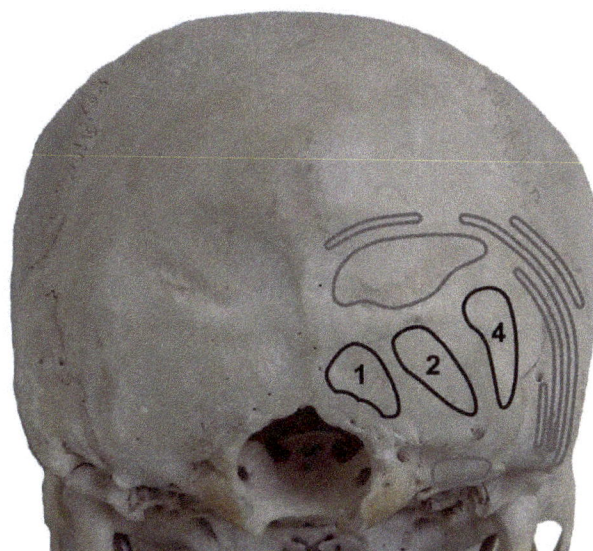

Skull from below and behind

1.2 Kneading the suboccipital muscles using the pad or tip of your thumb

- Stand, sit on a chair, lay on your back or kneel on the floor.
- Lift your left arm and grasp the top and back of your head with your hand.
- Lift your right arm, reach around the back of your head and place the tip or pad of your thumb on the muscles under the occiput and to the right side of the spine.

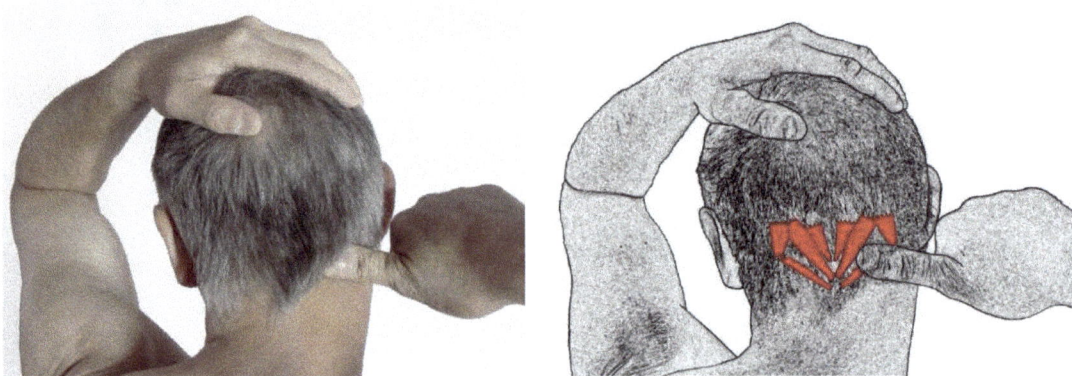

- Tilt your head backwards a bit to shorten and relax trapezius and the overlying fascia and allow better access to the deeper suboccipital muscles.
- Push into the muscles with your thumb while simultaneously flexing your head as you increase the pressure.

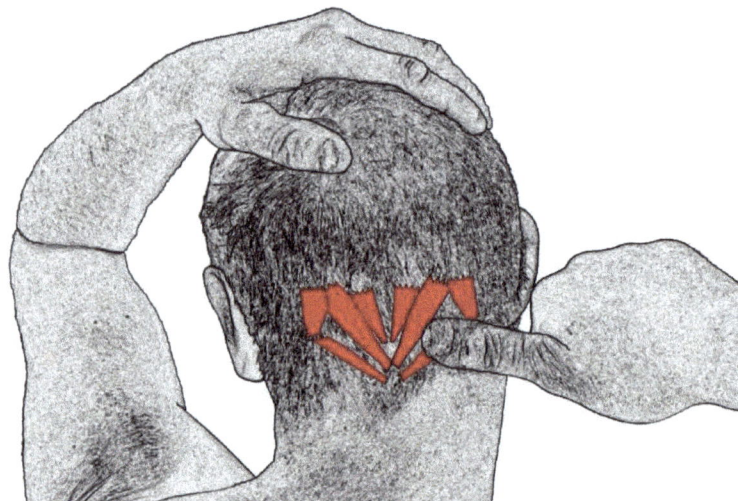

- Repeat the pushing action with your thumb while rotating your head to the left.
- Repeat the pushing action with your thumb while sidebending your head to the left.
- Repeat the pushing action with your thumb while combining flexion, rotation and sidebending of your head to the left.
- Place the tip of your thumb further from the midline when kneading the muscles concerned with rotation and sidebending.

- Push through the trapezius to the deeper suboccipital muscles.
- Work on an area just below the occiput and up to about 2 cm to the right of the midline of the back of your spine.

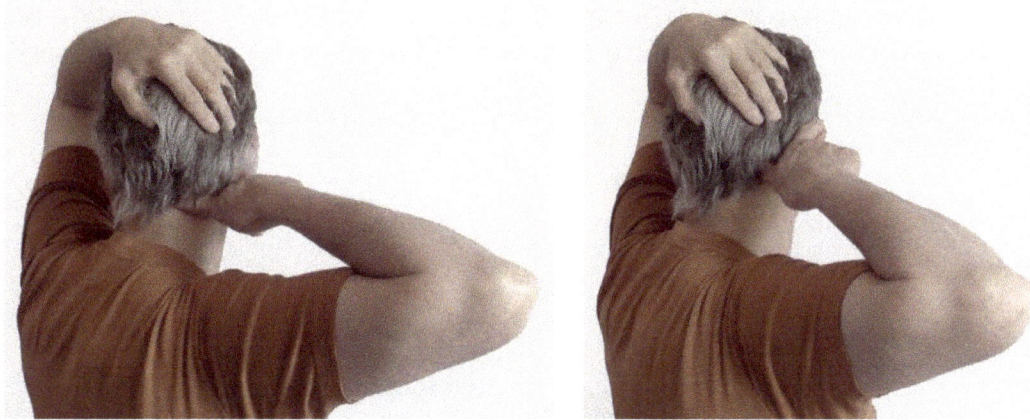

- Switch hands and repeat the technique on the left side of the spine.
- This is the only technique that can effectively treat the suboccipital and deep cervical muscles because strong localised pressure can be applied with your thumb.

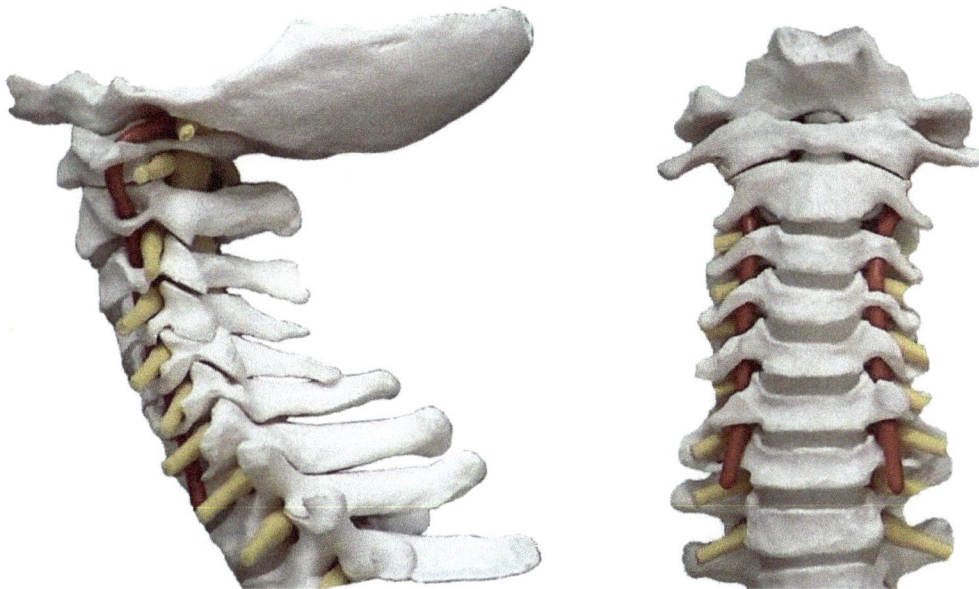

Cervical spine, nerves and blood vessels - side view (left) & anterior view (right)

THE CERVICAL SPINE

Massaging the cervical muscles can be useful for tension headaches, neck pain, muscle spasms such as acute torticollis, degenerative changes such as osteoarthritis, whiplash injuries for example from a motor vehicle accident and conditions linked with poor posture and frequent users of computers or mobile phones.

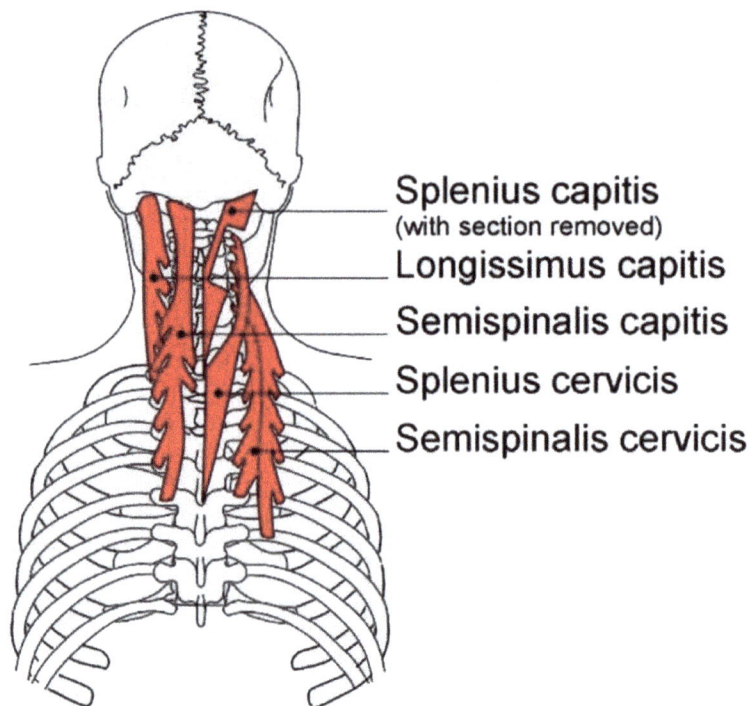

Splenius capitis
(with section removed)
Longissimus capitis
Semispinalis capitis
Splenius cervicis
Semispinalis cervicis

Posterior head, ribs, cervical and thoracic spine

The cervical spine consists of seven cervical vertebrae and cervical and shoulder muscles attaching on the occiput, upper rib cage, clavicle, scapula, sternum and cervical and thoracic spine.

The posterior cervical muscles are a group of short overlapping muscle running down the back of the cervical spine and configured in a zigzagging fashion. They lie beneath the upper trapezius and levator scapulae and at the side of the spine they are beneath the sternocleidomastoid. They control movement of the head and neck, and most are named according to where they attach.

The capitis muscles arise on the occiput and temporal bones of the skull and attach on the spinous and transverse process which project from the cervical and thoracic vertebrae below. The cervicis and semispinalis muscles pass between the spinous processes and transverse processes of cervical and thoracic vertebrae. Even deeper to these are multifidus, interspinales and intertransversarii muscles which pass between the spinous processes and transverse processes down either side of the whole spine.

The erector spinae muscles are the primary back muscles. They extend up into the cervical spine as iliocostalis cervicis, longissimus cervicis and spinalis

18

cervicis. They attach to the ribs and the transverse processes and spinous processes of cervical and upper thoracic vertebra. Deep cervical fascia covers and separates the individual muscles and attaches to the ligamentum nuchae and occipital bone above and to the thoracic and lumbar spine below.

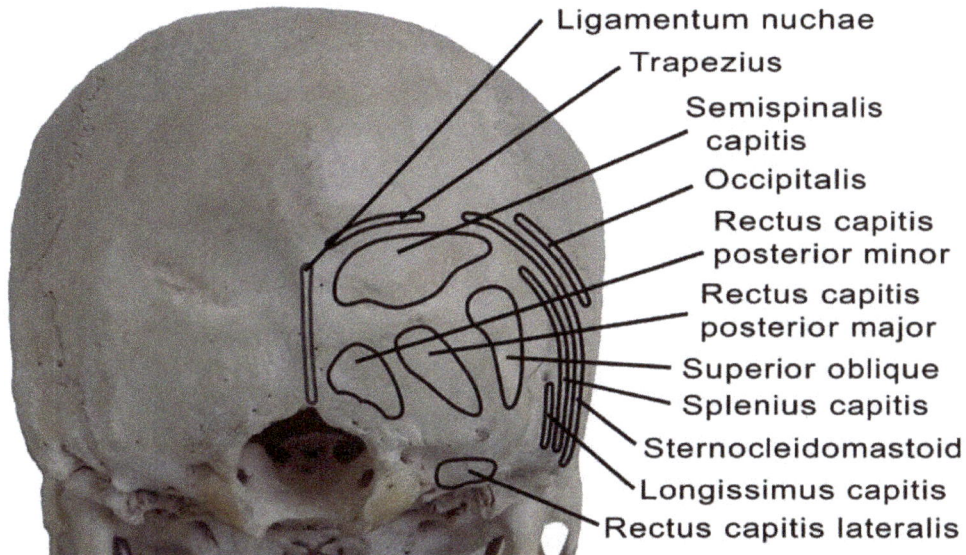

View of skull from below and behind showing muscle attachments of trapezius, sternocleidomastoid, posterior cervical muscles and suboccipital muscles

Upper trapezius arises on the occiput, ligamentum nuchae, a band of strong fibrous tissue running down the back of the neck, and the spinous process of C7 vertebra and attached at the end of the clavicle, at the tip of the shoulder.

The muscle tilts the head and neck sideways and backward and lifts and rotates the shoulders upwards.

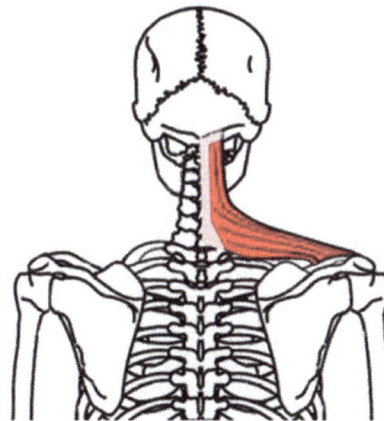

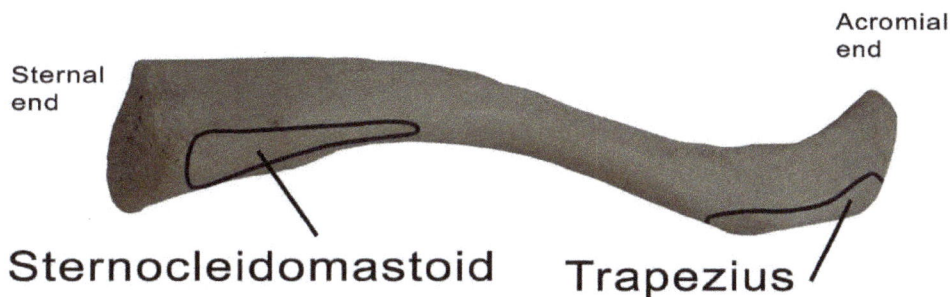

Right clavicle - superior view and upper trapezius attachment

1.3a Kneading or transverse friction of the upper trapezius and posterior cervical muscles using the tips of your hooked fingers

- Stand, sit on a chair or kneel on the floor.
- Reach behind your head with your left hand and grasp the back and top of your head.
- Reach behind your head with your right hand and place your fingertips against the middle of your occiput at the back of your head.
- Keep your fingers in a hooked finger position throughout the technique.

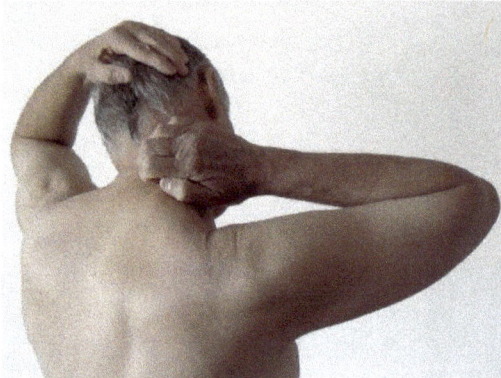

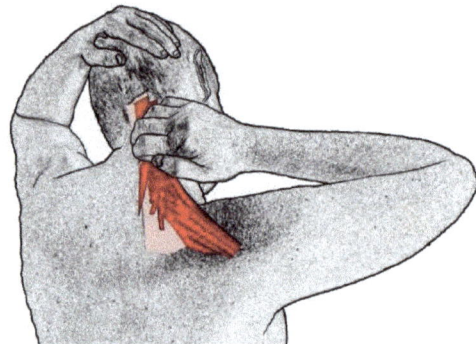

- Flex and sidebend your head to the left while simultaneously sliding your fingertips across the upper trapezius at the back and right of your occiput.
- Reposition your fingertips so they are just under the occipital bone and in the furrow running down the middle of the back of your cervical spine.
- Flex and sidebend your head to the left while simultaneously sliding your fingertips across the upper trapezius in line with the first cervical vertebra.
- Move your fingertips from the middle to the right of your cervical spine.

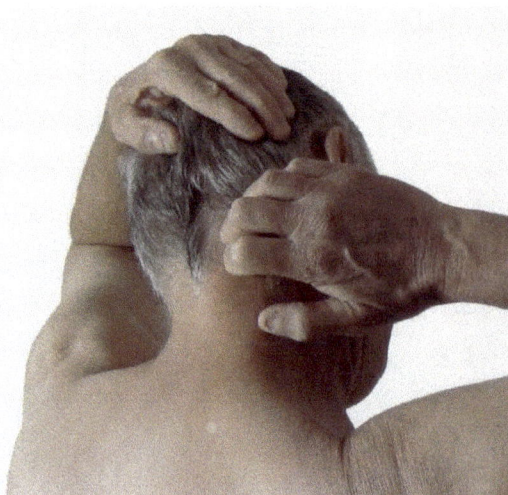

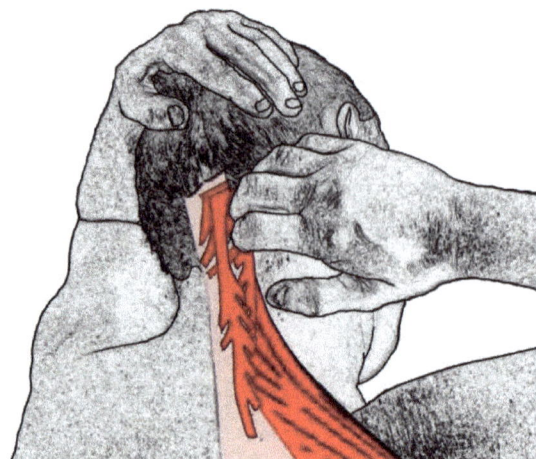

- Reposition your fingertips again just under the occipital bone.
- Tilt your head backwards to relax the upper trapezius muscle and get better access to the deeper posterior cervical muscles.

- Sidebend your head to the left and rotate your head to the right while simultaneously pushing the tips of your middle and index fingers through trapezius and into and across the deeper cervical muscles.
- Reposition your fingertips about one vertebra level further down the back of your cervical spine and repeat the action of moving your fingertips from the midline towards the right along short parallel strips.

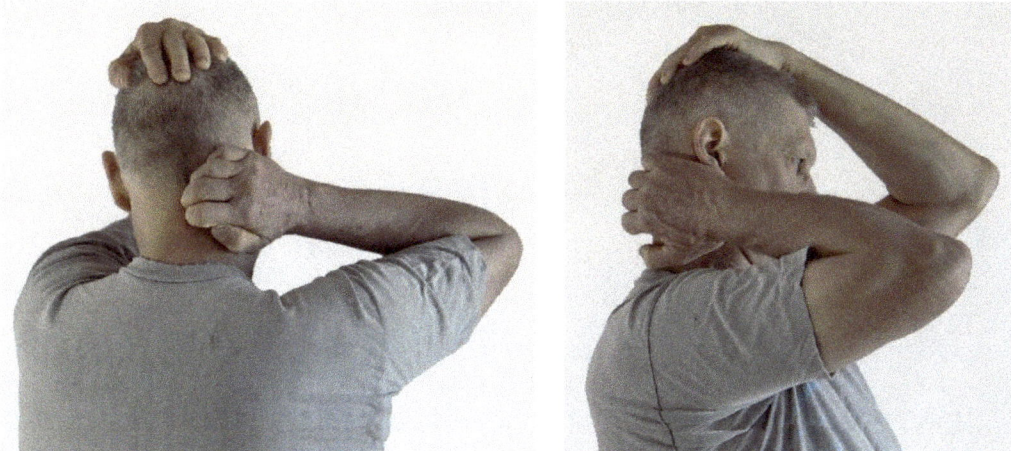

- Move your fingertips in an outwards direction but do not press on the sensitive nerves and blood vessels at the side of your neck.
- Work down the whole of the back and right side of your cervical spine and then swap hands and repeat the technique on the left side.
- Remember to tilt your head forwards to treat the upper trapezius and backwards to treat the posterior cervical muscles.

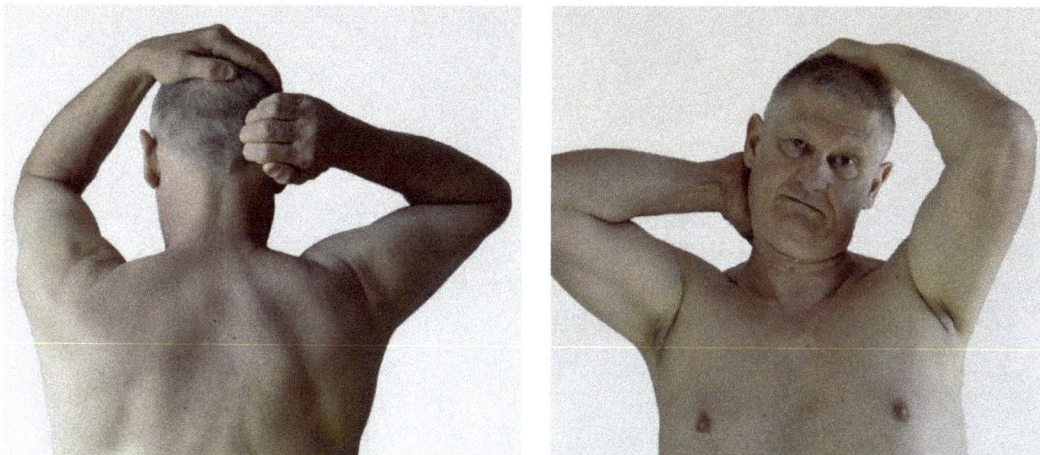

- Do not pull or push your head with your left hand and strain ligaments.
- Treat short tight muscles with cross fibre kneading and fibrous changes in muscles with transverse friction.

1.3b Kneading upper trapezius and posterior cervical muscles bilaterally

- Stand, sit on a chair, kneel on the floor or lay on your back on the floor with your head on a pillow and your spine straight.
- Reach around the back of your cervical spine with both hands and place your fingertips in the depression in the middle of the back of your spine.

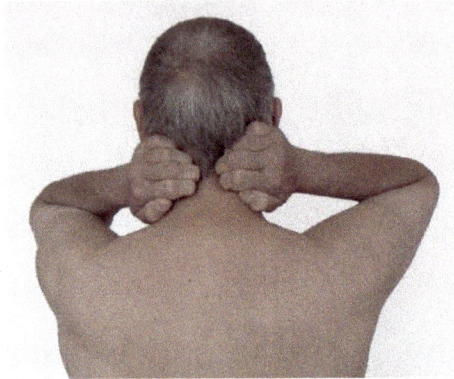

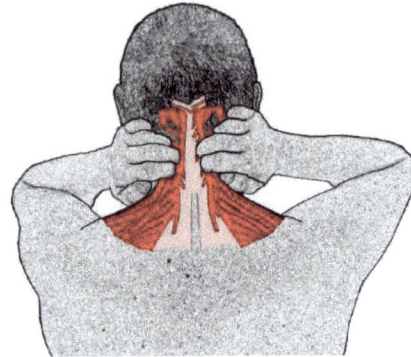

- Start at the muscle attachments on the occiput at the base of the skull.
- Press your fingertips into the back of your neck and then curl your fingers so your fingertips move apart and outwards against the inside of the two columns of muscles running down the back of your cervical spine.

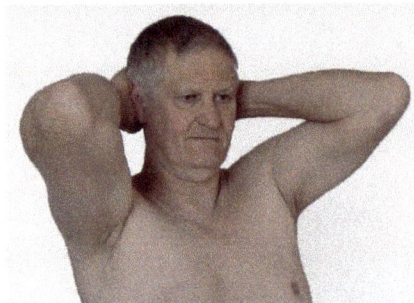

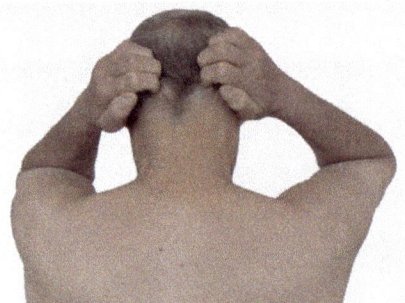

- Tilt your head forwards to knead the upper trapezius and tilt your head backwards to relax trapezius and knead the posterior cervical muscles.
- As you pull your fingertips across the two columns of muscles take care not to pull on the hairs at the back of your head.

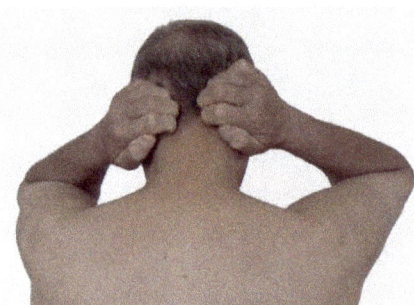

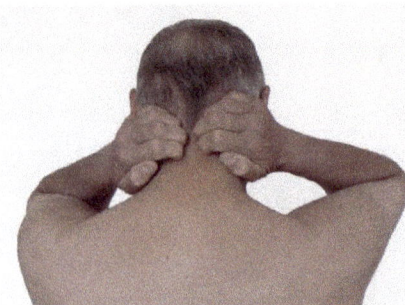

- Systematically work along strips down the length of the cervical spine from the highest fibres of the upper trapezius and suboccipital muscles to the start of the middle trapezius and the deeper cervical muscles arising from the thoracic spine.

1.3c Kneading the posterior cervical muscles and the cervical part of upper trapezius using the pads or tips of your fingers

- Stand or sit on a chair with your arms hanging at your side.
- Flex your left forearm at the elbow and reach around the back of your head and place the palm of your left hand behind your occiput, this is the bone at the base of your skull.
- Find the hard ridge that runs from right to left across the occiput and place your fingertips just under it and along the outer border of the muscles attaching here.

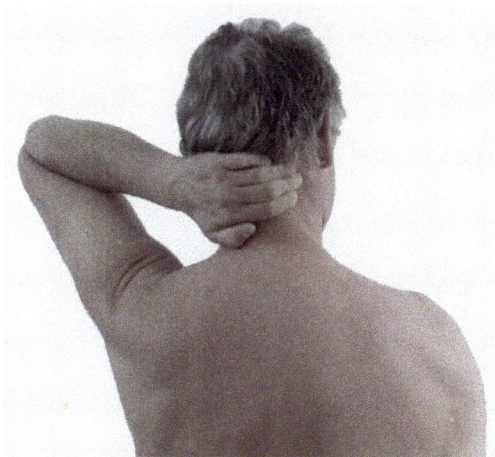

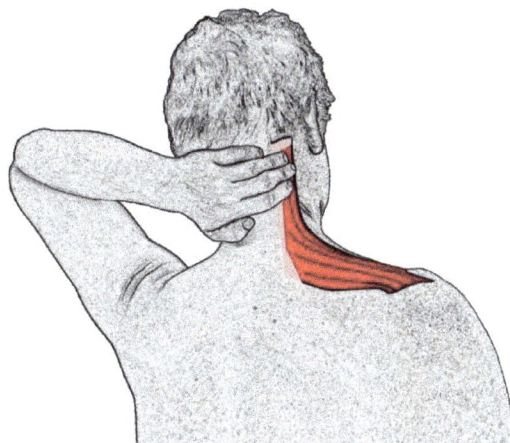

- Flex your fingers and hook your fingertips around the outer border of the upper trapezius and posterior cervical muscle.
- Slide your fingertips across the muscle while simultaneously sidebending your head to the left and flexing your head, just nodding it forward slightly.
- Follow a line just under the ridge with your fingertips and stop when you reach the midpoint of the occiput.

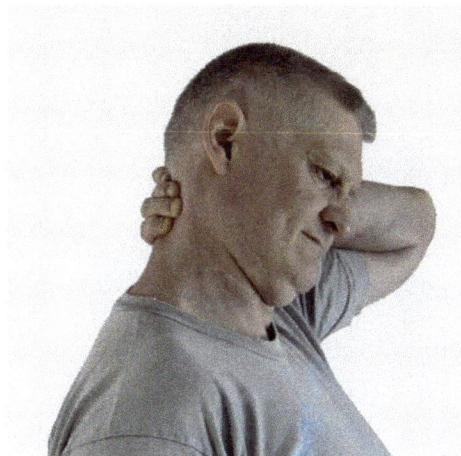

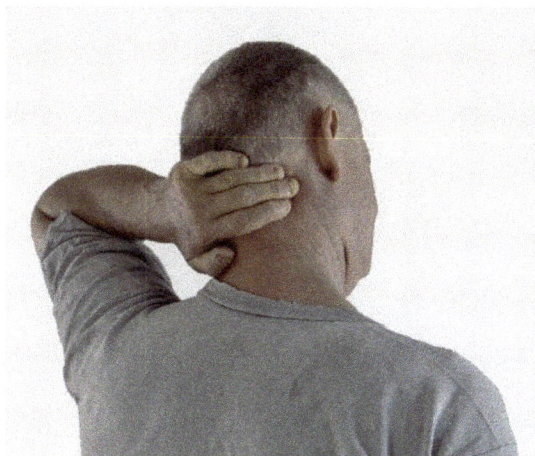

- Work systematically down the right side of the cervical spine along short parallel strips until your reach the bottom of your cervical spine.
- Use the weight of your right arm hanging by your side to stretch the muscle.

1.3d Kneading upper trapezius using the pads or tips of your hooked fingers

- Stand or sit on a chair with your arms hanging at your side.
- Flex your left forearm at the elbow and then reach across the front of your body and hook the fingers of your left hand over the top of your right shoulder.

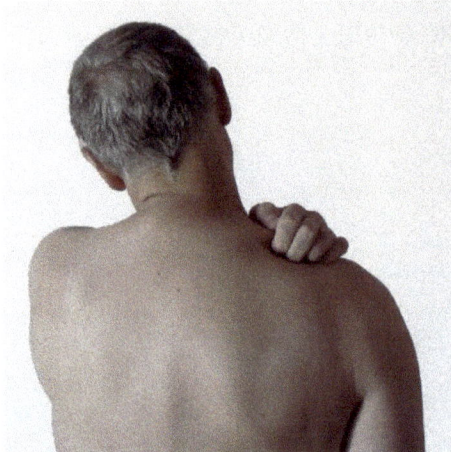

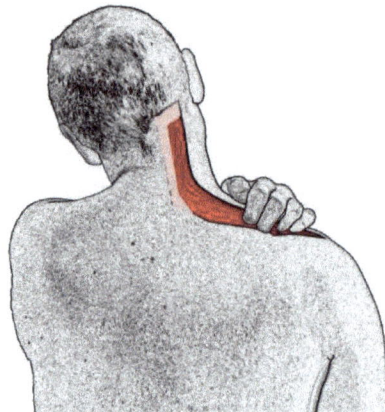

- Allow the weight of your right arm hanging at your side to pull the shoulder down and give the upper trapezius a mild stretch.
- Sidebend your head to the left to stretch the muscle a bit further.
- Start where the muscle attaches on the clavicle at the end of the shoulder.
- Push your fingertips or pad of your fingers into the muscle, then allow them to slide over the muscle, moving forwards over the shoulder towards the clavicle.

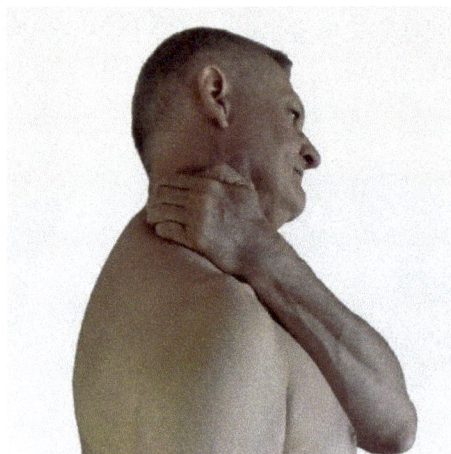

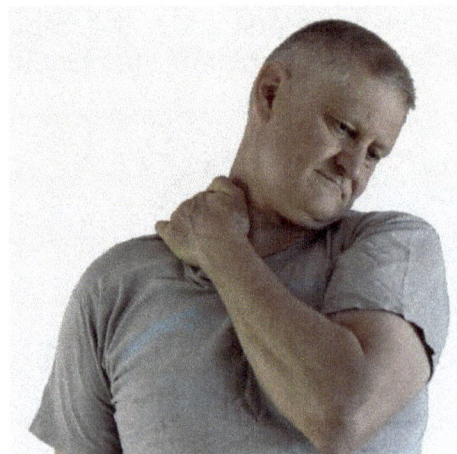

- Continue along short strips across the top of your shoulder to the bottom of your cervical spine.
- In the cervical area push your fingertips sideways from the depression in the middle of the spine across back and right side of your neck.
- Do not press into the side or front of the neck where there are sensitive blood vessels and nerves.

24

- Continue along short strips up the back of the cervical spine to the base of the skull.
- Move in a direction perpendicular to the muscle fibres.

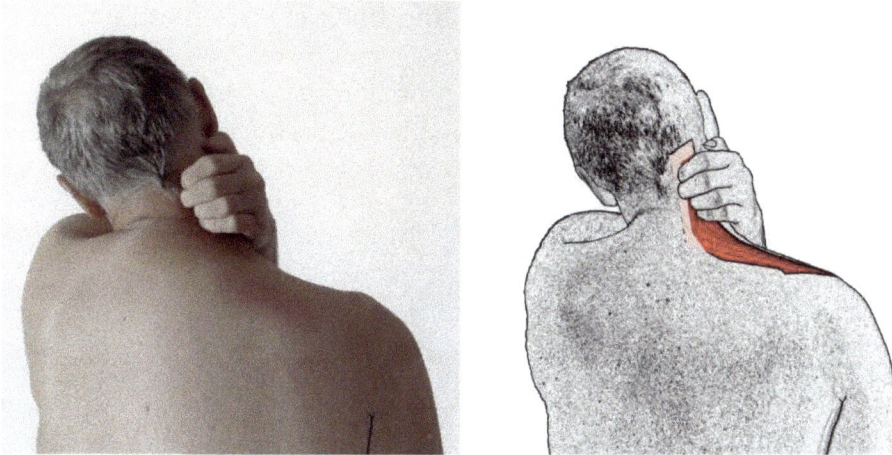

- This technique can be used up to about the second cervical vertebra.
- This technique can also be used to treat the posterior cervical muscles and levator scapulae which lie underneath upper trapezius.

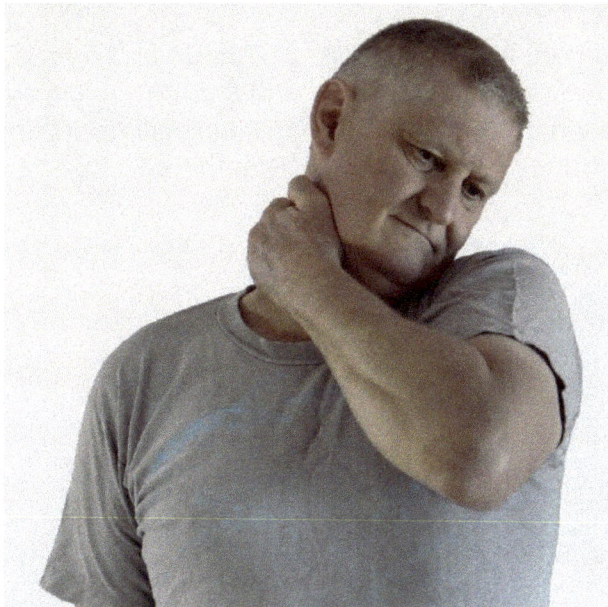

1.3e Kneading upper trapezius and posterior cervical muscles using the tip or pad of your thumb

- Stand, sit on a chair, lay on your back or kneel on the floor.
- Lift your left arm and grasp the top and back of your head with your hand.
- Lift your right arm, reach around the back of your head and place the pad of your right thumb on the muscles at the top and right side of your cervical spine and below your occiput.

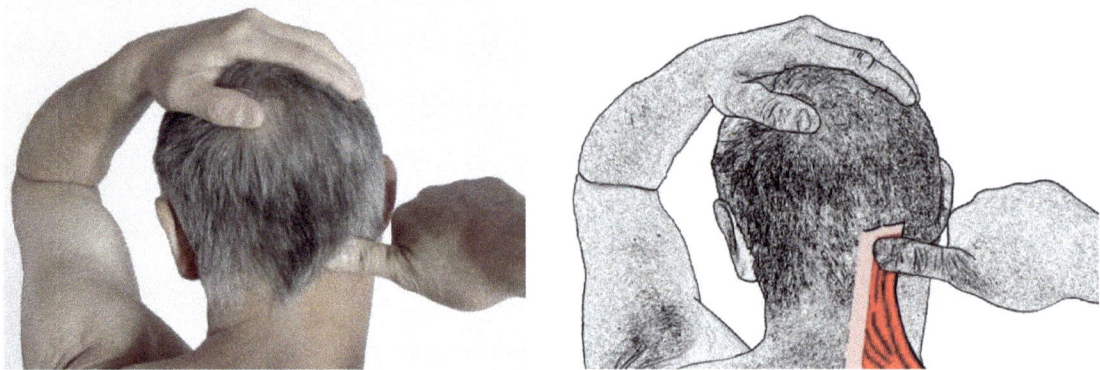

- The upper trapezius and the cervical muscles below run the entire length of the cervical spine.
- Push on the highest fibres of upper trapezius and with the pad of your thumb while simultaneously flexing and sidebending your head to the left.
- Work down the entire length of the right side of your cervical spine and then return to the top of the neck to treat the cervical muscles.

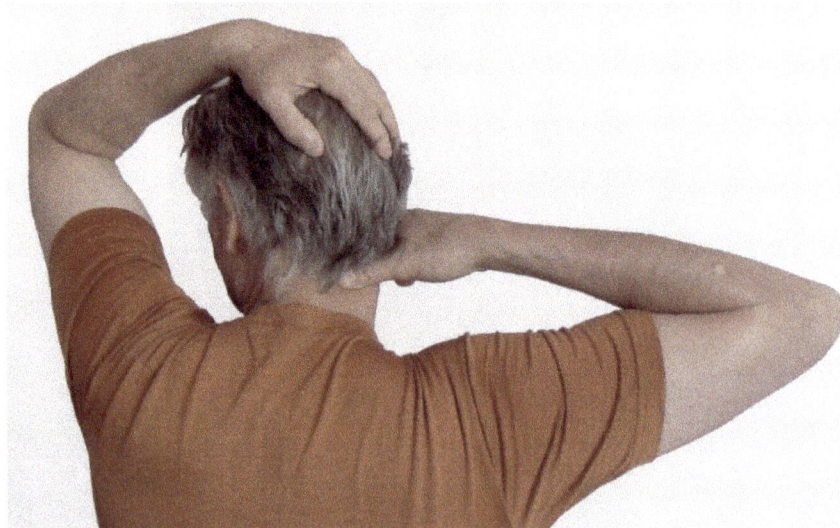

- Tilt your head forwards to treat the upper trapezius and tilt it backwards to relax trapezius and treat the deeper posterior cervical muscles.
- Push on the highest fibres of the cervical muscles and with the pad of your thumb while simultaneously rotating and sidebending your head to the left.
- Switch hands and repeat the techniques on the left side of the spine for the upper trapezius and then the posterior cervical muscles.

1.3f Kneading upper trapezius and the posterior cervical muscles using the tips of your hooked fingers

- Lay on your back on the floor, lift your head off the floor and grasp the back and top of your head with your left hand.
- Reach behind your head with your right hand and place your fingertips on the back of your head so they line up along the middle of the occiput.
- Return your head and hands to the floor so that the back of your occiput rest on your fingertips and the back of your right hand rests on the floor.

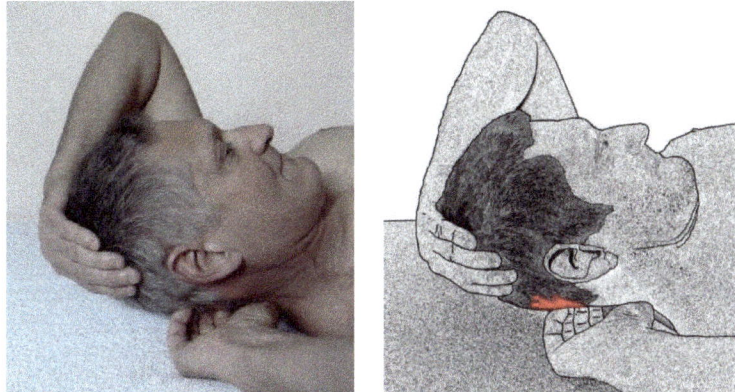

- If you have a stiff back, you may need to place your right hand on a firm pillow to raise your head and prevent hyperextension and neck strain. Flex and sidebend your head to the left while simultaneously sliding your fingertips across the trapezius at the back and right of your occiput.
- Relax your neck and allow the weight of your head to help push the muscles against your fingertips but take care not to pull your hair.
- Reposition your fingertips so they are just under the occipital bone and in the furrow running down the middle of the back of your cervical spine.

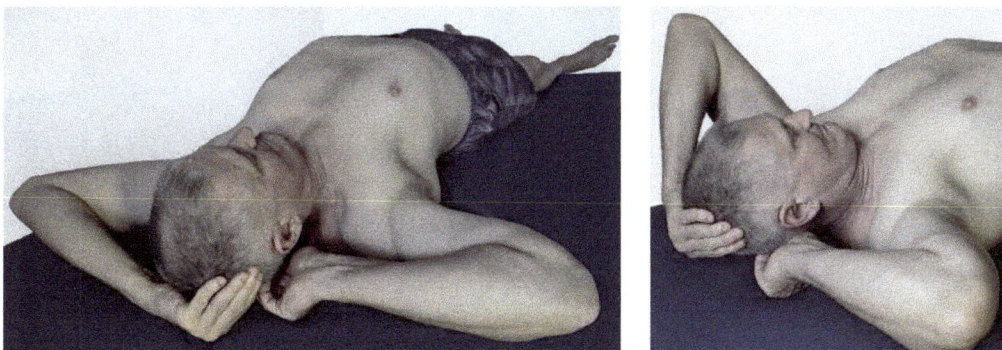

- Flex and sidebend your head to the left and slide your fingertips across the upper trapezius but this time across the fibres below the occiput.
- Slide your fingertips to the right of your cervical spine.
- Tilt your head backwards to relax upper trapezius and get better access to the deeper posterior cervical muscles.
- When treating the cervical muscles sidebend your head to the left and add rotation to the right, instead of flexion.
- Work down the right side of the neck, tilting the head backwards to treat the posterior cervical muscles and forwards to treat upper trapezius.

1.3g Kneading upper trapezius and upper posterior cervical muscles using the wadi or two balls in a net

- Lie on your back and raise your head off the floor.
- Reach behind the back of your head and support your head in your hand.

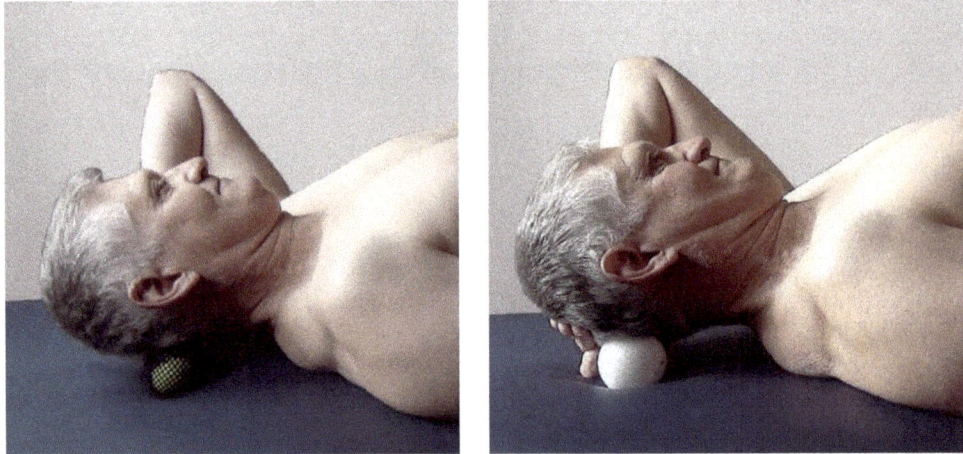

- Grasp the wadi or balls in the other hand and reach behind your head with your hand and the wadi or balls.
- Place the wadi or balls against the back of your head so one wheel or ball rests against right side of your occiput and the other rests on the left.

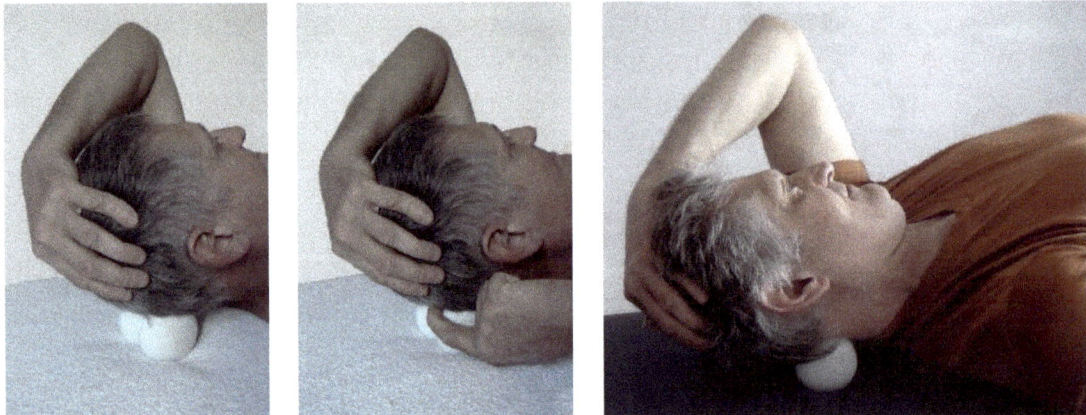

- Move your head from side to side over the wheels or balls and rotate your head if you want to put more pressure on one side of the spine.
- Work systematically along parallel strips from the occiput to about half-way down the cervical spine.

1.3h Kneading upper trapezius and posterior cervical muscles using the wadi or two balls in a net on their side

- Lie on your back and raise your head off the floor.
- Reach behind your head with your left hand and support it in your hand.
- Grasp the wadi or balls in the right hand so that your thumb and index finger sit in the valley between the wadi wheels or balls.
- Reach behind your head with your right hand holding the wadi/balls and place them on their side pressed against the middle of your occiput.

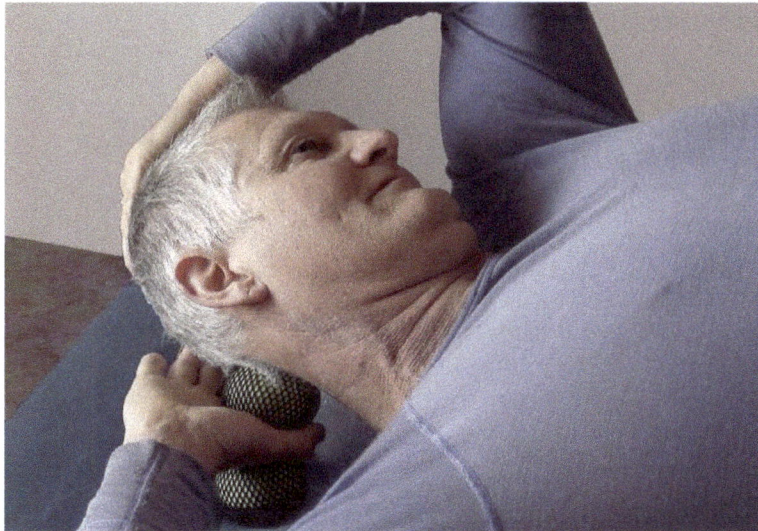

- Return your head and the wadi/balls to the floor.
- Flex your head, rotate it to the right and sidebend it to the left while simultaneously moving the contact point of the wadi/ball outwards and across the right upper trapezius overlying the occiput.
- Flex your wrist to tilt the wadi/balls and move it over the muscle. Let the natural weight of the head do most of the work.
- Reposition the wadi/ball with the contact just below the occiput and in the furrow running down the midline at the back of your neck.

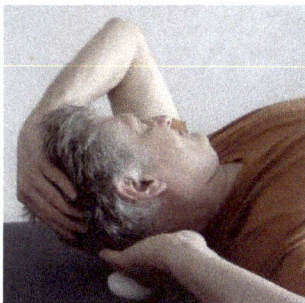

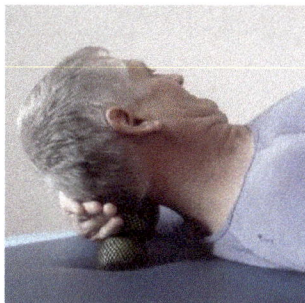

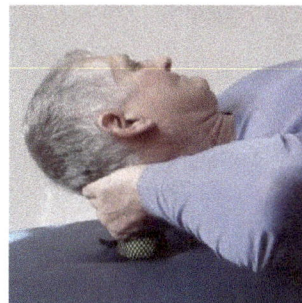

- Repeat the head and wrist movements and push the wadi/ball outwards against the inside of the trapezius and cervical column of the muscles.
- Tilt your head forwards to treat upper trapezius and backwards to relax upper trapezius and treat the deeper posterior cervical muscles.
- Continue down the right side of the cervical spine to about C5 vertebra.

Sternocleidomastoid

Massaging sternocleidomastoid can be useful for neck pain, tension headaches, strains from overhead work such as painting a ceiling, muscle spasms such as acute torticollis, degenerative changes such as osteoarthritis, whiplash injuries for example from a motor vehicle accident, conditions linked with poor posture, as well as asthma, sinusitis, bronchitis, pneumonia and influenza.

Sternocleidomastoid has two parts, one arises from the top of the sternum and attaches on the occiput and the other arises from an area on top of the clavicle, near the sternum and attaches on the mastoid process just behind the ear.

Actions: When working with some muscles it takes the head and neck forwards but when working with other muscles it tilts the head backwards. When one sternocleidomastoid muscle contracts it sidebends the head and neck to one side and rotates the head to the other, but when both work together with other muscles they produce level rotation.

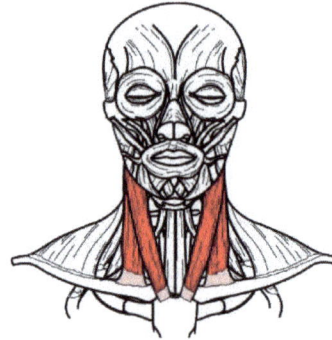

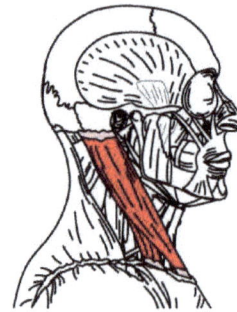

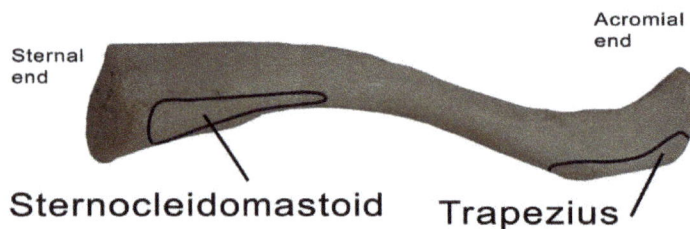

Sternal end   Acromial end

Sternocleidomastoid   Trapezius

Right clavicle - superior posterior view and muscle attachments

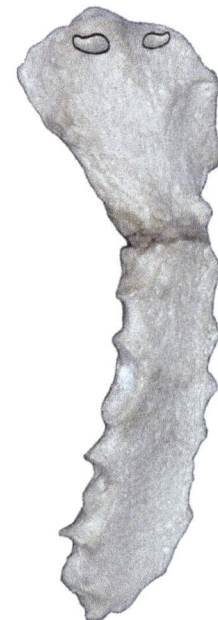

Sternum

1.4 Kneading sternocleidomastoid using the pads of your fingers

- Stand or sit on a chair with your arms at your side.
- Flex your right forearm at the elbow and then reach up to your right ear and place your fingertips behind the sternocleidomastoid muscle.
- Hook your fingers around the muscle, close to where it attaches on the mastoid process, the large bone at the base of the skull, just behind and under the ear.
- Sidebend your head a little to the left and rotate it a little to the right.
- Press into the muscle with the pads of your fingers while simultaneously increasing the sidebending and rotation of your head and neck.
- You can also take your head backwards a bit while tucking in your chin.

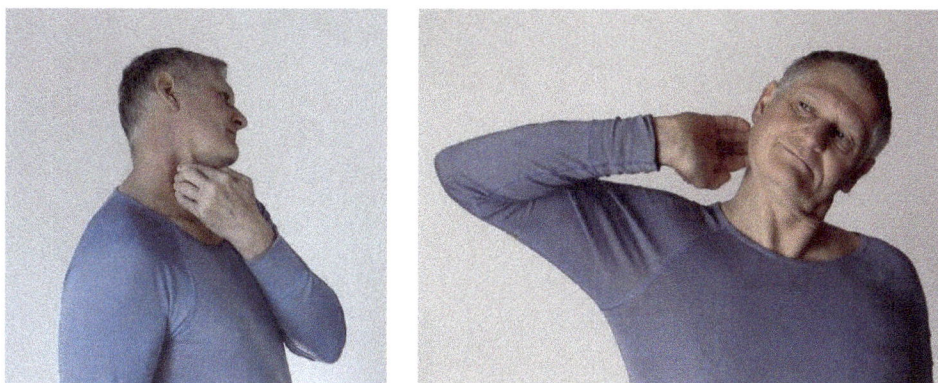

- Move down the muscle at about one-centimetre intervals until you get about half-way down the neck and then change hands.
- Reach across the front of your body with your left hand and hook your fingers around the back of sternocleidomastoid muscle at about the half-way point.
- Continue pressing forwards and into the muscle at about one-centimetre intervals with the pads of your fingers while sidebending and rotating your head and neck.
- Stop when you get to where the muscle attaches on the clavicle.

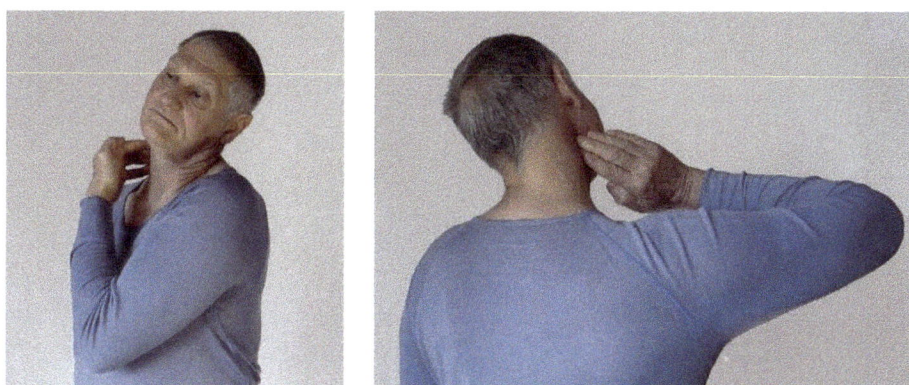

- As you work down the muscle, slide your finger a short distance forwards and across the muscle - but do not go over the muscle and do not press into the side or front of the neck where there are sensitive blood vessels, nerves and other structures.

Scalene

Massaging scalene can be useful for thoracic outlet syndrome, where the anterior scalene muscle becomes tight and short affecting nerve function and circulation to the upper limbs; whiplash injuries; respiratory diseases such as asthma and bronchitis; torticollis and muscle spasms; postural problems such as the forward head posture and dowager's hump; a scoliosis or reversed cervical lordosis or any alteration in spinal alignment; anything resulting in the shortening of the scalene muscles for example bad sitting habits. Most problems are a combination or lifestyle and genetic factors.

Anterior Scalene arises from the transverse processes at the side of vertebrae C3 to C6 and attaches on the upper surface of rib 1.
It lies behind sternocleidomastoid.

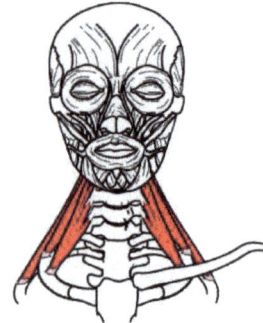

Middle Scalene arises from the transverse processes at the side of vertebrae C2 to C7 and attaches on the upper surface of rib 1.

Posterior Scalene arises from the transverse processes at the side of C5 to C7 and attaches on the upper surface of rib 2.

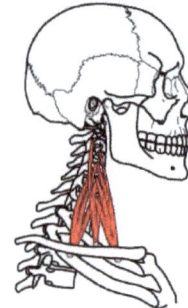

The scalene raise the upper ribs and sidebend the cervical spine to the same side.

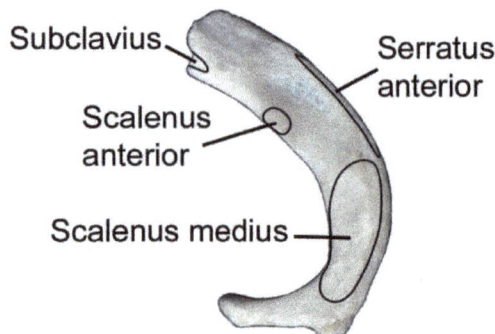

Subclavius
Serratus anterior
Scalenus anterior
Scalenus medius

Right Rib 1 - superior view

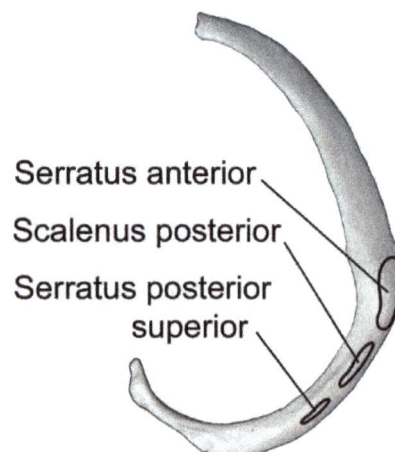

Serratus anterior
Scalenus posterior
Serratus posterior superior

Right Rib 2 - superior view

1.5 Kneading scalene muscles using the tips and pads of your fingers

- Stand or sit on a chair with your arms at your side.
- Flex your right forearm at the elbow and then reach up the right side of you neck and place your fingers around the back of the scalene muscles.
- To find the scalene, first locate the mastoid process, the large bone just behind the ear, then slide the pads of your fingers down the side of the neck to the first bony landmark, the transverse process of C1.
- From C1 the smaller transverse processes of all the other vertebra follow a straight line, a ridge of little bumps running down the side of the neck.

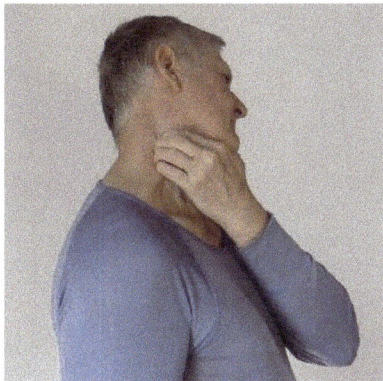

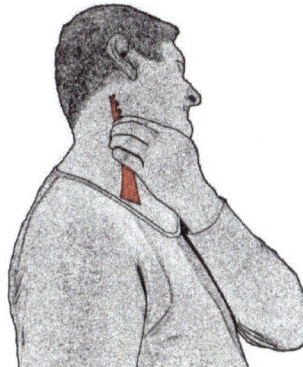

- With the fingertips hooked around the back of the scalene muscle-bony ridge, take your head backwards by tucking in your chin and sidebend your head a short distance to the left.
- Slide your fingertips over the ridge as you increase the chin tuck.
- Move down the muscle at about two-centimetre intervals until you get about half-way down the side of the neck and then change hands.
- Reach across the front of your body with your left hand and hook your fingers around the back of the scalene ridge at about the half-way point.
- Keep your head and neck sidebent to the left and chin tucked in.

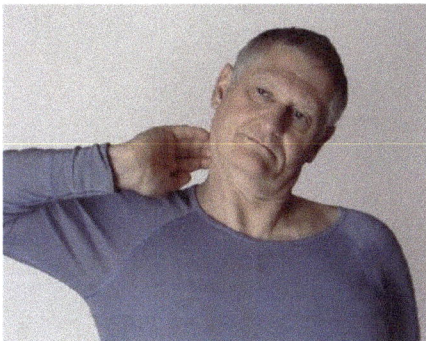

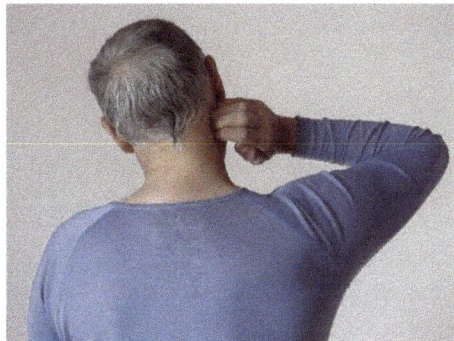

- Slide your fingertips forwards and across the scalene muscle-bony ridge with a rake like action again while increasing sidebending of the head.
- Tuck you chin in after each sliding action and keep it tucked in while you reposition your hand to start the manoeuvre again.
- Work down the side of the neck until your reach the end of the muscle attaching on the first rib.
- Take care not to press into the sensitive blood vessels and nerves in front of the neck.

Levator scapulae

Levator scapulae arises from the transverse processes at the sides of the cervical vertebrae C1 to C4 and attaches right at the top of the inner border of the scapula, between the spine of scapula and the superior angle. The fibres twist so that the lowest fibres on the scapula become the highest on the spine. The muscle is deep to trapezius.

Levator scapulae lifts the scapula and hence the shoulder and rotates it downwards. When the scapula is fixed, it rotates and sidebends the cervical spine to the side.

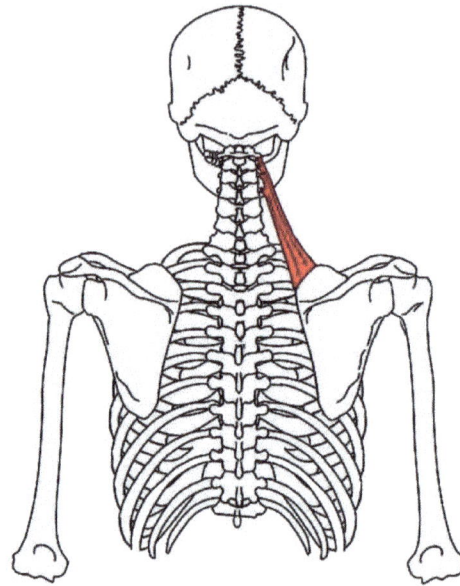

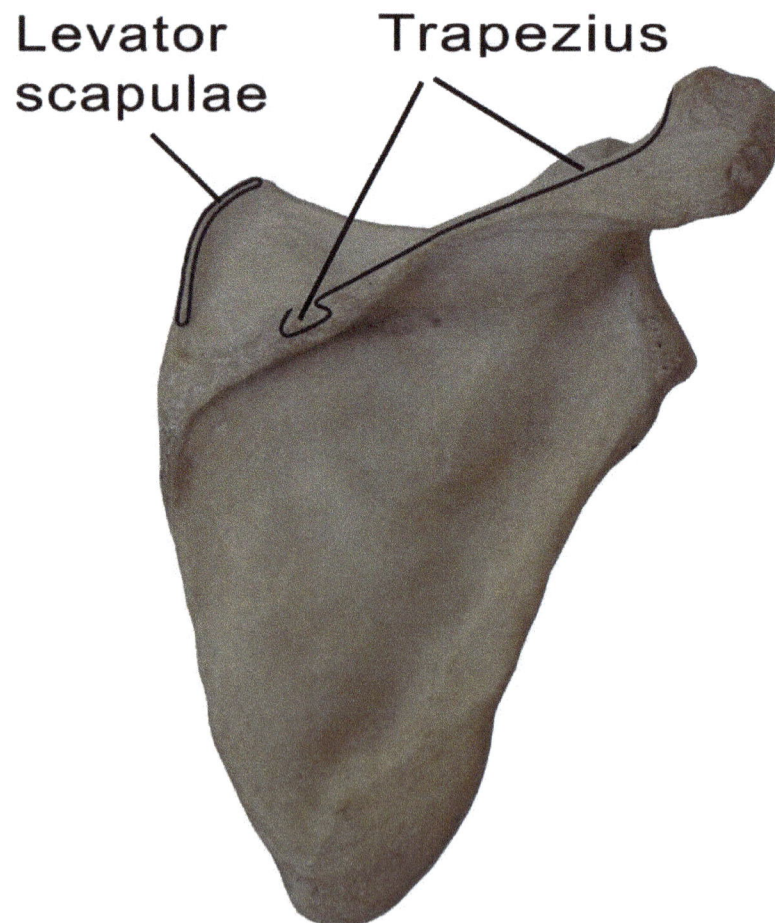

Levator scapulae   Trapezius

1.6a Kneading levator scapulae using your fingertips

- Sit straight on a chair, reach down the side of the chair with your right hand and grasp a suitable part of the chair to fix the right shoulder in a depressed position.
- Reach across the front of your body, over your right shoulder and as far behind your right shoulder as you can with your left hand.

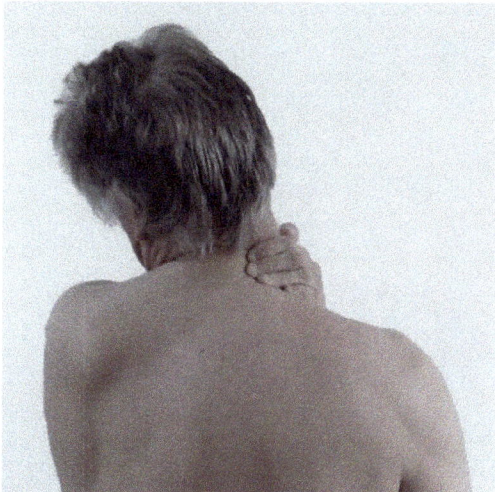

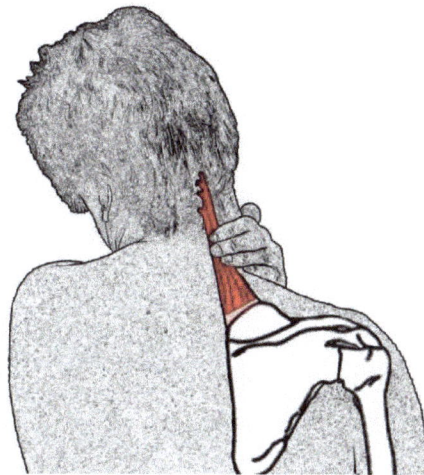

- Place your fingertips on the top and back of your rib cage, just above the point levator scapulae arises at the top of the inner border of the scapula.
- Levator scapulae is under trapezius so flex your fingers and push your fingertips through trapezius and then hook them around levator scapulae.
- Sidebend and rotate your head and cervical spine a short way to the left.
- Pull with your fingers and then slide your fingertips across the muscle while simultaneously sidebending and rotating your head to the left.

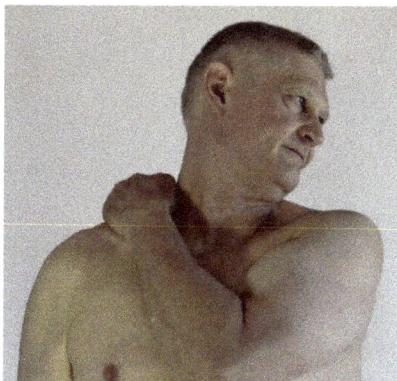

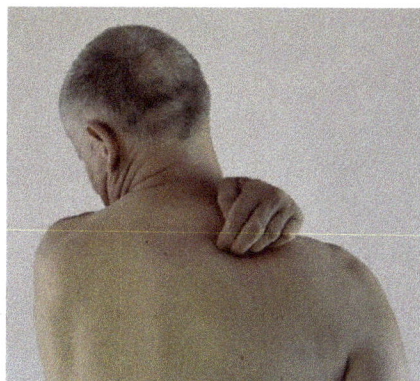

- Start at the inner upper border of the scapula and work up the back of the neck until the levator scapulae passes under, blends with cervical muscles, and becomes difficult to feel.
- Move across short parallel strips as the muscle is not very wide.
- Keep your right shoulder depressed.
- This technique can be done kneeling on the floor and depressing and fixing the shoulder by holding your ankle with one hand.
- As the muscle is situated deep under trapezius you will need to press hard - the technique can be a little challenging on the fingers.

1.6b Kneading levator scapulae using the wadi or a blunt pointy object

- Sit straight on a chair, reach down the side of the chair with your right hand and grasp under the seat of the chair to fix the right shoulder in a downward position.
- Grasp the wadi or pointy object in your left hand, reach across the front of your body, over your right shoulder and as far behind your shoulder as you can.

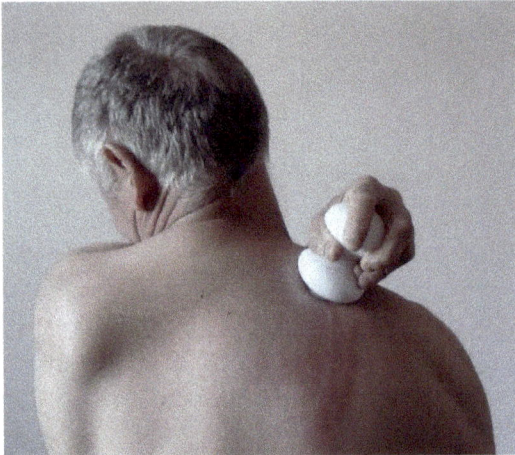

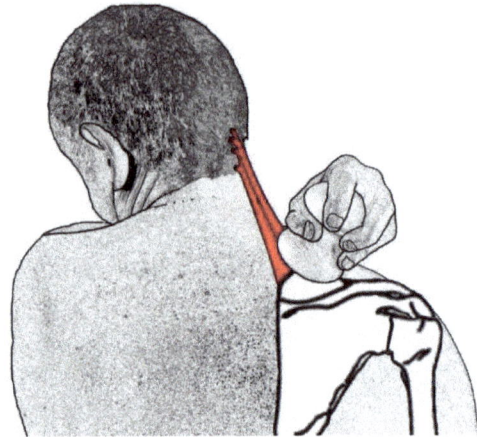

- Place the edge of the wadi just below the point where levator scapulae muscle arises at the top of the inner border of the scapula.
- Press the edge firmly against your rib cage because the muscle is situated deep under the trapezius.
- Sidebend and rotate your cervical spine to the left as you slide the edge of the wadi upwards and outwards across the muscle.

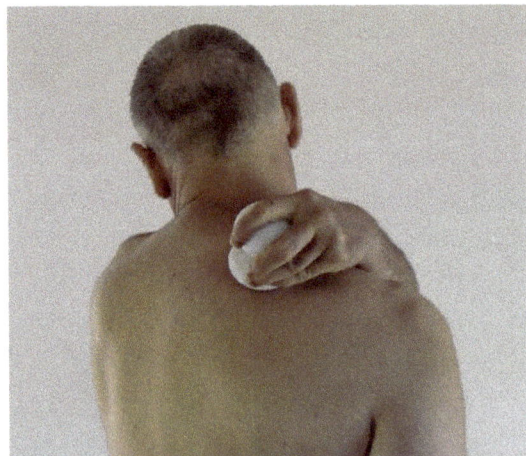

- Work up the muscle from where it starts on the inner upper border of the scapula to where it merges with other muscles at the base of the neck.
- Move across short parallel strips because the muscle is relatively narrow.
- Keep your right shoulder down with a firm hold on the side of the chair.
- This technique can be done kneeling on the floor and holding your ankle to fix your shoulder in a downward position.

THE THORACIC SPINE AND SHOULDERS

Massaging the middle trapezius, rhomboids and levator scapulae muscles at the top and back of the thoracic spine and shoulders can be useful for people who spend a long time sitting using a computer or mobile phone.

Massaging these muscles can be useful for shoulder pain and tension, overuse syndromes, torticollis, whiplash injuries, a dowager's hump, scoliosis, reversed or increased thoracic kyphosis, round shoulders, tension headaches, high levels of stress, the effects of asthma and bronchitis, muscle spasms, postural fatigue caused by prolonged sitting and bad sitting habits.

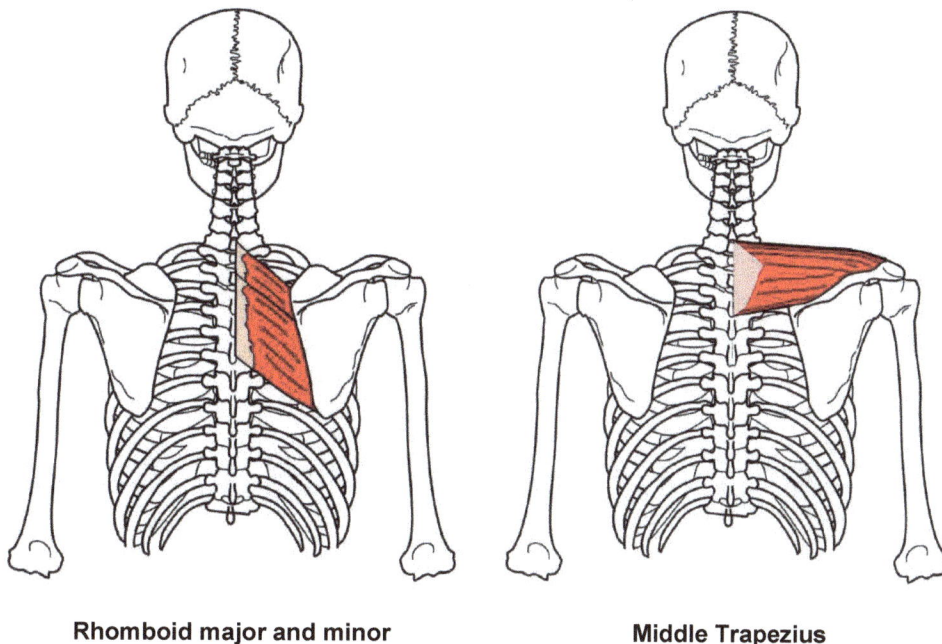

Rhomboid major and minor   **Middle Trapezius**

Middle trapezius arises on the spinous processes and ligaments of vertebra C7 to T3 and attaches on the spine and acromion process of the scapular. It acts to pull the shoulders backwards.

Rhomboid major and minor arise from the spinous processes of vertebrae C7 and T1 to T5 and attach onto the inner border of the scapula. It acts to pull the shoulders backwards and rotate them downwards.

1.7a Kneading middle trapezius and rhomboid major and minor using the tips of your hooked fingers or the pads of your fingers

- Stand or sit on a chair.
- Flex your left forearm at the elbow and then reach across the front of your body, over your right shoulder and as far down the right side of thoracic spine as you can.
- Hook the fingers of your left hand over the spine of your scapula, which you can feel as a bony ridge running across the right side of your back.
- Use this bony ridge to pull your hand further down the back.

- Slide the fingers along the spine of the scapula until they drop over the inner edge of the scapula and onto the ribs.
- Flex your right shoulder about 90 degrees so your arm is horizontal and straight out in front of you, and then reach forwards and away from your body with your right hand.

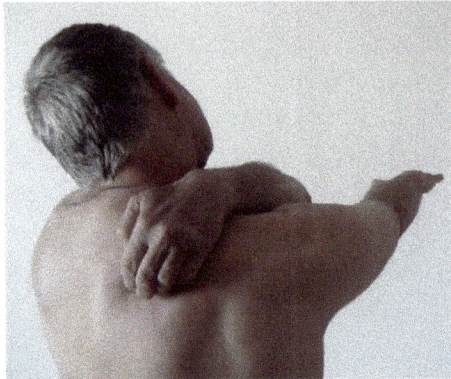

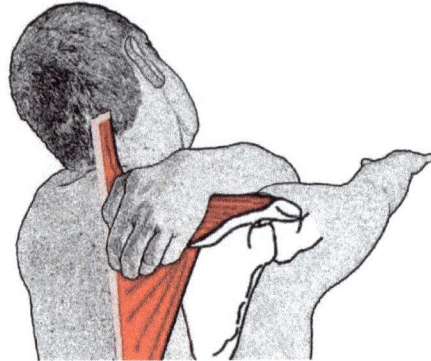

- Raising and reaching away with the arm takes the scapula away from the spine and stretches middle trapezius and rhomboid fibres.
- Sidebend your head to the left to stretch the muscle fibres further.

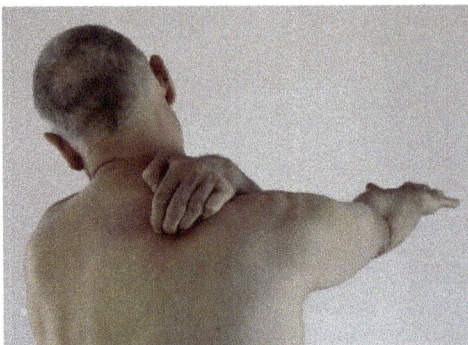

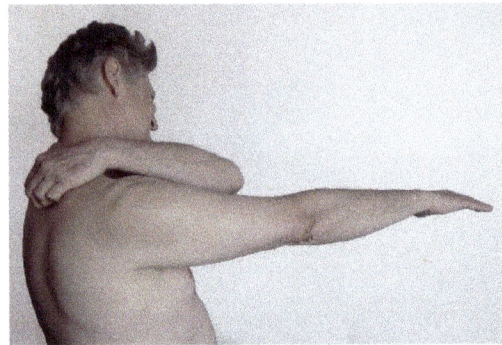

- Press the pads or tips of your fingers into the muscles and then slide them up towards the top of the shoulder while simultaneously increasing the reaching action of your arm and the sidebending of your head.
- Slide your fingertips upwards and outwards and diagonally across your back and towards the end of your right shoulder so your kneading is perpendicular to the muscle fibres.

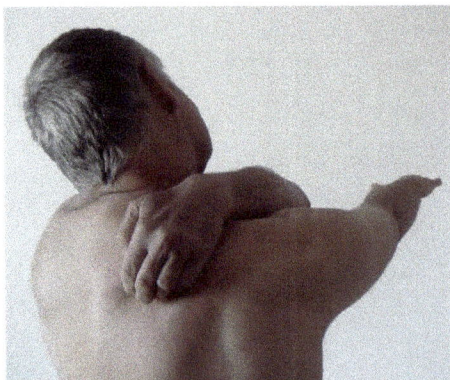

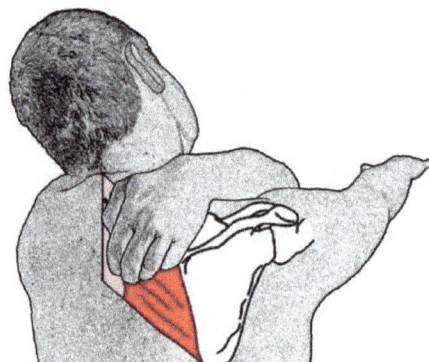

- This technique can be done with your arm hanging loosely at your side.

1.7b Kneading middle trapezius and rhomboids using a small, rolled-up towel or two balls in a net

- Lie on your back on a mat or carpeted floor with your head on a small pillow.
- Flex your right hip and knee and then roll onto your left side.
- Place a tightly rolled-up towel or two balls in a net against the back of your rib cage between the spine and the bottom of the right side of your scapula and orientated so it is parallel with the spine.

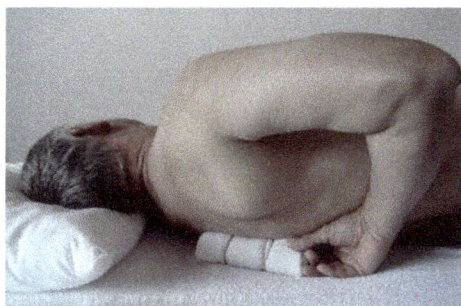

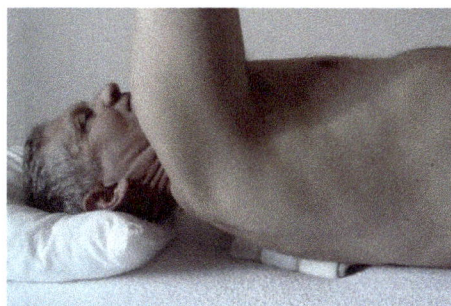

- Start with the rolled-up towel next to the spine, in the depression between your spinous processes and the inner column of spinal muscles.
- Hold the rolled-up towel in position against your back and then return your back and the rolled-up towel to the floor.
- Allow your trunk to relax over the rolled-up towel but keep your right hip and knee flexed.

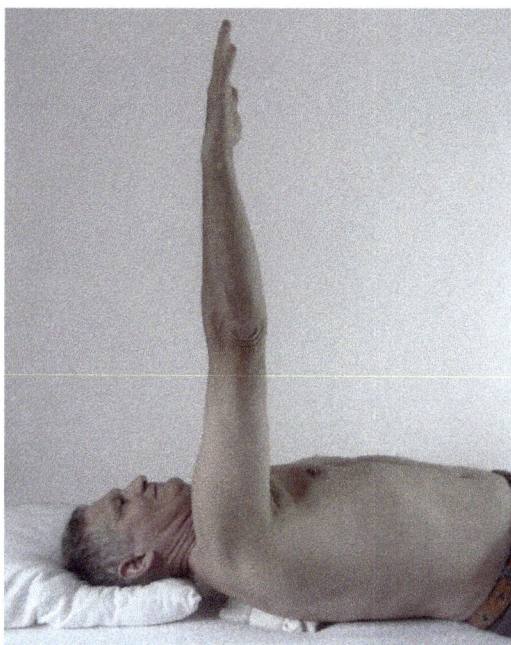

- Flex your right arm 90 degree so it is vertical.
- Sidebend your head to the left to stretch the muscle fibres.
- Move your right knee a short distance to the right to put more body weight over the rolled-up towel and increases pressure on the muscle.

- Reach up to the ceiling with your right hand to move your scapula away from the spine and stretch the muscles while it is pinned to your ribcage by the rolled-up towel.
- Now combine the previous two actions with deep breathing: Take a deep breath in and then exhale and move your knee to the side and reach upwards with your hand.

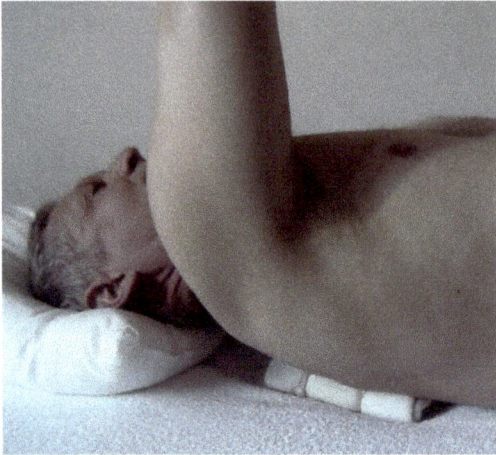

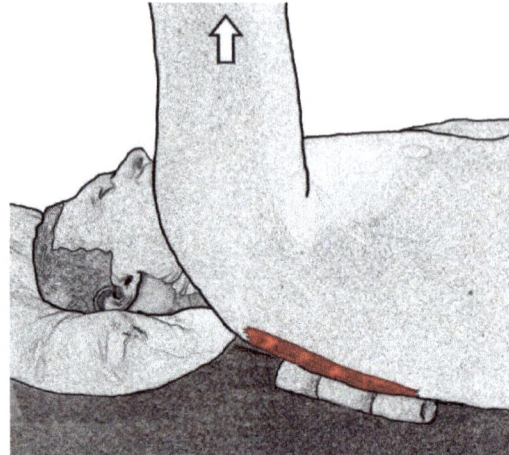

- After three breaths return your right knee and arm to a more relaxed position, then roll onto your left side again.
- Place the rolled-up towel halfway between your spine and the border of your scapula and then roll back to the floor and repeat the technique.
- Place the rolled-up towel so it is even further from your spine and is against the inner border of the scapula and repeat the technique again.

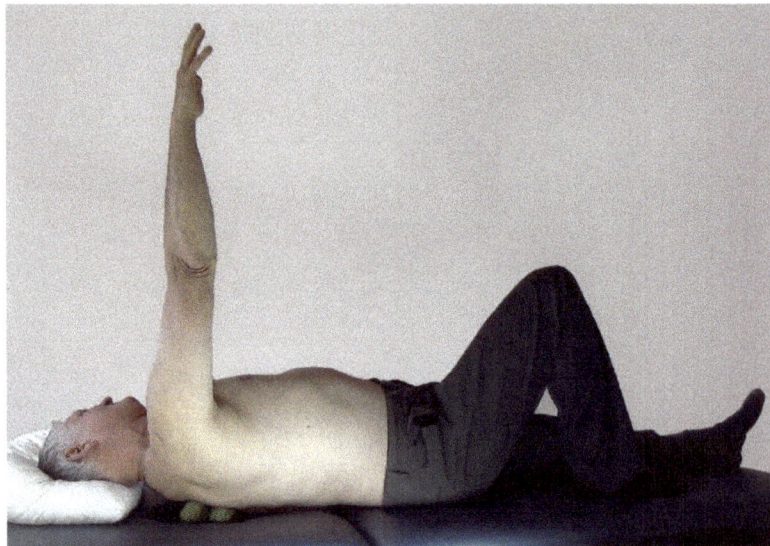

- Move the rolled-up towel up the spine and then repeat the technique in the three positions just described - next to the spine, halfway between the spine and the scapula and next to the border of the scapula.
- The technique becomes impractical above a certain level of the thoracic spine because it is too difficult to use your body weight effectively.
- This technique can also be done using two balls in a net.

THE THORACIC SPINE AND RIB CAGE

Combining deep breathing and rib mobilising, stretches muscles of the thoracic spine and rib cage and can be useful for pain in these muscles; whiplash injuries; muscle spasms; scoliosis or abnormal spinal alignment; postural fatigue; joint degeneration; and respiratory diseases such as asthma and bronchitis.

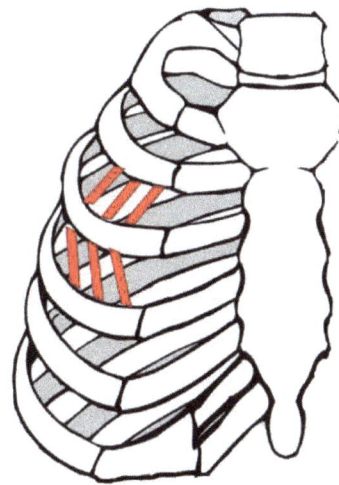

The **intercostal muscles** arise from the lower border of ribs 1 to 11.
The **external intercostal muscles** run obliquely, downwards and forwards to the upper border of the rib below. Their action is to produce inspiration.
The **internal intercostal muscles** are deeper and run obliquely, downwards and backwards, to attach on the upper border of the rib below. Their action is to produce expiration.

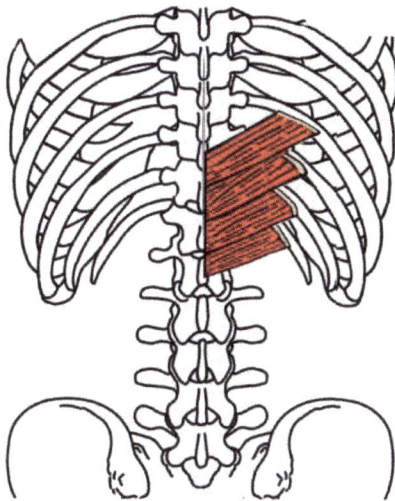

Serratus posterior inferior   Anterior intercostal muscles

Quadratus lumborum arises on the back of the pelvis and runs vertically to the bottom of rib 12, and obliquely to the tip of transverse processes of lumbar vertebrae L1 to L4. A third layer may be present running from L1 to L4 transverse processes bottom of rib 12. The muscles help fix the lower ribs for respiration.

Serratus posterior inferior arises from the spinous processes of T11 to L2 and the adjacent ligaments and passes upwards and outwards to attach on the under surface of ribs 9 to 12. The muscles help depress the ribs for forced exhalation.

Serratus posterior superior arises from the back of C7 to T3 vertebrae and attaches on the upper surface of ribs 2 to 5. It lies deep to the rhomboids. The muscles help elevate the ribs for forced inhalation.

1.7c Mobilising technique for increasing exhalation of the rib cage

- Lie on your left side and flex both hips and knees.
- Flex your left hip 90 degrees and flex your right hip a bit less so your right knee is just behind your left knee.
- This will allow the right side of your pelvis to tilt downwards and pull on the lower ribs.
- Keep the back of your pelvis perpendicular to the floor.
- Lift your upper body off the floor and rest on your left elbow and forearm.

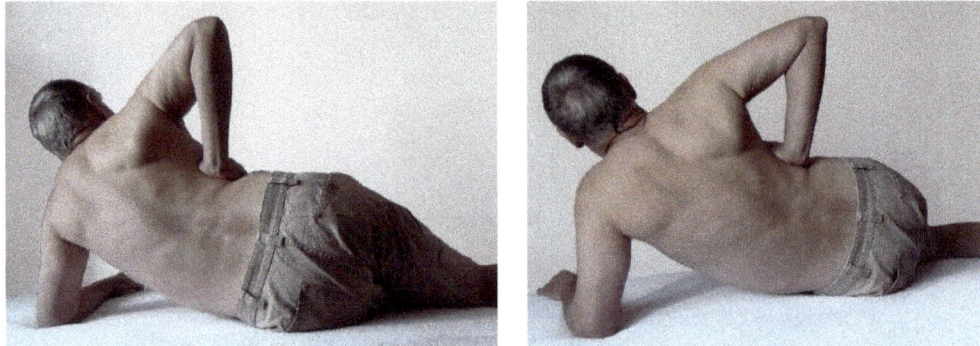

- Your left elbow is flexed 90 degrees and directly under your left shoulder.
- Allow your lower thoracic spine to drop towards the floor so your spine is sidebent right.
- This facilitates exhalation of the ribs on the right.
- Place the heel of your right hand on the right side of your rib cage.
- Start with your hand at the bottom of the rib cage and as near to the spine as possible.
- Your fingers should point forwards and wrap around your ribs.

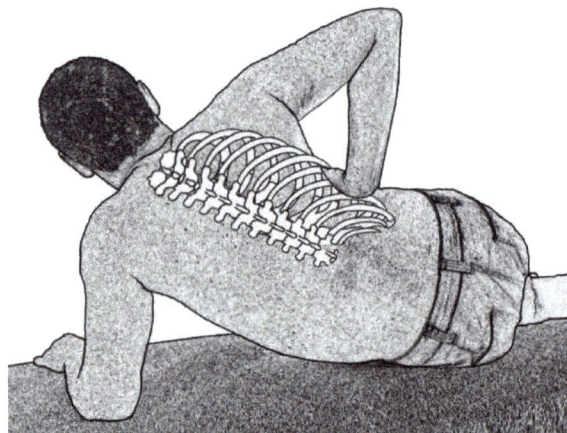

- Take a deep breath in, then exhale and push against your lower ribs with your right hand.
- Pushing helps depress the lower ribs and increase sidebending for greater exhalation.
- Work up the rib cage to the arm pit, one rib at a time.
- As you go higher up the rib cage flex your right elbow.
- Turn onto your right side and repeat the technique for the left rib cage.

1.7d Mobilising technique for increasing inhalation of the rib cage

- Lie on your left side with your head on a small pillow and flex both hips and knees about 90 degrees.
- Reach forwards and away with your left hand and slide your left shoulder forwards.
- This rotates your spine to the right and sidebends it to the left.
- Keep the back of your pelvis perpendicular to the floor.
- Raise your right arm over your head until it rests against the right side of your head.

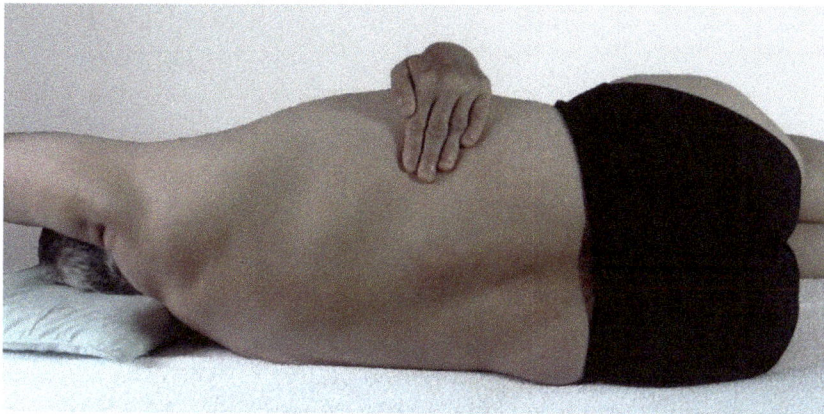

- Reach across the front of your body with your left hand and then over the side of your body and place your fingertips on the side of rib 12 at the bottom of the rib cage.
- Try to get your fingers as close as possible to your spine.
- Take a deep breath in and then exhale and push rib 12 downwards towards the full exhalation position with your left hand.
- Inhale and reach your right hand away from your head while you continue to hold down rib 12 with your left hand.
- Work up the rib cage one rib at a time until you reach the arm pit.

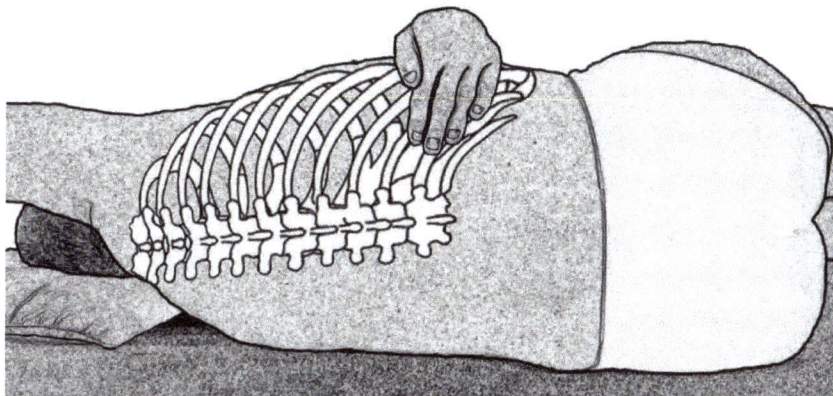

- As you go higher up the ribs the type of rib movement changes.
- In the lower rib cage there is more bucket handle movement so you should press downwards and inwards, whereas in the upper rib cage there is more pump handle movement so you should press downwards and backwards.

THE THORACIC AND LUMBAR SPINE

Massaging the muscles of the thoracic and lumbar spine can be useful for lower and upper back pain from muscle and ligament injuries including whiplash injuries, muscle spasms, scoliosis, increased or reversed thoracic kyphosis or any alteration in spinal alignment, intervertebral disc and joint degeneration (osteoarthritis), postural fatigue and sciatica. Massaging these regions of the spine can help sedentary as well as manual workers and is especially beneficial for people who spend time sitting using a computer or mobile phone

Muscles of the spine

The major muscle group in the thoracic and lumbar spine is the **erector spinae** which is made up of nine muscles of varying lengths, size and attachments, and the composition of these muscles and their tendon varies throughout the spine.

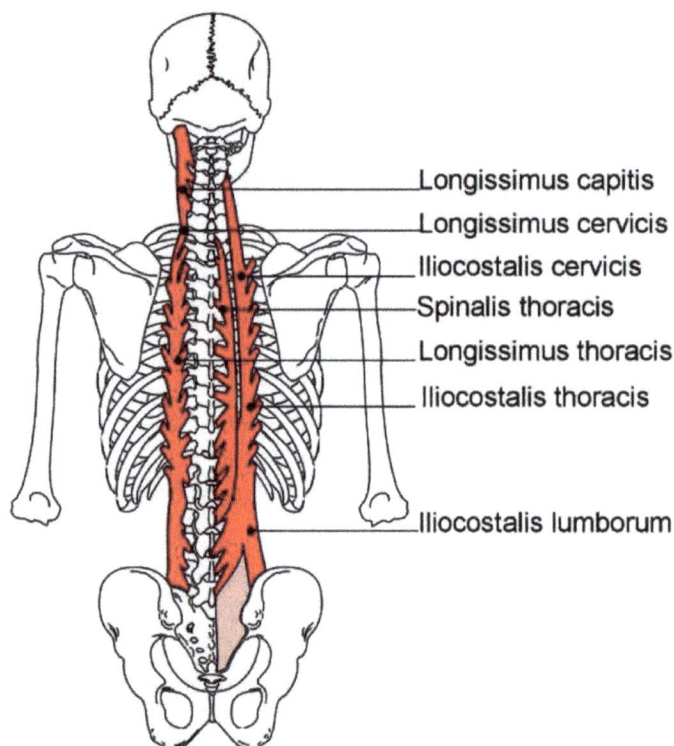

Longissimus capitis
Longissimus cervicis
Iliocostalis cervicis
Spinalis thoracis
Longissimus thoracis
Iliocostalis thoracis

Iliocostalis lumborum

Erector spinae, pelvis, spine, ribs, head and shoulders   **Spine and pelvis**

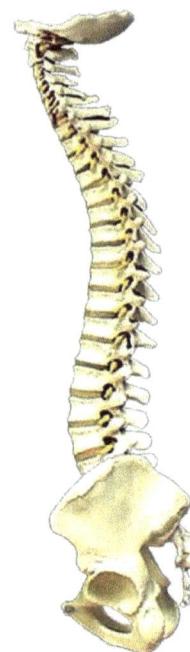

The erector spinae arise on the sacrum as a broad thick tendon, and in the lumbar becomes a thick muscle. In the thoracic it separates into three distinct columns: iliocostalis, longissimus and spinalis. A depression, the paravertebral gutter, runs the length of the thoracic and lumbar spine between the bulk of the muscle mass and the bony spinous processes. When both right and left sides of the muscle contracts there is extension (backward bending). When one side contracts there is extension, side bending and rotation of the spine and head.

Iliocostalis the outer column includes: iliocostalis lumborum which runs from the pelvis to the ribs; iliocostalis thoracis and iliocostalis cervicis, which run from rib to rib and rib to vertebra.

Longissimus the middle column includes longissimus thoracis and cervicis which run between vertebra; and longissimus capitis, which run from vertebra to skull.

Spinalis the inner column includes: spinalis thoracis and spinalis cervicis which run between vertebra; and spinalis capitis, which runs from vertebra to skull.

Other spinal muscles include **semispinalis thoracis** and **semispinalis cervicis**, which run from vertebra to vertebra, and **semispinalis capitis**, which also attaches on the skull. **Interspinales**, which run from one spinous process to another and are present between C2 and T3, and T11 and L5.

Intertransversarii, which run from one transverse process to another and are present between C1 and T1, and between T10 and the sacrum. **Multifidus** arises on the sacrum and extends as high up as C2. **Rotatores** are the deepest muscles and are most developed in the thoracic spine.

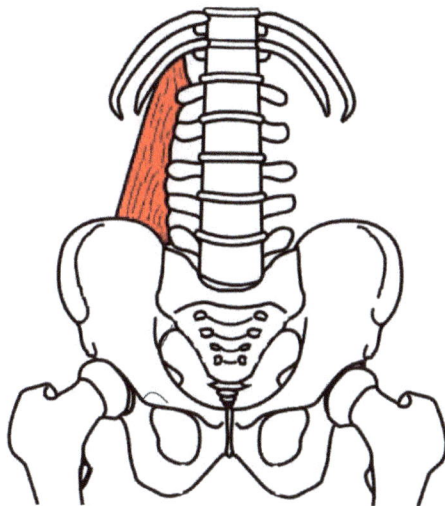

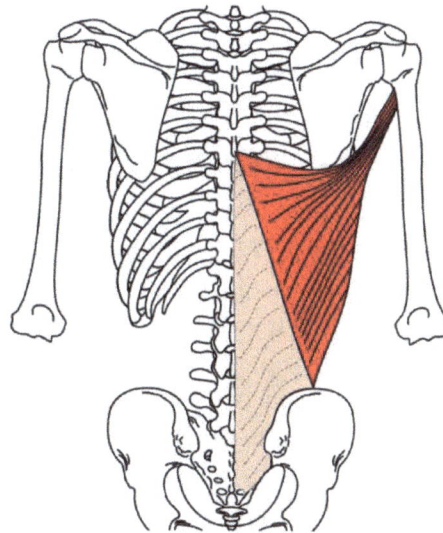

Quadratus lumborum   Latissimus dorsi and thoracolumbar fascia

The **thoracolumbar fascia** extends from the cervical spine to the sacrum. It also attaches on ribs, the iliac crest of the pelvis, transverse and spinous processes of vertebra, spinal ligaments and deep fascia. In the lumbar it is thick and strong and has three layers. It encloses and intermeshes with muscles in the lumbar region and merges with abdominal fascia.

The **latissimus dorsi** muscle attaches on the upper outer border of the thoracolumbar fascia as well as the spine and ribs and on the upper part of the humerus at the front of the shoulder. **Serratus posterior inferior** and **serratus posterior superior** run from vertebrae to rib.

Quadratus lumborum arises on the back of the pelvis. Some fibres run vertically and attach at the bottom of rib 12, and other fibres run obliquely and attach on the tip of transverse processes of lumbar vertebrae L1 to L4. A third layer may be present running from L1 to L4 transverse processes to the bottom of rib 12. Most of the muscle lies deep to erector spinae. When it acts on one side quadratus lumborum produces lumbar sidebending. When it acts on both sides it fixes the lower ribs to enable full respiration.

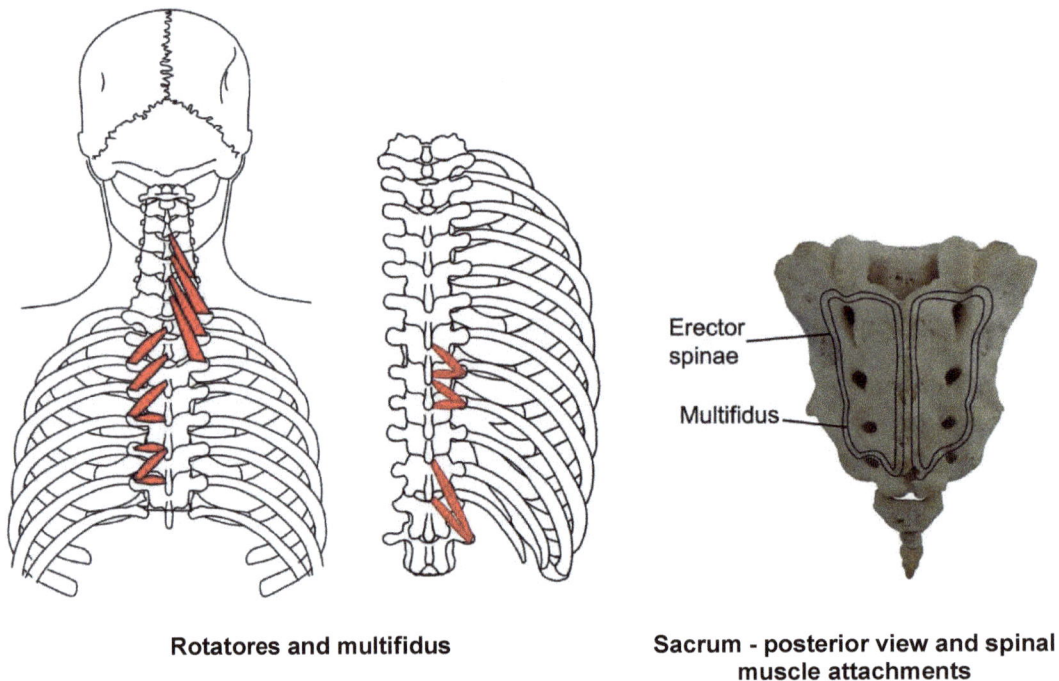

Rotatores and multifidus

Sacrum - posterior view and spinal muscle attachments

Erector spinae

Multifidus

Contraindications for inhibition of the spine techniques

The following group of techniques are contraindicated for some groups of people and a range of diseases and health problems. Do not do any of the thoracic and lumbar inhibition techniques if you are under 14 years of age, overweight or very pregnant, have recently had back surgery or a spinal fracture, or have extreme back stiffness because of osteoarthritis or ankylosing spondylitis or a severe kyphosis, scoliosis, or acute symptoms such as extreme back pain or swelling, or active rheumatoid arthritis or a history of osteoporosis, haemophilia, spina bifida or cancer, or have a spondylolisthesis. Consult a qualified health professional if you are unsure whether you have something that could be a problem for you doing the techniques or if you need a diagnosis.

These techniques require good shoulder integrity. Rotator cuff problems can be made worse from doing these inhibition techniques because they involve taking the arms over the head. Do not do these techniques while you have a rotator cuff injury, have had rotator cuff surgery or think you may be vulnerable to a rotator cuff injury. Avoid these techniques or modify them if you are genetically hypermobile (extremely flexible) or vulnerable to dislocation of the shoulder.

If you have any of these health issues the techniques can be done more safely without an applicator. They can be highly effective when done just lying on your back on a mat on the floor. People with an increased kyphosis or who have a hypermobile neck may need to do these techniques with a pillow behind their head. If through doing these techniques over time you become more flexible in the thoracic spine then you can gradually reduce the height of the pillow until you have no pillow and later move to a small, folded towel before eventually trying the rolled-up towel, two balls in a net and the wadi. The most important thing is to avoid allowing your head to drop back into a hyperextended position.

1.8a Inhibition of muscles of the thoracic spine using muscle contraction, relaxation and breathing over a rolled-up towel

<u>Start position</u> There are two ways to lie on the rolled-up towel - method A and B.

- Grasp the tightly rolled-up towel in your right hand.
- **A**. Sit on the floor, on a carpet or mat.
- Reach behind your back with the rolled-up towel and place it across the middle of your back at right angles to your spine.
- Hold the rolled-up towel in place across your back and lie on the floor over the rolled-up towel.
- **B**. Lie on the floor with your hips and knees flexed.
- Move your knees to the left and allow the right side of your body to raise off the floor.
- Place the rolled-up towel behind your back so it runs across it.
- Holding the rolled-up towel in place, move your legs back to the upright position and return the right side of your body and the rolled-up towel to the floor.
- Adjust the rolled-up towel so it is straight and perpendicular to the spine.

Most people have a convex curvature or kyphosis in the middle of their thoracic spine, and they should place the rolled-up towel at the apex of their kyphosis. If you cannot find your kyphosis or do not have one, then place the rolled-up towel in the middle of your thoracic spine or where it is stiff and inflexible.

A.

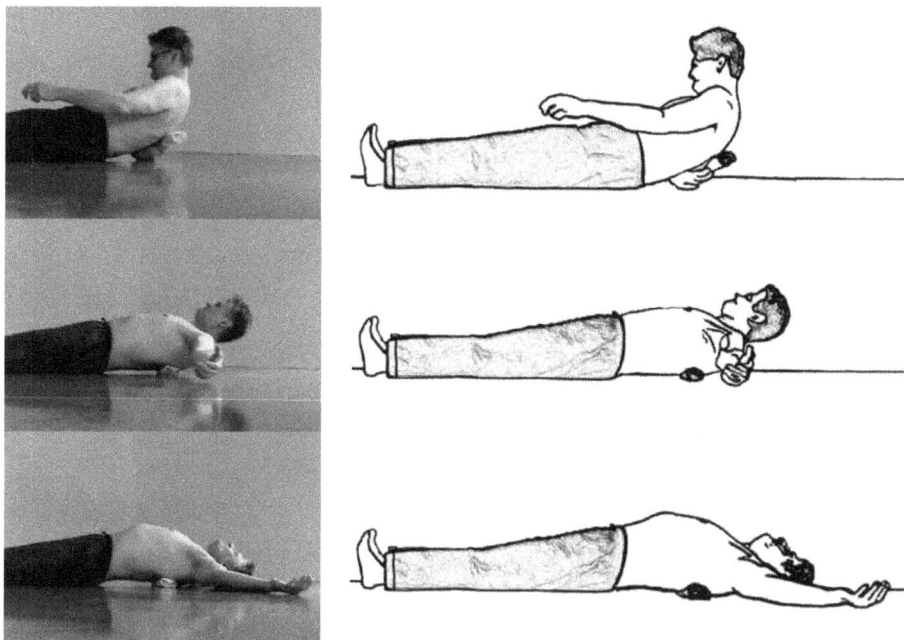

- Move your feet and arms apart, turn your palms upwards, tuck your chin in and relax over the towel.
- Take a deep breath, hold it in for a few seconds and then exhale, let go of your muscles and relax your whole body.
- Repeat the deep inhalation, exhalation and relaxation of your body two or three more times, each time with your arms wider.

1.8b Inhibition of the muscles on both sides of the thoracic spine using a bilateral upper limb rotation stretch over a rolled-up towel

Begin by adopting the start position described in technique 1.8a. The tense and relax method is followed by the dynamic stretching method in each technique.

- Move both arms apart until they are at right angles to your body.
- Take a deep breath, hold it in and rotate your arms in opposite directions.
- Rotate one arm outwards (external rotation) until your thumb points down into the floor and simultaneously rotate the other arm inwards (internal rotation) until your other thumb also points into the floor.
- Full outward rotation means going 90 degrees past the palm up position.
- Full inward rotation means going 90 degrees past the palm down position
- Turn your head towards the arm that is outwardly rotated.

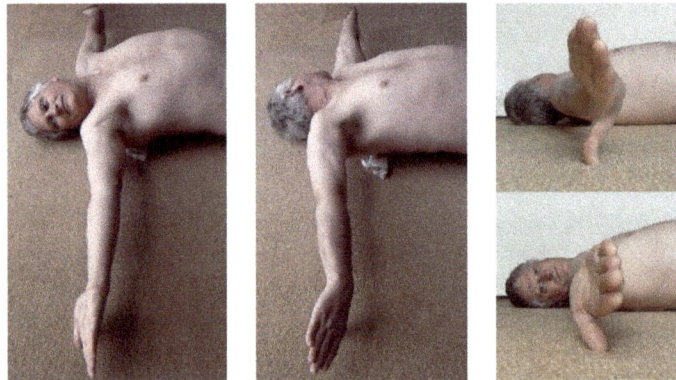

- Tense your muscles at the end of the rotation movements and then exhale and let go of your muscles and allow your body to relax and sink onto the rolled-up towel and into the floor.
- Take in another deep breath and hold it in.
- Rotate your arms in the opposite direction, tense your muscles again, then exhale let go of your muscles and relax your whole body.
- Repeat the technique in each direction two or three times and then move the rolled-up towel one vertebra higher or lower.
- Focus on the apex of the thoracic convexity or where there is most stiffness but cover the thoracic spine from about T5 to T12.

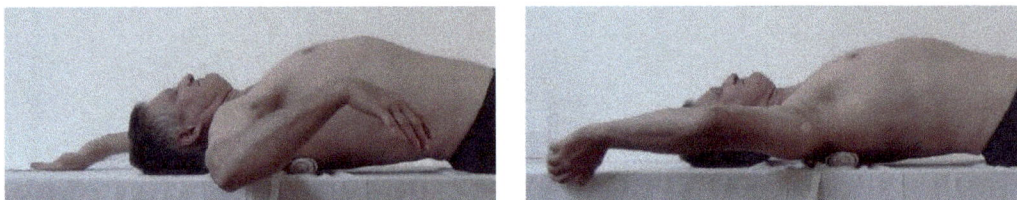

- The dynamic stretching method involves keeping both arms moving.
- Rotate one arm outwards while you rotate the other arm inwards.
- Pause at the end of the movement to increase the muscle contraction.
- Try this technique with your arms flexed 90 degrees at the elbow.
- Touch the floor with both elbows, then with both elbows and one hand and then with both elbows and both hands simultaneously.

1.8c Inhibition of the muscles of the thoracic spine using a unilateral upper limb longitudinal stretch over a rolled-up towel

Begin by adopting the start position described in technique 1.8a.

- Take both arms over your head and feel a change in the weight distribution of your body over the rolled-up towel and an increase in pressure on your back muscles.
- Move your arms slowly and cautiously over your head, especially if you are round shouldered, stiff in your spine or have not warmed up.
- Take a deep breath and hold it in.
- Reach along the floor and away from your head with one arm.

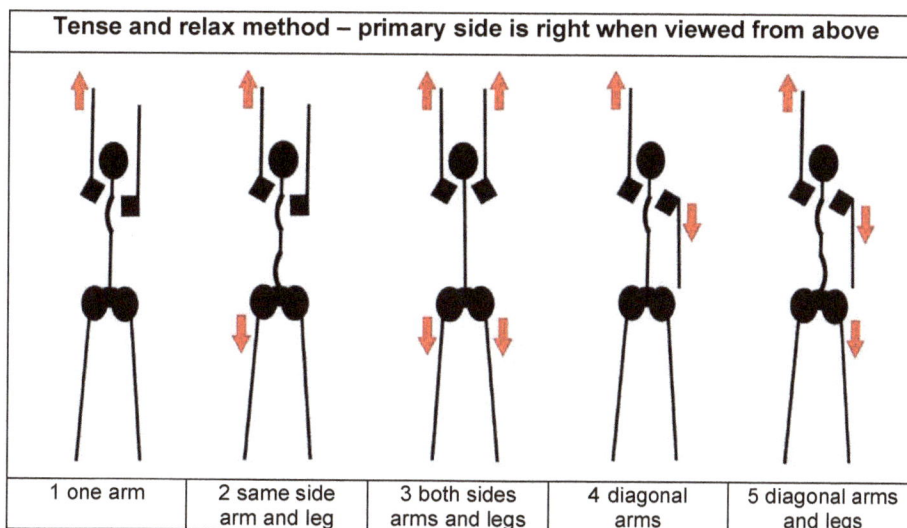

Tense and relax method – primary side is right when viewed from above				
1 one arm	2 same side arm and leg	3 both sides arms and legs	4 diagonal arms	5 diagonal arms and legs

- Longitudinal movement of the right arm is achieved by elevating and tilting your scapula and sidebending the thoracic spine to the left.
- Stretch from your shoulder to your fingertips and keep your arm straight.
- Hold the stretch for a few seconds, then exhale and relax.
- Allow your arm to drop towards the floor and your body to sink onto the rolled up towel and into the floor.
- Repeat this stretch two or three times, going a little harder each time and then repeat the stretch with the other arm.
- This is the tense and relax, one arm technique - see chart stick-body 1.

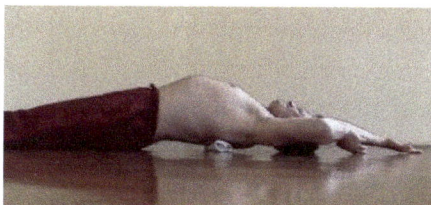

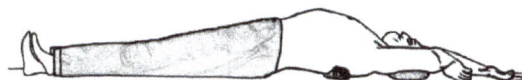

- An alternative to the tense and relax method is the dynamic stretch.
- Reach away with one arm and then the other and always keep moving.
- Increase your muscle contraction at the end of each stretch.
- Alternate between left and right several times, then move the rolled-up towel one vertebra level higher or lower, and repeat the technique.

49

1.8d Inhibition of the muscles of the thoracic spine using a unilateral upper and lower limb longitudinal stretch over a rolled-up towel

Begin by adopting the start position described in technique 1.8a.

- Take both arms over your head and feel an increase in pressure on your back muscles from the rolled-up towel.
- Take care not to strain your shoulders by moving too quickly - warm up.
- Dorsiflex your right foot by pointing your heel away and lifting your toes.
- Take a deep breath and hold it in.
- Reach away, along the floor and above your head with your right arm and reach away and along the floor with your right leg.
- Stretch down one side of your body - from your shoulder to your fingertips and from your hip to your heel.
- Longitudinal movement of the right leg is achieved by sidebending your lumbar spine to the left and tilting your pelvis and hips.
- Keep your right knee and elbow straight.
- Do not point your toes - better leg movement is achieved by dorsiflexing your foot and pushing away from your heel.

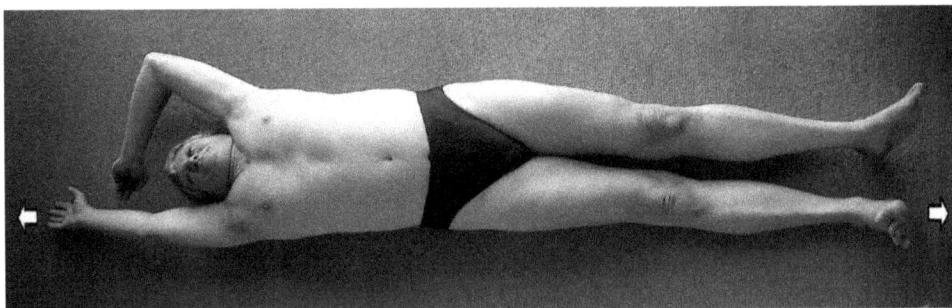

- Hold the stretch for a few seconds, then exhale and relax.
- Allow your arm and leg to drop towards the floor and your body to sink onto the rolled up towel and into the floor.
- This is the tense and relax, same side arm and leg technique and longitudinal arm and leg stretch - see chart stick-body 2.
- Do these actions two or three times and then repeat them two or three times with your arm and leg on the left side of your body.
- An alternative to the tense and relax method is the dynamic stretching method which involves keeping your arms and legs moving.
- Reach with your right arm and leg simultaneously and then reach with your left arm and leg simultaneously.
- Alternate movement between the left and right side of your body, several times without stopping.
- Increase your muscle contraction at the end of each movement.
- After massaging the muscles at this vertebral level, sit up or roll over, then move the rolled-up towel one vertebra level higher or lower and repeat the technique.
- Cover the whole thoracic spine but focus on areas of tightness and where the thoracic curvature is greatest.

1.8e Inhibition of the muscles of the thoracic spine using a bilateral upper and lower limb longitudinal stretch over a rolled-up towel

Begin by adopting the start position described in technique 1.8a.

- Take both arms over your head and feel an increase in pressure on your back muscles from the rolled-up towel.
- Take care not to strain your shoulders by moving too quickly - warm up.
- Contract your quadriceps so your kneecaps move towards your head.
- Dorsiflex your feet by pointing your heel and lifting your toes.

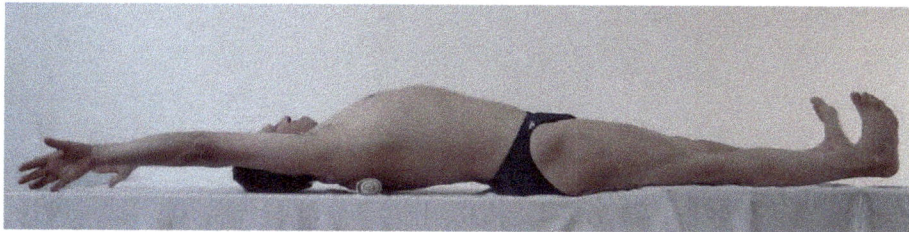

- Take a deep breath and hold it in.
- Simultaneously reach away, along the floor and above your head with both arms and along the floor with both legs.
- Stretch from the shoulders to the fingertips and the hips to the heels.
- Stretching both sides means there is no spinal sidebending and no hip movement, but there is muscle contraction and deep breathing acting on the rib cage and tension followed by relaxation affecting the spine.
- Keep your elbows and knees straight and push away with both heels.
- Dorsiflex your feet and point your heels - not your toes.
- Hold the tension for a few seconds, then exhale and relax.
- Allow your arms and legs to drop towards the floor and your body to sink onto the rolled up towel and into the floor.
- This is the tense and relax, both sides arms and legs technique and longitudinal arms and legs stretch - see chart stick-body 3.

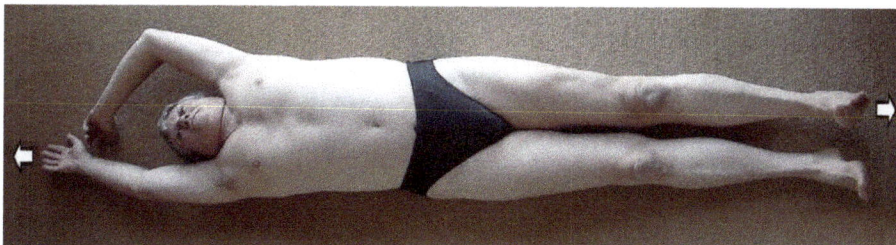

- Do these actions two or three times then sit up or roll over and move the rolled-up towel one vertebra higher or lower, and repeat the technique.
- Cover the whole thoracic spine but focus on areas of tightness.
- An alternative to the tense and relax method is the diagonal dynamic stretching method which involves keeping both arms and legs moving.
- Here the right arm and left leg alternate with the left arm and right leg.
- Reach away with your right arm and left leg simultaneously and then reach away with your left arm and right leg simultaneously.
- Repeat these alternating movements several times without stopping.

1.8f Inhibition of the muscles of the thoracic spine using a bilateral upper limb diagonal stretch over a rolled-up towel

Begin by adopting the start position described in technique 1.8a.

- Take your right arm over your head and notice how it changes the weight distribution of your body over the rolled-up towel and increases pressure on the muscles on the right side of your spine.
- Move your arm cautiously to avoid straining your shoulder.
- Keep your left arm at your side.
- Take a deep breath and hold it in.

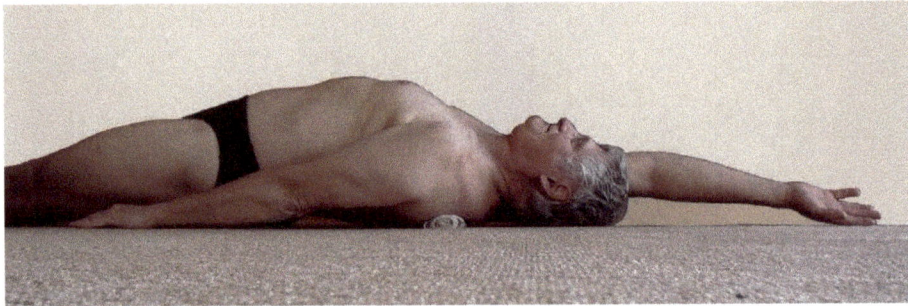

- Reach upwards, along the floor and away from your head with your right arm and simultaneously reach downwards, along the floor and towards your foot with your left arm.
- Reaching upwards with your right arm involves right scapula elevation and upward tilt, reaching downwards with your left arm involves left scapula depression and downward tilt and both contribute to the thoracic spine sidebending to the left.
- Stretch from the shoulders to the fingertips and keep both arms straight.
- Hold the stretch for a few seconds, then exhale, relax and allow both arms to drop towards the floor and your body to sink onto the rolled up towel and into the floor.

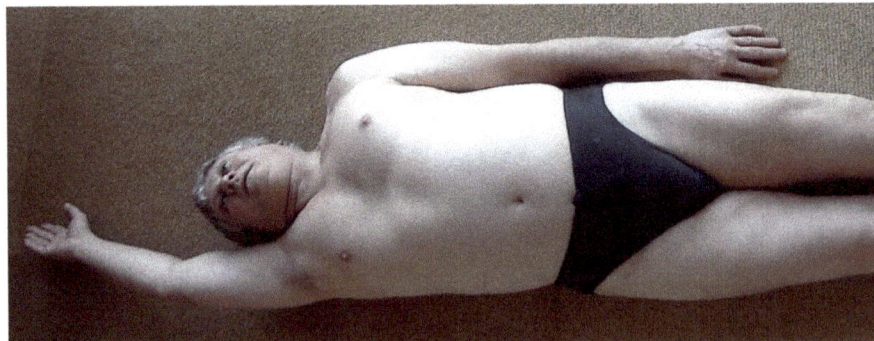

- This is the diagonal arms stretch (see stick-body 4).
- Repeat the stretch two or three times, a bit harder each time, then repeat it with your left arm over your head and your right arm by your side.
- Sit up or roll over, then move the rolled-up towel one vertebra level higher or lower and repeat the technique.

1.8g Inhibition of the muscles of the thoracic spine using a bilateral upper and lower limb diagonal stretch over a rolled-up towel

Begin by adopting the start position described in technique 1.8a.

- Take your right arm over your head and feel an increase of pressure from the rolled-up towel on the muscles on the right side of your spine.
- Keep your left arm at your side.
- Contract your quadriceps so your kneecaps move towards your head.
- Dorsiflex both feet by pointing your heels away and lifting your toes.
- Take a deep breath and hold it in.

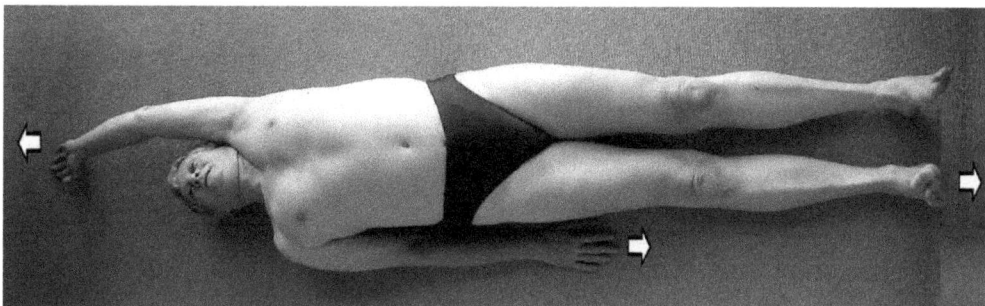

- Simultaneously reach along the floor and above your head with your right arm and reach along the floor and towards your left foot with your left arm and reach away and along the floor with your left leg.
- Reaching with the left leg is achieved by sidebending the lumbar spine left and tilting the pelvis and hips.
- Keep your knees and elbows straight.
- Hold the stretch for a few seconds, then exhale and relax.
- Allow your arm and leg to drop towards the floor and your body to sink onto the rolled up towel and into the floor.

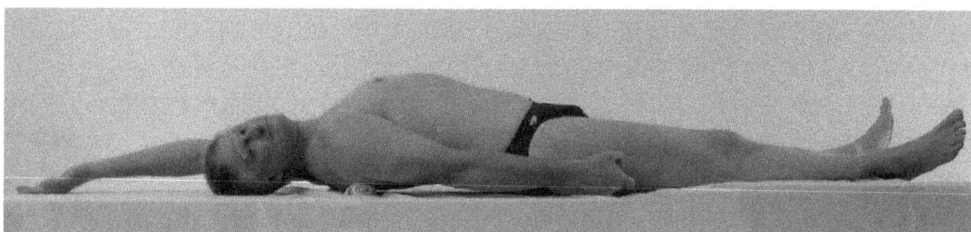

- This is the diagonal arm and leg stretch (see stick body 5. in diagram) - stretching one side of your body upwards and stretching the other side of your body downwards.
- Do these actions two or three times and then reposition your arms with the left arm above your head and your right arm at your side and repeat the stretch two or three times on this side.
- Sit up or roll over and move the rolled-up towel one vertebra level higher or lower and repeat the technique.
- Cover the whole thoracic spine but focus on areas of tightness and where there is the most thoracic curvature.

<u>1.8h Inhibition of the muscles on one side of the thoracic and lumbar spine using body mass over a rolled-up towel or two balls in a net</u>

- Grasp the rolled-up towel in your right hand.
- Lie on the floor with your hips and knees flexed.
- Move your knees to the left and allow the right side of your body to raise off the floor.
- Place the rolled-up towel behind your lower thoracic spine, positioned so it runs across it.

The 'two balls in a net' technique is similar to the 'rolled-up towel' technique, except for the placement of the balls and the area of the spine that each cover.

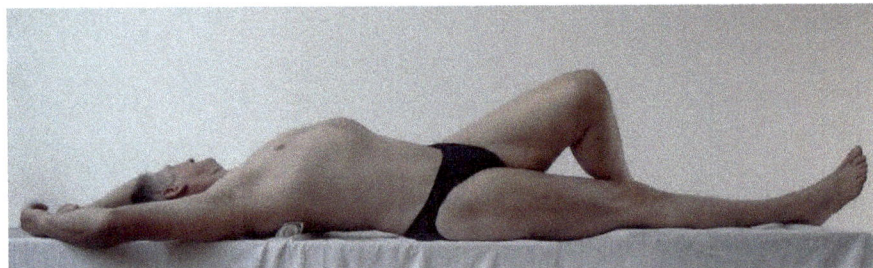

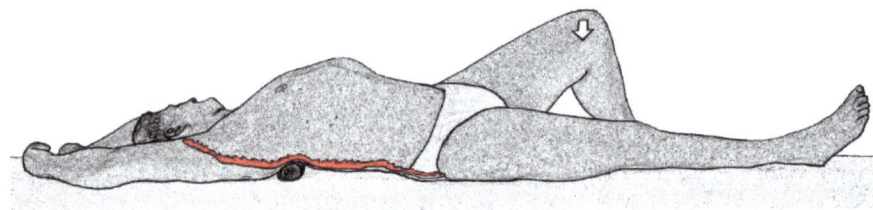

The balls are placed on one side of the spine, whereas the rolled-up towel sits across the spine. The balls sit in the depression at the side of the spine, whereas the rolled-up towel rests on bones in the middle of the spine and on muscles either side of the spine. The two balls can either be placed in a head to toe direction down one side of the spine or perpendicular to the spine with one ball in the depression next to the spine and the other resting on the muscles further away from the spine.

The rolled up towel technique is best used on the muscles of the thoracolumbar and thoracic spine up to about T5. It also works on the muscles of the sacrum, lumbar and thoracic spine. The two balls in a net technique is best used on the muscles of the lumbar spine. It also works on the muscles of the sacrum and thoracic spine up to about T9. Adjust the position of your arms above your head to get the right amount of pressure on the muscles without causing discomfort.

- Keeping the rolled-up towel in place, return the right side of your body and the rolled-up towel to the floor but keep your hips and knees flexed.
- Adjust the rolled-up towel so it is straight and perpendicular to the spine.
- Straighten your right leg but keep your left hip and knee flexed.
- Take a deep breath in, then exhale and move your left knee to the right.
- Stop moving when you feel the rolled-up towel pushing on the muscles of the spine and hold the position.

- Take a deep breath over a three to five seconds period and as you inhale feel an increase in pressure from the rolled-up towel on the muscle.
- As you exhale take more of your body weight over the rolled-up towel by moving your left knee further to the right and relax your back muscles.
- Repeat the breathing, movement and inhibition two or three times.
- Reposition the rolled-up towel one vertebra level higher or lower, either by wriggling over the rolled-up towel or by flexing both hips and knees, turning onto your right side and placing the rolled-up towel in the new location with your left hand.

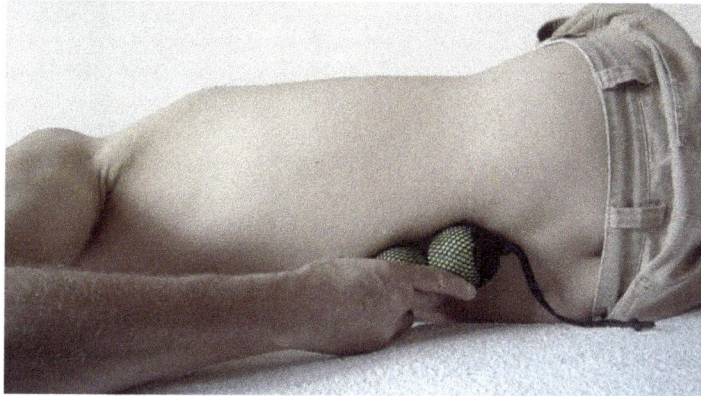

- Straighten your left leg and bend your right leg and repeat the technique on the left side of the spine.
- Repeat the technique until both sides have been massaged.
- The outer ball can be useful as a handle for moving the two balls in a net.
- Using either of the two placements described above, start with the balls at the bottom of the right side of the lumbar spine.
- Take a deep breath in, then exhale and move your left knee to the right until you feel an increase in pressure on the muscles of the spine.

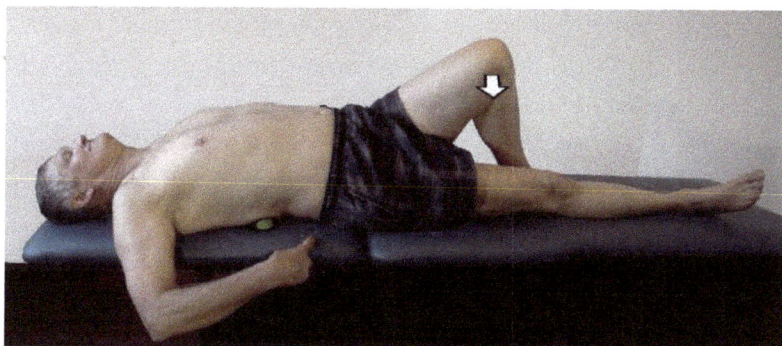

- Hold this position for three to five seconds as you inhale and feel the increase in pressure of the balls on the muscles.
- Exhale, relax and take more of your body weight over the balls by moving your left knee further to the right.
- Repeat the breathing, movement and inhibition two or three times and then reposition the balls one vertebra level higher or lower.
- With the balls technique it is easier to work up one side of the spine and then work up the other.
- Repeat the technique until both sides have been massage.

1.8i Inhibition of the muscles on both sides of the lumbar and thoracic spine using two balls in a net

- Lie on your back, on a carpet or mat on the floor.
- Grasp the balls in your right hand.
- Flex your hips and knees and then lift your pelvis off the floor.
- Place the two balls behind your lower back, one on each side of the lower lumbar spine and then return your pelvis, lumbar and the balls to the floor.
- Straighten your hips and knees and return your legs to the floor.
- Take a deep breath in and contract your buttocks and abdominal muscles to tilt your pelvis backwards towards the floor and flatten the lumbar spine.

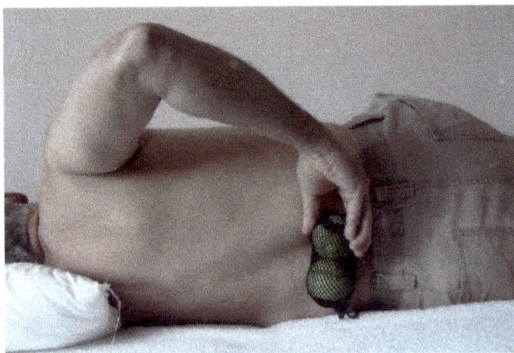

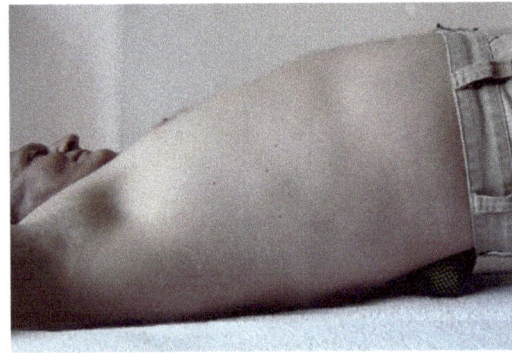

- Allow the balls to press into the back muscles for three to five seconds and then exhale and relax.
- The pelvic tilt and ball pressure both stretch and relax the back muscles.
- Flex your hips and knees, then lift your pelvis off the floor, reposition the balls one vertebra level higher up the spine and then return your pelvis and the balls to the floor, straighten your legs and repeat the pelvic tilting.
- Work up the lumbar spine and into the thoracic spine to about T8 vertebra level and then place the balls at the bottom of the lumbar spine for the second part of this technique.

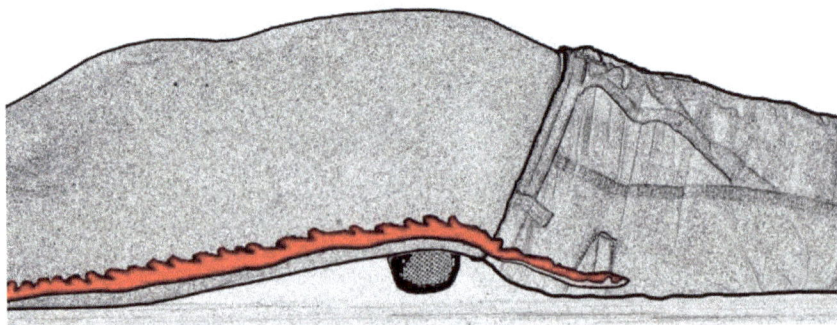

- Take another deep breath in and tilt your pelvis backwards towards the floor then depress the right side of your pelvis by reaching down and away with the heel of your right foot while simultaneously elevating the left side of your pelvis.

- The depression-elevation actions create localised lumbar sidebending and rotation to the left and treats a greater number of back muscles including the deep muscles.

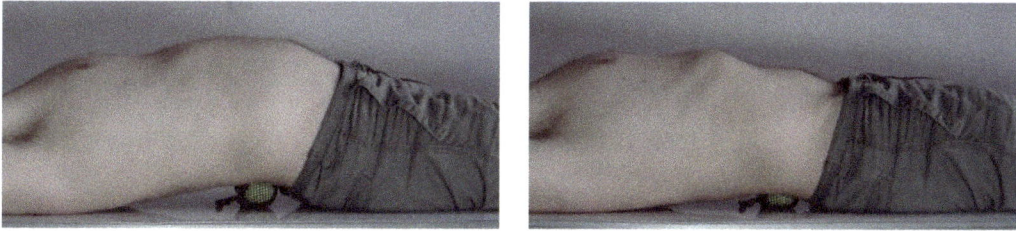

- Allow the balls to press into the back for three to five seconds and then exhale and relax.
- Repeat the depression-elevation actions of the pelvis on the other side to create localised lumbar sidebending and rotation to the right.
- Work up the lumbar and thoracic spine, as far as about T8 with the inhibition actions.
- The outer columns of muscles can be treated by loosening the cord of the net, so the balls are positioned further apart.

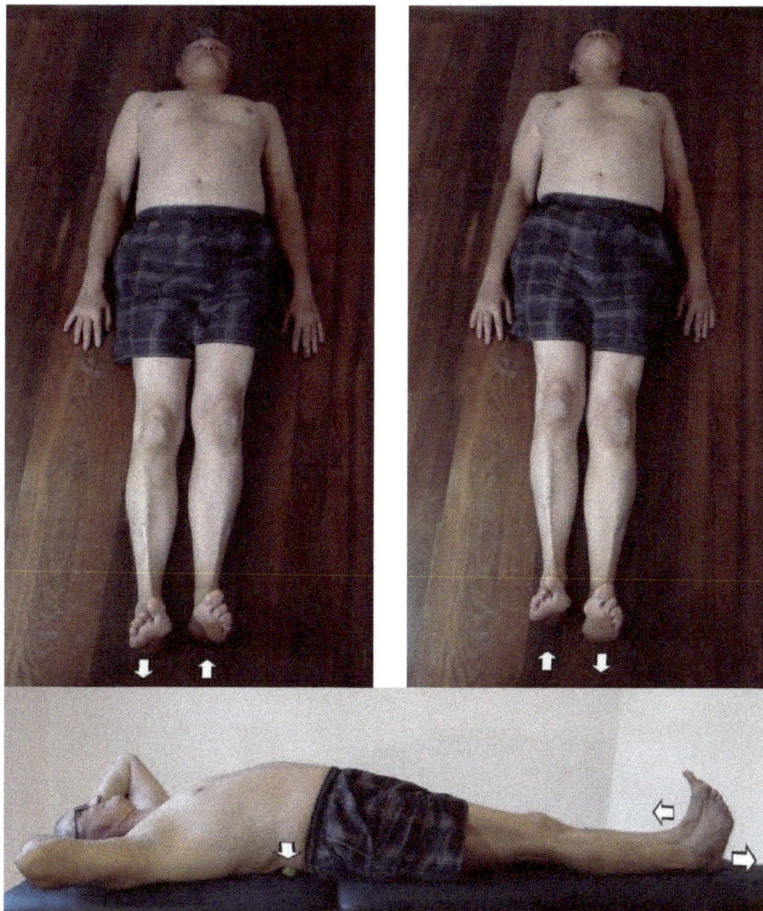

- A basic version of this technique can be done by just relaxing over the balls, deep breathing and letting the weight of the body sink onto the balls.

1.8j Inhibition of the muscles on one side of the sacrum, lumbar and lower thoracic spine rolling on two balls in a net

- Grasp the balls in your right hand.
- Lie on your back on a carpet or mat on the floor.
- Flex your hips and knees and then move your knees to the left so that the right side of your pelvis comes off the floor.
- Place the two balls behind your back, aligned in a head-to-toe direction down the right side of your lumbar spine.

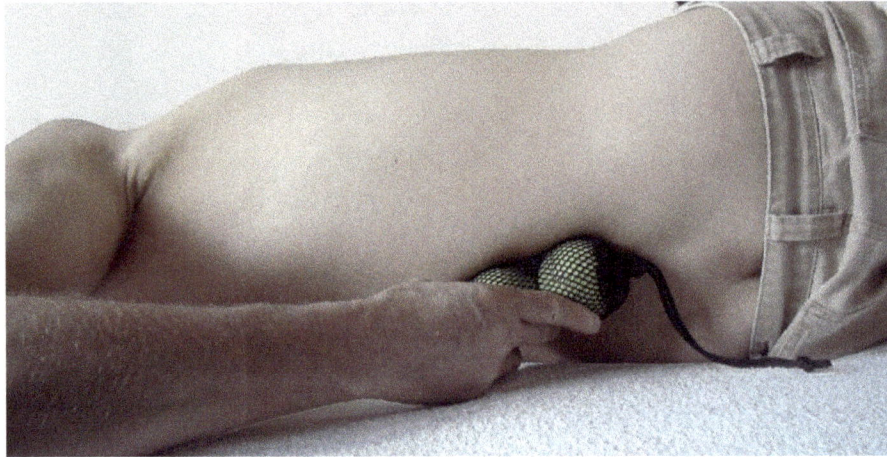

- Place the bottom ball against the back of the right side of your sacrum and place the top ball in the depression between the lumbar vertebra L5 and the innermost column of muscles.
- Maintaining the position of the balls, return your pelvis, spine and the balls to the floor, but keep your hips and knees flexed.
- The full weight of your pelvis rests on the balls, carefully balanced over the right side of your sacrum and lower lumbar spine.

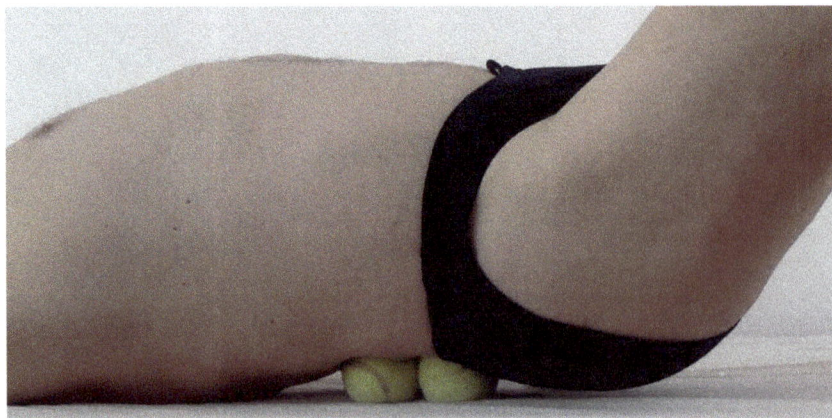

- Keep the back of your head, thoracic spine, rib cage, shoulders and arms in contact with the floor and your pelvis horizontal.
- Move your pelvis sideways over the balls so the bottom ball rolls over the muscles attaching on the sacrum and the ligaments of sacroiliac joint and

the top ball rolls over the inner column of back muscles on the right of the L5 vertebra.

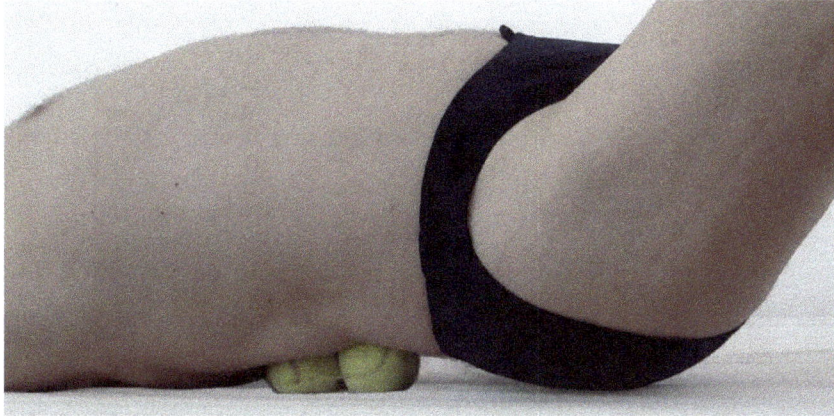

- Lift your pelvis off the floor and reposition the balls one or two vertebra levels higher.
- Return your body and the balls to the floor and repeat the sideways movement of the pelvis over the balls.
- Sometimes moving too quickly will cause the muscles to tense up so roll slowly over the muscle columns so the muscles relax.
- About half-way up the lumbar spine it may be necessary to lift the left side of the pelvis and tilt it to the right to treat the outer column of erector spinae and quadratus lumborum.

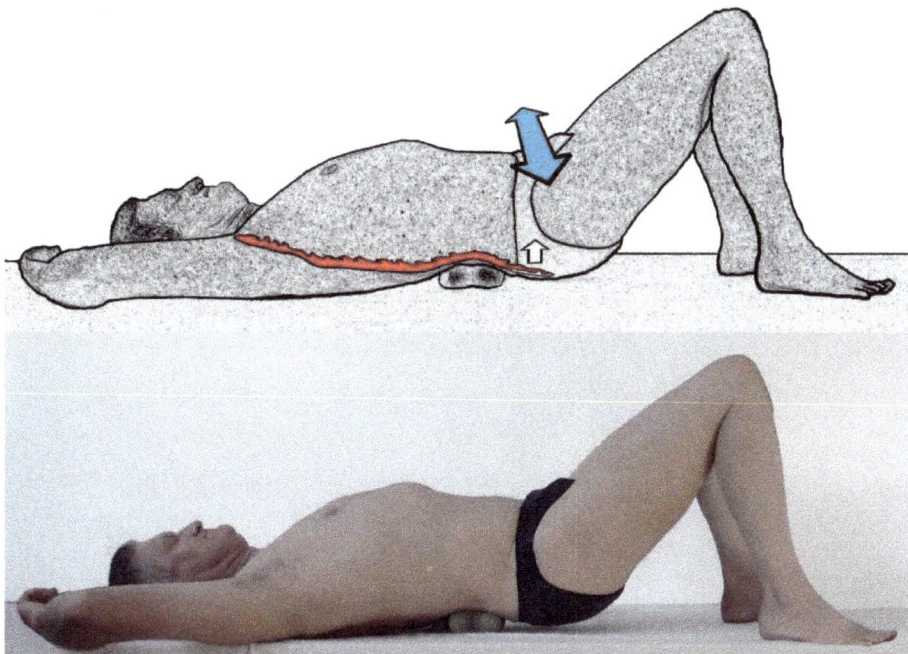

- Repeat the rolling action, steadily working up the lumbar to the lower thoracic spine.
- Do not go above the lower thoracic spine because the weight of the body on one side of the spine can be extremely uncomfortable.

1.8k Inhibition of the muscles of the lumbar and lower thoracic spine using the wadi on its side

- Grasp the wadi in your right hand.
- Lie on your back, on a carpet or mat.
- Flex your right hip and knee but keep your left leg straight.

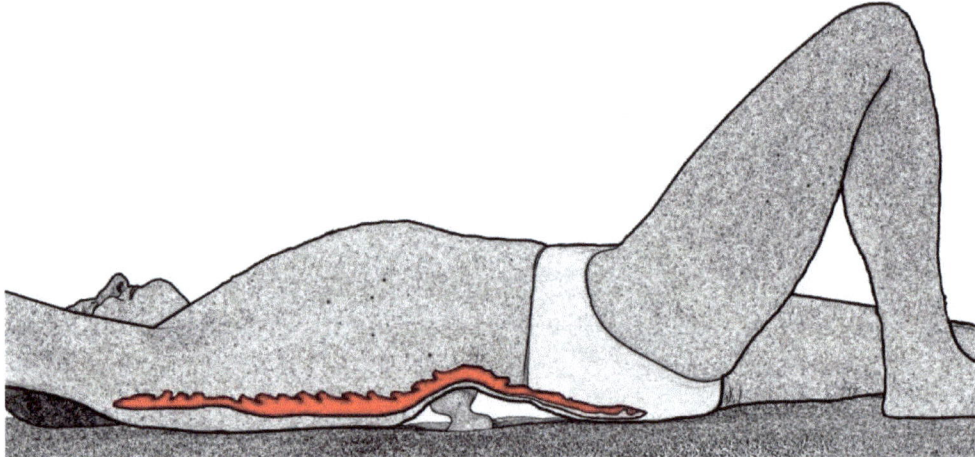

- Move your right knee to the left so that it passes over your left thigh and allows the right side of your pelvis and lumbar spine to come off the floor.
- Place one end of wadi against the right side of your back so the apex of the dome sits in the depression between the bones and the innermost column of spinal muscles.

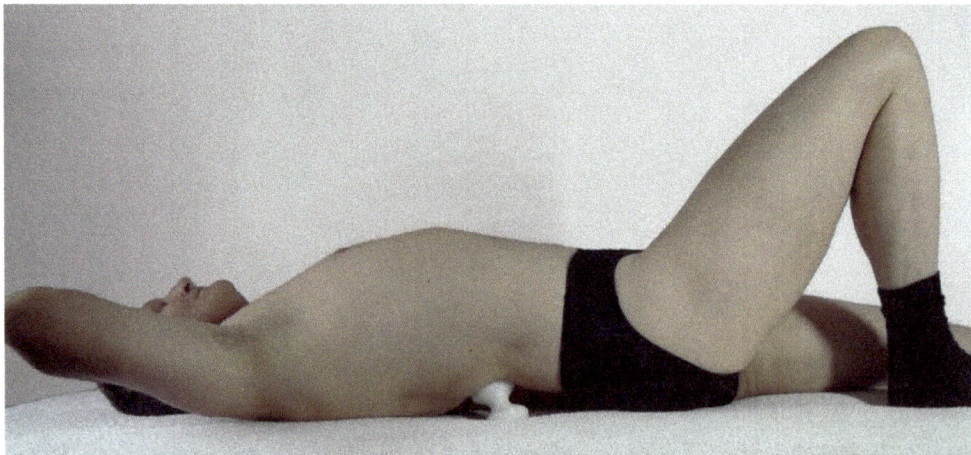

- Hold the wadi against your back with the thumb and index finger of your right hand and tilt it away from the spine so that it presses into the muscle rather than against the bone.
- Move your right knee to the right so the right side of your pelvis and lumbar spine and the wadi return to the floor.
- The wadi now rests on its side between the floor and muscles on the right side of your spine and your right thigh is close to the vertical position.

60

- Take a deep breath in.
- As you exhale increase wadi pressure on the muscle by moving your right knee to the right to put greater body mass over the wadi and by tilting the wadi into the muscle with your right hand.

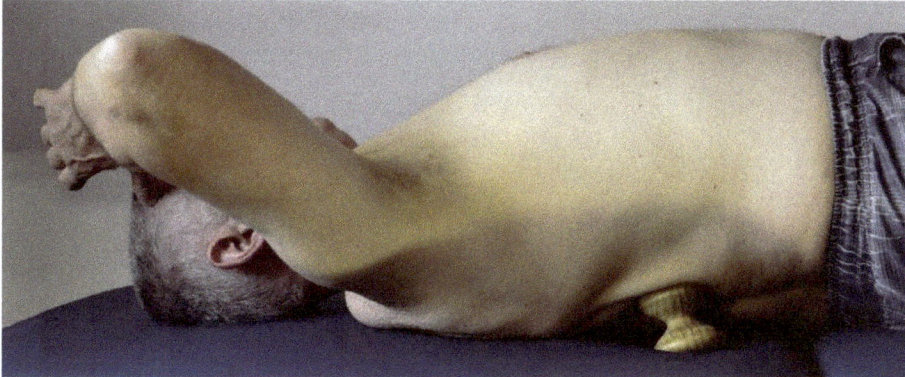

- This part of the technique treats the innermost columns of back muscles (erector spinae) and the deep layer of back muscles (multifidus and rotatores).
- Systematically work along the right side of the spine one vertebral level at a time and then repeat the technique on the other side of the spine.
- To treat the outermost column of back muscles as well as quadratus lumborum place the wadi further away from the spine and angle it towards the spine.

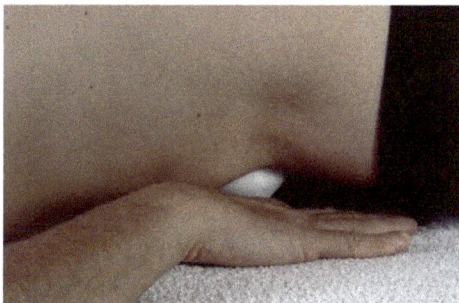

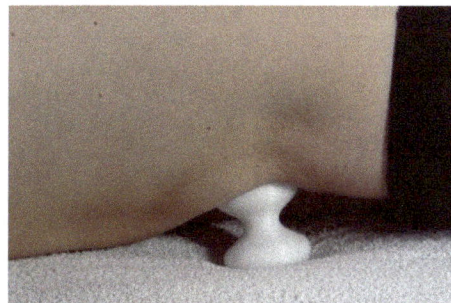

- This technique is useful for the lumbar and into the thoracic spine up to about T8.
- Take care not to press into the ribs or vertebrae.

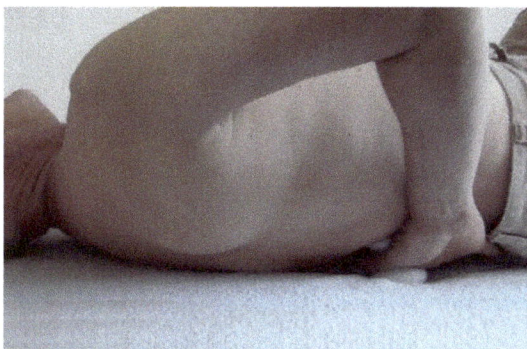

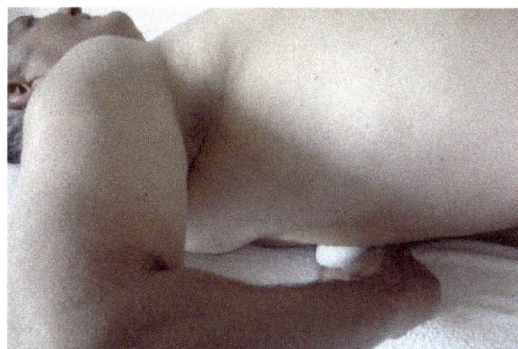

THE SACROILIAC SPINE

Massaging muscles overlying the sacrum may be helpful for lower back pain for example if they are strained by lifting heavy objects or with unprepared or weak muscles. Massaging the sacroiliac ligaments can be useful if they are strained. Rotating and sidebending the spine in a forward bent position can strain them.

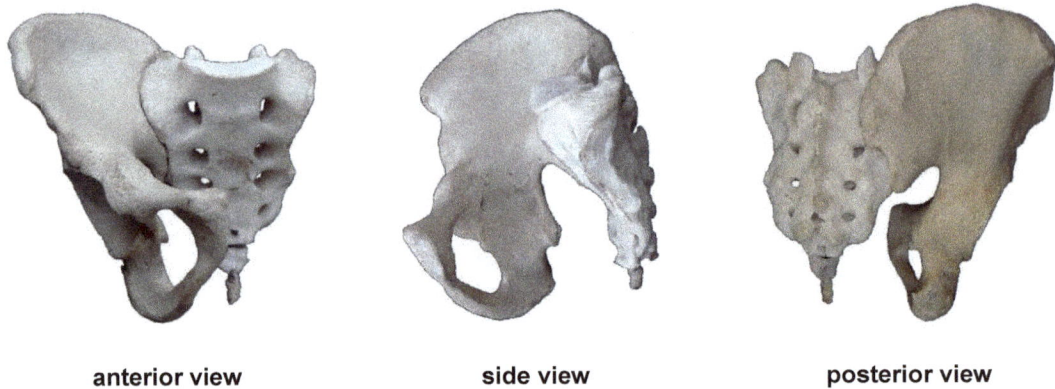

anterior view   side view   posterior view

The sacroiliac ligaments

The primary ligaments of the sacroiliac joint are the posterior sacroiliac ligament, interosseous sacroiliac ligament, sacrotuberous ligament and the sacrospinous ligament.

The **posterior sacroiliac ligaments** are long and short ligaments running between the sacrum and ilium. They are superficial to the stronger interosseous sacroiliac ligaments and the sacroiliac joints. The short posterior sacroiliac ligament arises on an inner lip in the rear of the iliac crest and attaches on an area on the superior posterior sacrum. The long posterior sacroiliac ligament arises on posterior superior iliac spine and attaches on the outside of the sacrum.

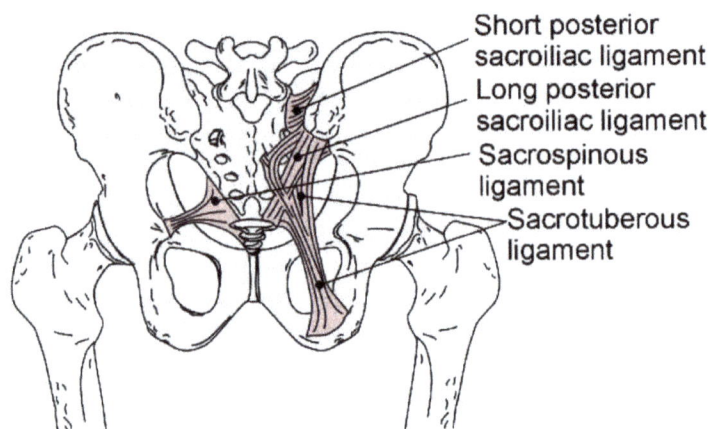

Short posterior sacroiliac ligament
Long posterior sacroiliac ligament
Sacrospinous ligament
Sacrotuberous ligament

The pelvis and ligaments - posterior view

The sacroiliac joints are strong, L-shaped, weight bearing synovial joints between the sacrum and the two ilium bones of the pelvis. They are covered by two different kinds of cartilage, hyaline cartilage over the sacrum and fibrocartilage over the iliac surface. Strong ligaments help maintain the stability of the joint. There is a small amount of movement at the SI joints, ranging between individuals from 2 to 10 degrees.

1.9 Friction of the posterior sacroiliac ligament using the wadi on its side

- Lie on your back, with your hips bent and then lift your pelvis off the floor.
- Grasp the wadi between the thumb and index finger of one hand and place the apex of one dome against the sacroiliac ligament at the top of the sacroiliac joint.

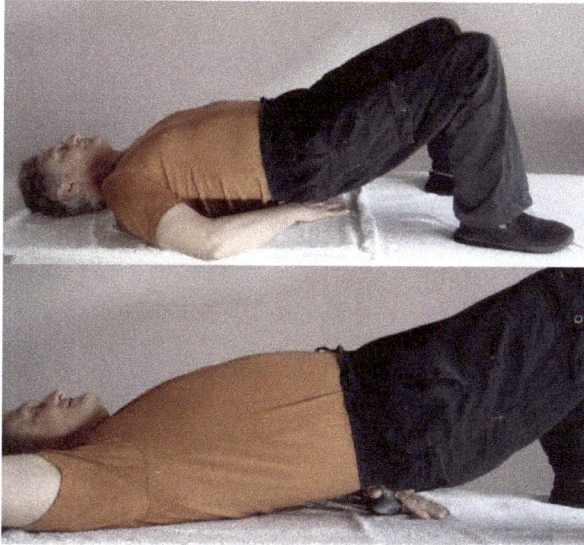

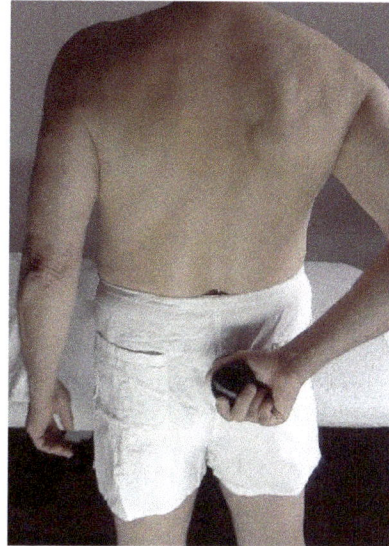

- Lower your pelvis and the wadi to the floor.
- The wadi is on its side with the apex of one dome on the floor and the other pressed against the ligament.
- Keep your pelvis horizontal and the sacrum against on the wadi.
- Flex your hips and knees and move your pelvis over the floor and wadi.

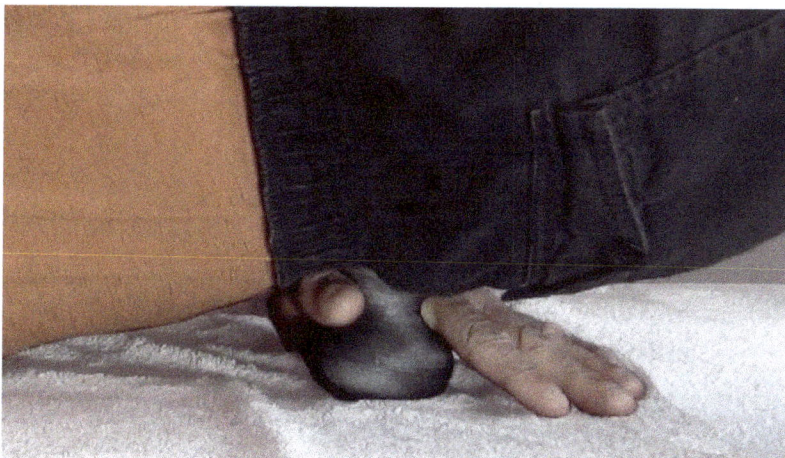

- Hold the wadi firmly in your hand, pinned to the floor and tilted so the apex of the dome of the wadi is directed onto the ligament.
- Apply friction over one area of ligament, then move the wadi up or down the sacroiliac joint and apply friction over on another.
- Repeat the friction down one sacroiliac joint and then do the other.

Part B The upper limbs

THE SHOULDER

Supraspinatus and capsular ligaments

Massaging the supraspinatus muscle and tendon can be useful when there is pain, restriction and weakness from a muscle strain, rotator cuff strain, tendinitis, tendinopathy, sub-acromial bursitis, shoulder impingement or frozen shoulder. Massaging the capsular ligaments can be useful when there is a restriction due to a frozen shoulder. Also, massage infraspinatus, trapezius, levator scapulae, middle deltoid, biceps, triceps, pectoralis major and minor, serratus anterior and the rhomboids when these problems exist.

Supraspinatus arises from the supraspinatus fossa, passes under the acromion process and its tendon attaches on the top of the greater tubercle of the humerus. The muscle is under trapezius. The tendon also merges with the capsule of the shoulder joint. It is the tendon most frequently strained in the shoulder.

The muscle initiates shoulder abduction - taking the arm away from the side of the body and helps stabilise the shoulder joint.

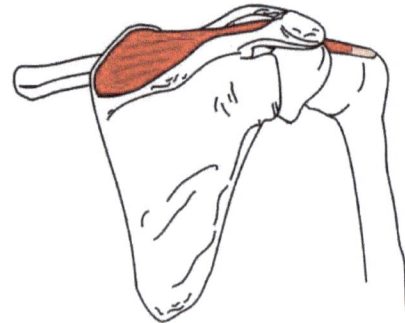

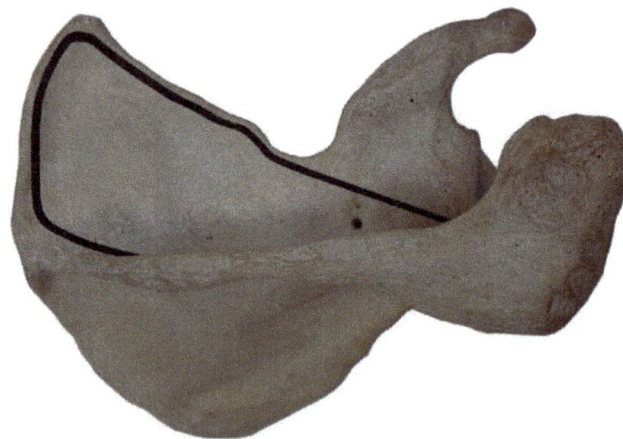

Supraspinatus - superior posterior view

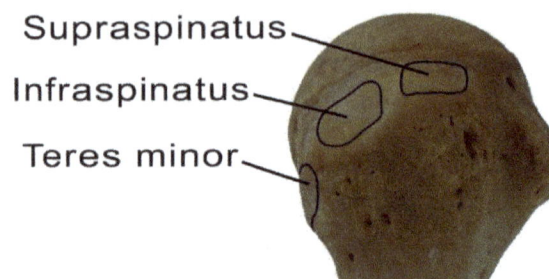

Head of humerus - side view

64

2.0a Kneading supraspinatus using the tips of your hooked fingers

- Stand, sit on a stool or kneel on the floor.
- Flex your right forearm at the elbow, then internally rotate your right arm at the shoulder and place your hand and forearm behind your back as far to the left as you can reach.
- Flex your left forearm at the elbow and then reach across the front of your body and over your right shoulder and place your left hand on top of the shoulder with your fingers on the spine of the scapula - the ridge of bone running horizontally behind your right shoulder.

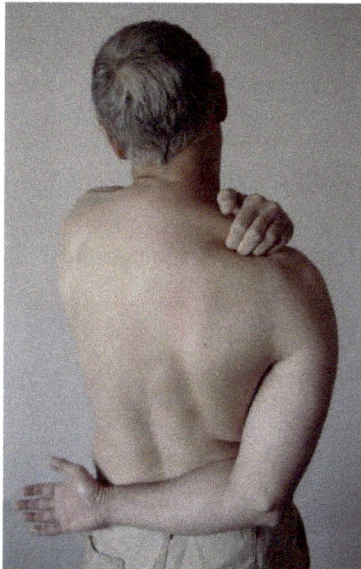

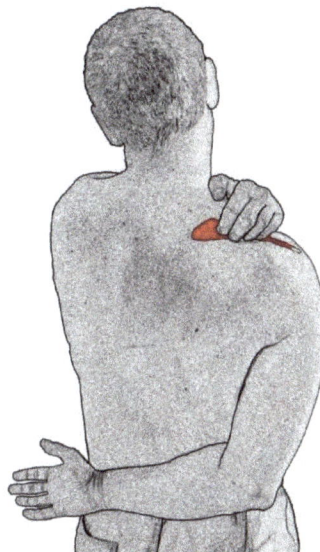

- Slide your left hand forwards over your shoulder until your fingertips drop off the spine of the scapula and into the shallow depression behind the trapezius muscle on top of the shoulder.
- Flex your fingers into a hooked position and press your fingertips into the depression.
- This depression is the supraspinatus fossa and contains supraspinatus.

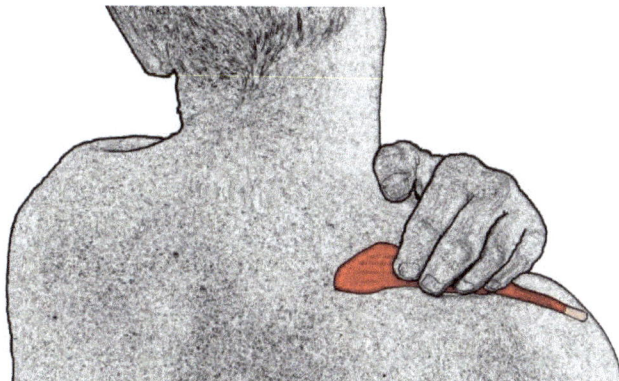

- Start with your fingernails right up against the spine of the scapula and your fingertips pressed against the muscle deep in the depression and near to the thoracic spine.
- Keep your wrist and hooked fingers firm and pull across the muscle in a forward direction while simultaneously moving your right hand left.

- Use the elasticity and moisture of the skin to move across the muscle.
- When the elasticity and moisture of the skin is exhausted, reposition the fingers further along the muscle, with the fingernails up against the spine of the scapula.
- Stop when you feel the bunching of the trapezius fibres at the top of the shoulder.
- Work along the entire length of the muscle, from the thoracic spine end to where the muscle disappears under the bone or acromion process near the tip of the shoulder.

2.0b Transverse friction over the supraspinatus tendon using your fingertips

- Stand or sit on a chair.
- Flex your right elbow about 90 degrees and keep it by your side.
- Move your elbow backwards so that your shoulder rolls forwards to expose as much of the supraspinatus tendon as possible.
- Keep your elbow close to your side and do not allow your arm to rotate.

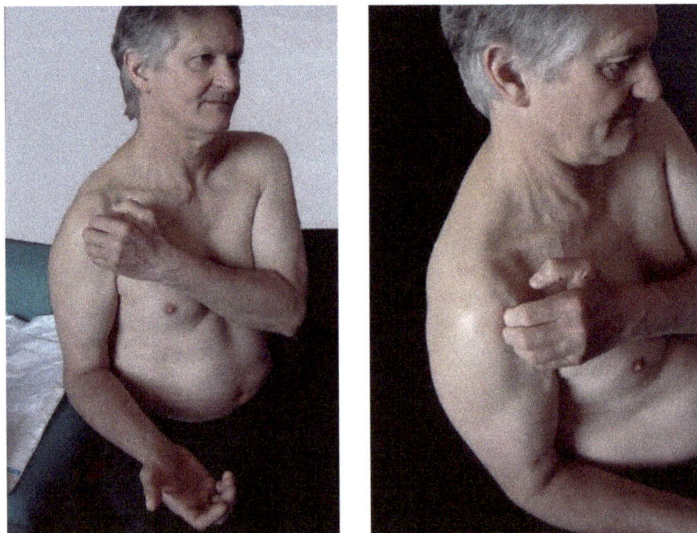

- Reach across the front of your body with your left hand and place your fingertips on the top of your shoulder, then move them to the end of the shoulder until they drop off the acromion process and onto the head of the humerus and the rotator cuff tendon.
- Use transverse friction on the tendon, which attaches over the top and front of the head of the humerus, an area of one or two square centimetres.
- Also use a lighter pressure over the depression for the biceps tendon in front of the shoulder, as a biceps tendinitis may be associated with a rotator cuff strain.
- Points of tenderness may indicate the location of the problem.
- Slide over the bone, not the skin, and take care not to tear the skin.
- Cease the transverse friction after about 30 seconds.
- There may be a small bruise on the area the next day, but this is OK.

2.0c Transverse friction over the anterior capsular ligament of your shoulder using the tip of your thumb

- Stand or sit on a chair.
- Flex your right elbow about 90 degrees and keep it near your side.
- Reach across the front of your body with your left hand and place the tip of your thumb in the crease at the front of your shoulder.

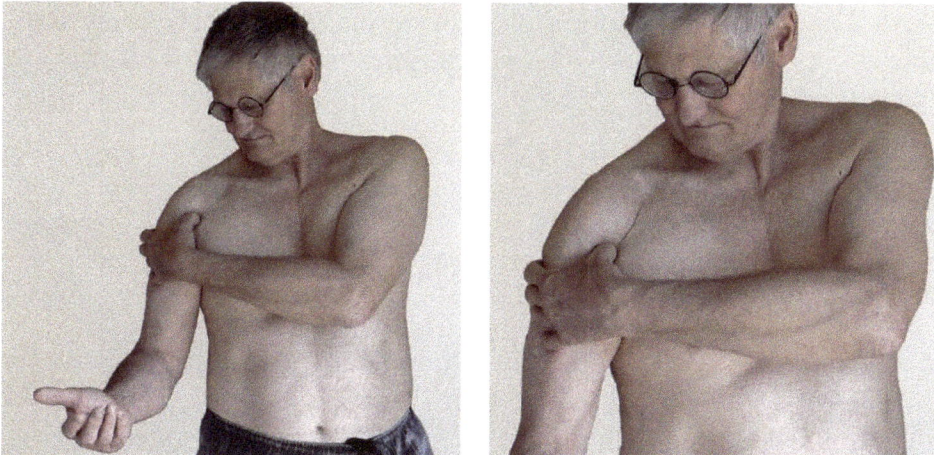

- Hook your fingers around the back of your shoulder and grasp your shoulder between the pads of your fingers and the tip of your thumb.
- Use transverse friction on the capsule, which runs about five centimetres down the front of your shoulder.
- Use the pressure of your fingers against the pressure of your thumb.
- Points of tenderness may indicate the location of the problem.

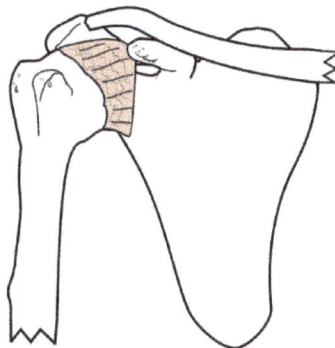

Anterior capsule and ligaments of shoulder

- Work from the top to the bottom of the shoulder down the depression between the anterior deltoid and pectoralis major muscles.
- Stay on the outside of the coracoid process, the small bump in front of your shoulder.
- Complete the transverse friction over a period of about 30 seconds.

Infraspinatus and Teres minor

Massaging infraspinatus and teres minor can be useful when there is pain and restriction from a muscle strain, a rotator cuff strain, tendinitis, tendinopathy, bursitis, shoulder impingement or frozen shoulder. It can help if there is restricted shoulder internal rotation because the muscles have become fibrous, tight and short as a result of postural fatigue or repetitive loading or overloading This is common in people who do repetitive work or are heavy users of their tools, such as house painters who push strongly outwards with their arm, four-wheel car drivers who must make many steering changes and tennis players with a strong backhand.

Infraspinatus arises from the infraspinatus fossa and its tendon attaches to the middle facet of the greater tubercle of the humerus. The tendon also merges with the capsule of the shoulder joint.

The muscle produces external rotation and horizontal extension of the shoulder and helps stabilise the shoulder joint.

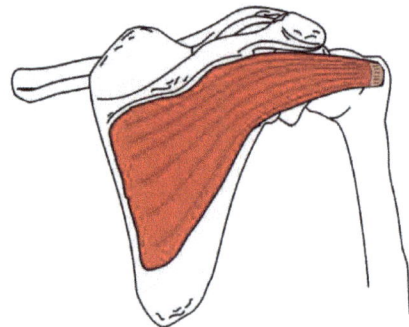

Teres minor arises from a flat strip which runs along the back of the scapula near the outer border. The tendon attaches on the lower part of the greater tubercle of the humerus and merges with the capsule of the shoulder joint. The muscle is palpable but its upper part is underneath posterior deltoid.

The muscle produces external rotation and assists with adduction and extension of the shoulder and pulls the humeral head down and provides stability during abduction.

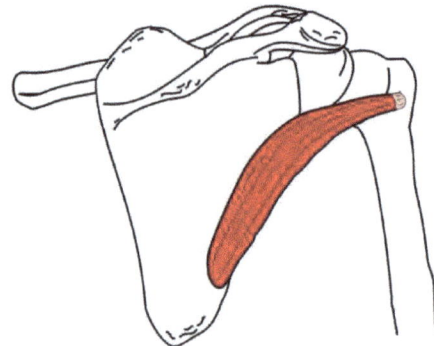

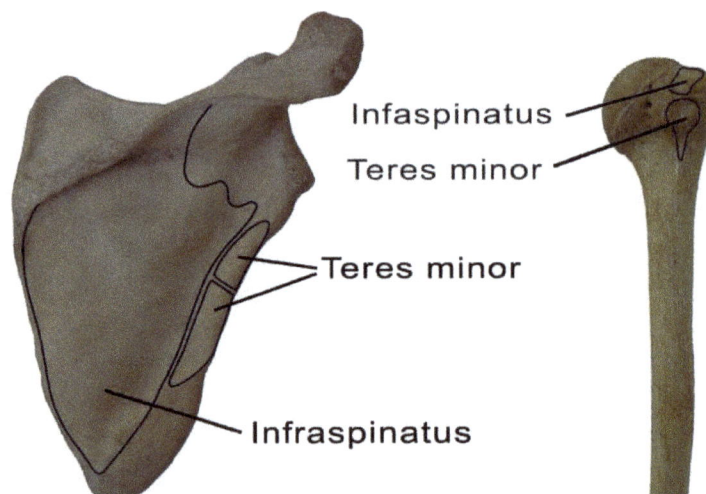

Scapula and humerus - posterior view

2.0d Kneading infraspinatus and teres minor using the weight of your body over the wadi or two balls in a net

- Stand with your back to a wall.
- Flex your right forearm at the elbow, then inwardly rotate your right arm at the shoulder and place your hand as far behind your back as possible.
- Grasp one of the two balls in the net with your left hand.
- Flex your left forearm at the elbow, and reach across the front of your body, over your right shoulder and down the back of your scapula with your left hand and the balls.

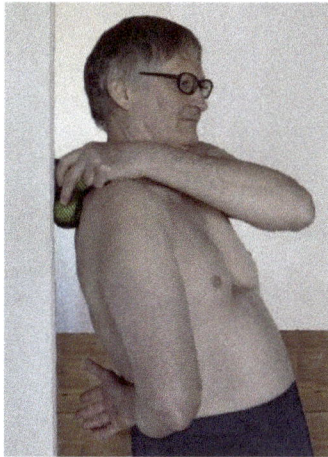

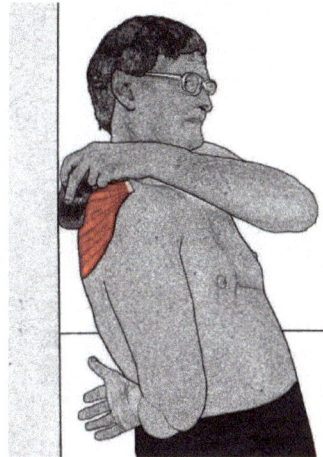

- Rest the front of your wrist on top of your shoulder and hang one of the balls down the back and over the spine of the scapula.
- Grasp one of the balls and position the other ball or dome over the teres minor or infraspinatus muscle in the infraspinatus fossa of the scapula.
- Lean back on the wall so the ball is between the muscle and wall.
- Flex and extend your knees so your body moves up and down and the muscle slides over the ball or dome.

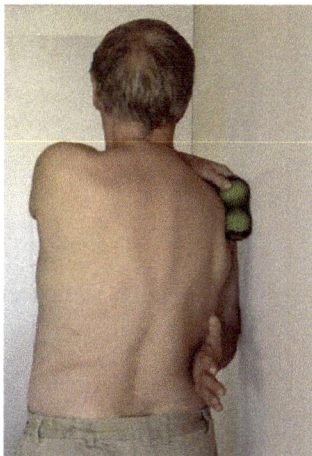

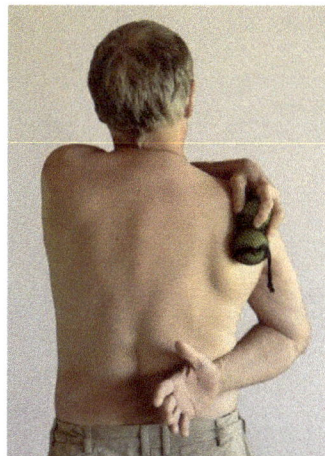

- Use this up down movement for kneading across the muscle fibres.
- If part of the bony surface is sensitive or if the muscle is tight and painful to treat, then you should reduce your body weight over the ball or dome.
- Systematically knead the whole surface of the muscles.
- Repeat the technique on the muscle on the other side if necessary.

Deltoid

Massaging deltoid is useful when there is pain from a muscle strain or rotator cuff strain, tendinitis, tendinopathy, sub-deltoid or sub-acromial bursitis, shoulder impingement or frozen shoulder. Middle deltoid pain can occur when there is a chronic rotator cuff problem because the muscle must compensate for supraspinatus muscle weakness, which has to initiate lifting of the arm sideways.

Deltoid gives the shoulder its rounded shape and has three parts, **anterior deltoid**, **posterior deltoid** and **middle deltoid**, all of which insert on the deltoid tuberosity in the middle of the outside shaft of the humerus via a short thick tendon.

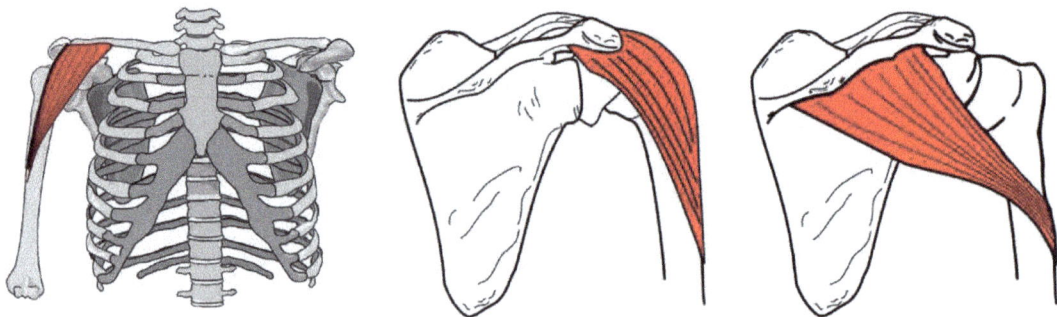

Anterior deltoid   **Middle deltoid**   **Posterior deltoid**

Anterior deltoid arises on the top, front and end of the clavicle. Middle deltoid arises on the edge and top of the acromion process. Posterior deltoid arises under the spine of the scapula.

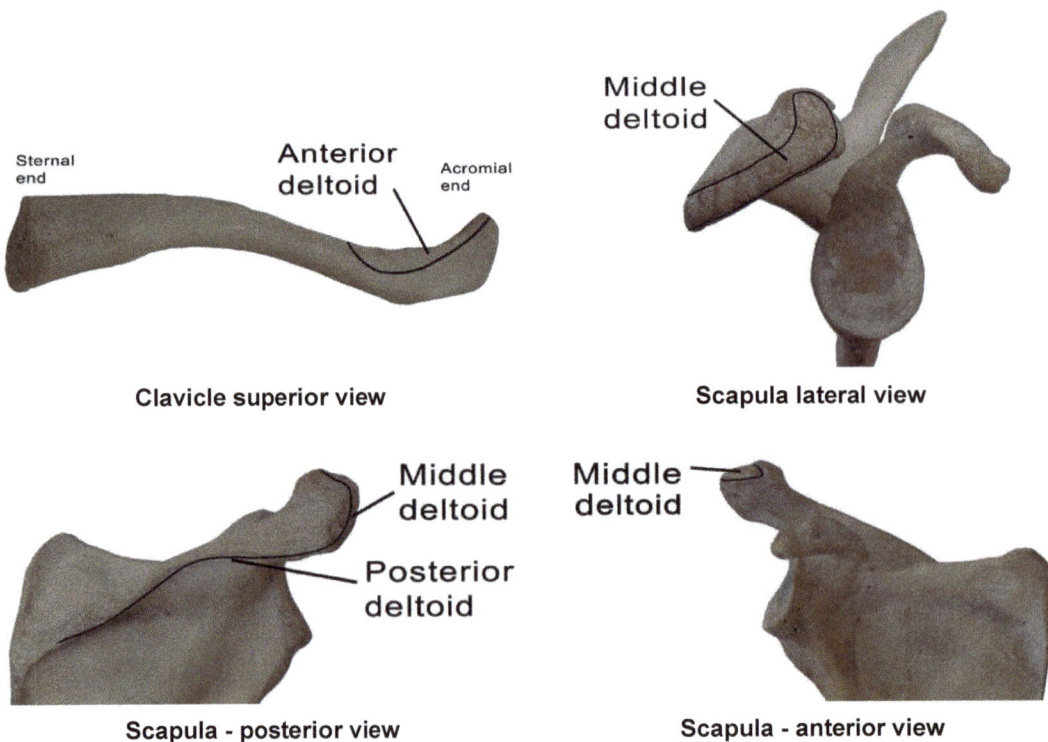

Clavicle superior view

Scapula lateral view

Scapula - posterior view

Scapula - anterior view

2.1a Kneading anterior deltoid using the tip of your thumb

- Stand, sit on a stool or kneel on the floor.
- Flex your right forearm at the elbow then rotate your right arm outwards at the shoulder.
- Reach across the front of your chest and right shoulder with your left hand and hook your fingers around the side and back of your shoulder.
- Place the tip of your thumb at the start of the anterior deltoid, about a third of the way from the end of the shoulder down the front of the clavicle.

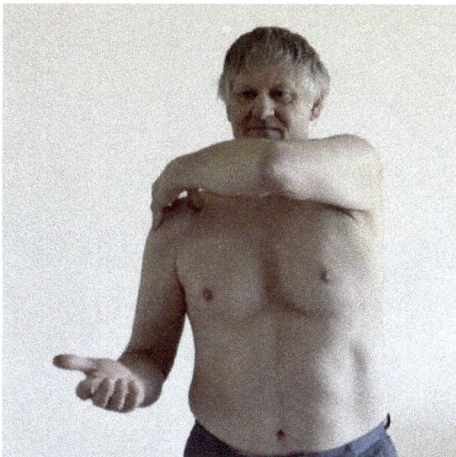

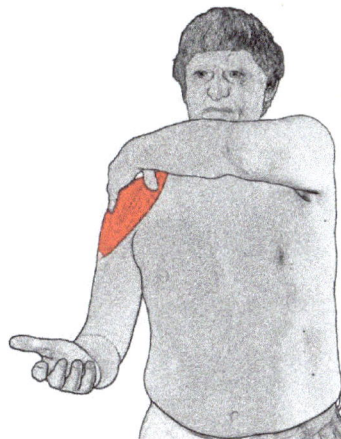

- Grasp your shoulder between your fingers and thumb.
- Move the tip of your thumb across the muscle in an outwards direction following a line under the clavicle.
- Push into the muscle with your thumb and pull with your fingers while simultaneously moving your right elbow backwards and rotating your arm outwards, which is shoulder extension and external rotation.
- Knead the uppermost fibres of anterior deltoid and then work down the arm along parallel but progressively shorter strips until the muscle tapers at the deltoid tubercle.

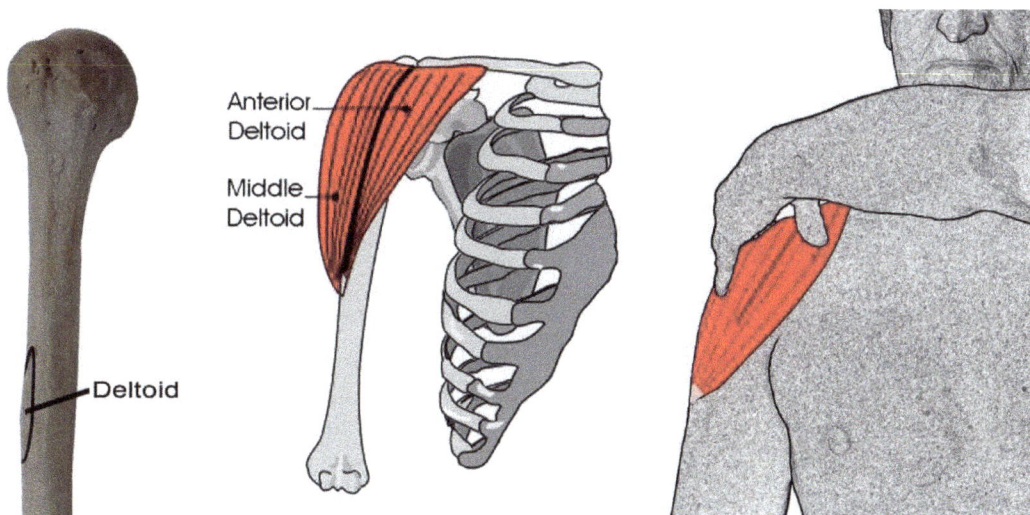

2.1b Kneading anterior deltoid using the tips of your hooked fingers

- Sit, stand or kneel on the floor and flex your right forearm at the elbow.
- Reach across the front of your chest and right shoulder with your left hand and place your index finger on a small flat area of bone at the end and top of your shoulder - this is the acromion process of the scapular.

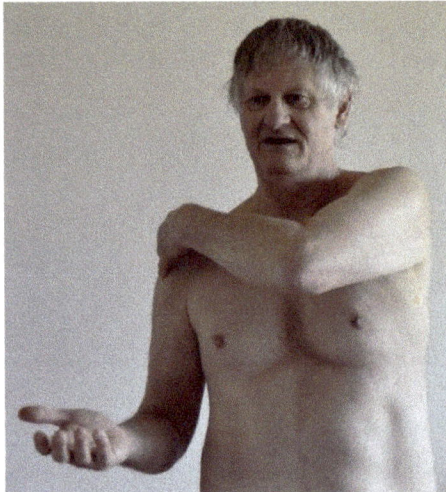

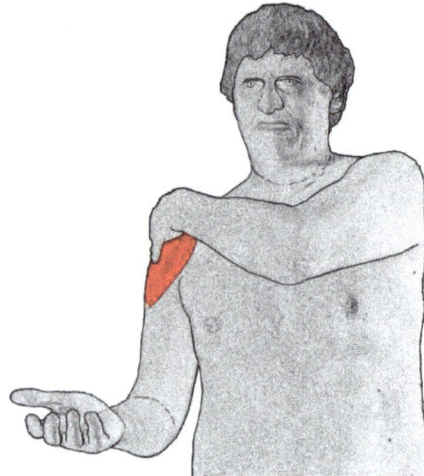

- Move your finger a one or two millimetres towards your neck and feel where the flat area rises to a bump - this is the end of your clavicle.
- Feel the line of the acromioclavicular joint between the flat acromion process and the bump forming the end of your clavicle.
- The edge of anterior deltoid attaches at the end of this line and extends about a third of the way along the clavicle at the front of your shoulder.

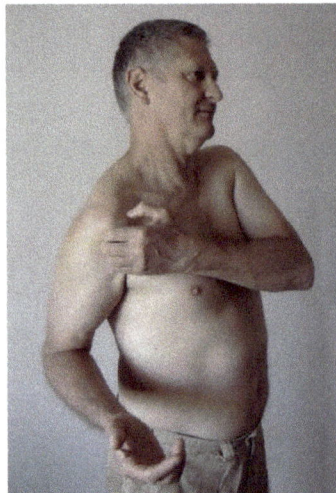

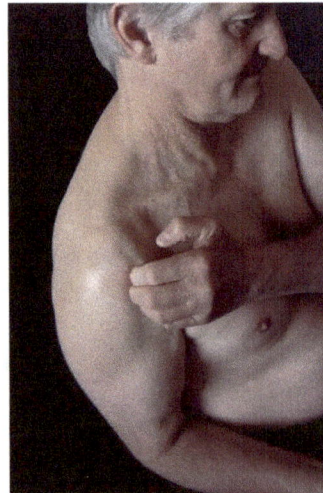

- Flex the fingers of your left hand into a fixed hooked position and press your fingertips against the outer border of the muscle.
- Move across the muscle fibres with a raking action of the fingertips, following a line under the clavicle, where the muscle attaches while simultaneously moving your right arm backwards and rotate it outwards.
- After kneading the uppermost fibres of anterior deltoid then work down the arm along parallel strips until the muscle tapers and ends at its attachment on the deltoid tubercle.

2.1c Kneading middle deltoid using the tips of your hooked fingers

- Stand, sit on a stool or kneel on the floor.
- Flex your right forearm at the elbow, then internally rotate your right arm at the shoulder and move your hand towards your abdomen.
- Reach across the front of your chest and right shoulder with your left hand and grasp the cup shaped area at the tip of the shoulder.

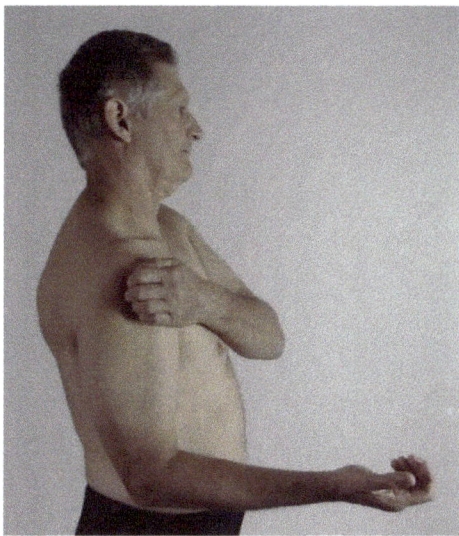

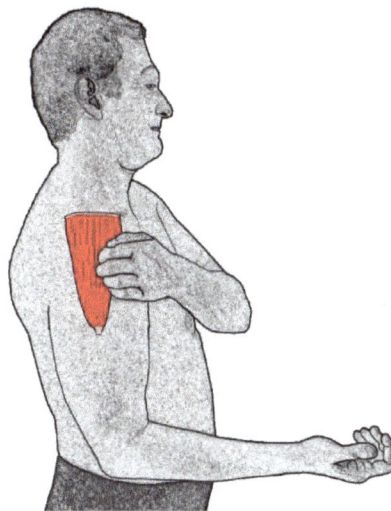

- Your fingers should be over the acromion process and your thumb over the clavicle.
- Flex the fingers of your left hand into a fixed hooked position and press your fingertips against the muscle.
- This should be where the top of the middle deltoid starts.

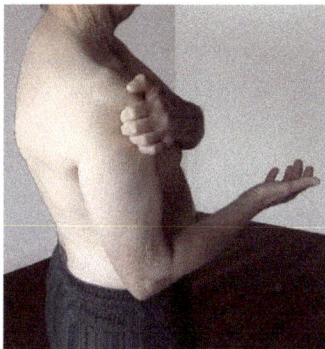

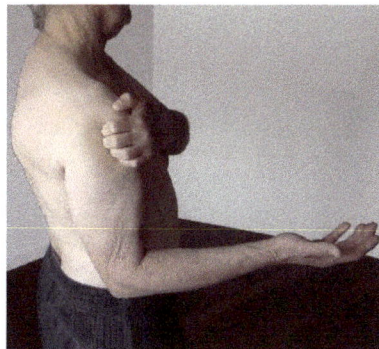

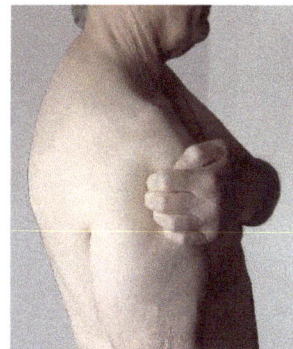

- Work across the muscle fibres in a forwards direction with a raking action of the fingertips while simultaneously externally rotating your right arm
- Keep your right elbow at the side of your body as you rotate your arm.
- Knead the uppermost fibres of middle deltoid first by following the bony ridge that forms the edge of the acromion process.

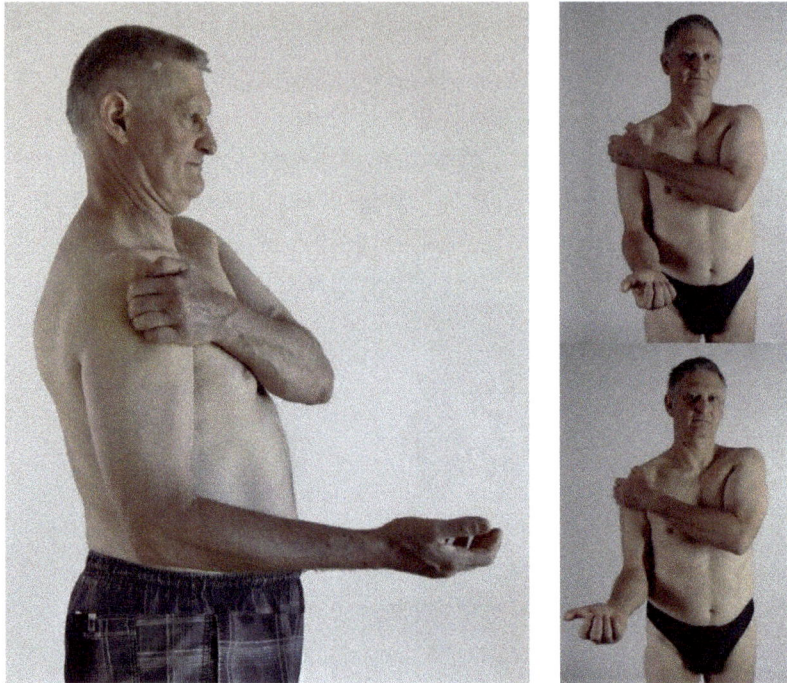

- Work down the arm, parallel with the ridge until the muscle ends on the deltoid tubercle.
- The muscle is wider at the top and tapers to its tendon attachment about halfway down the outside of your arm.

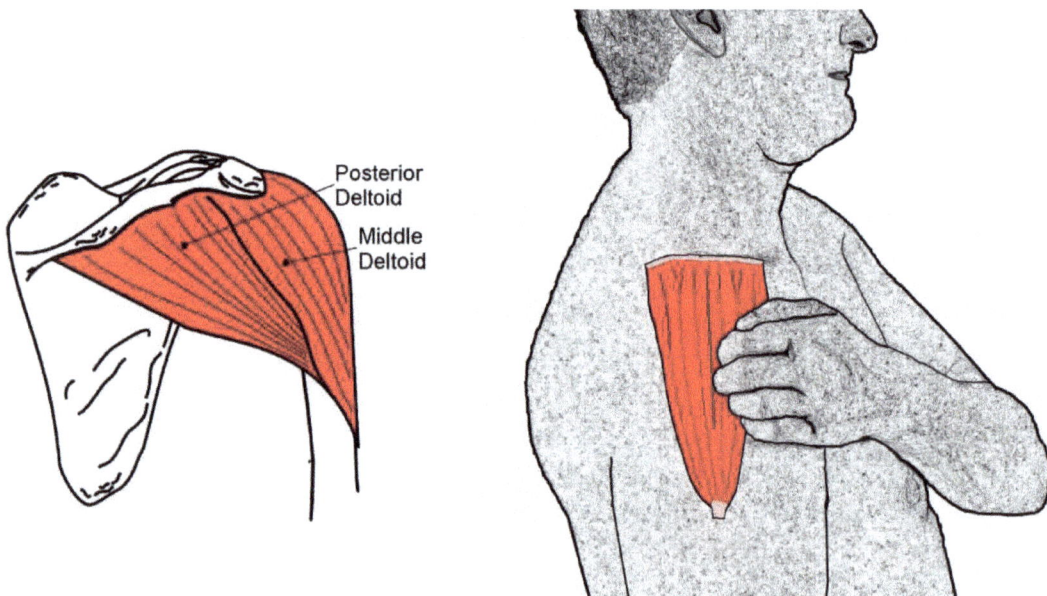

Posterior Deltoid

Middle Deltoid

2.1d Kneading posterior deltoid and teres minor using the tips of your hooked fingers

- Stand, sit on a chair or kneel on the floor.
- Flex your right forearm at the elbow, reach across the front of your body and place your palm against the left side of your rib cage.
- Flex your left forearm at the elbow, reach across the front of your body and over and behind your right shoulder with your left hand and place your fingers on the bony ridge running across the top of your back, which is the spine of your scapular.
- The posterior deltoid arises under the spine of the scapular.

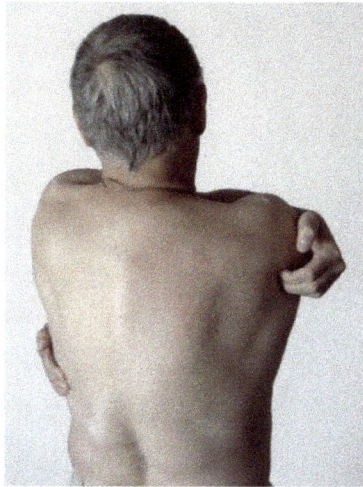

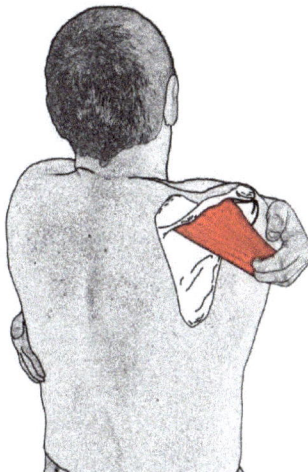

- Flex the fingers of your left hand so they are in a hooked position.
- Press your fingertips on the muscle, at the place it starts, at the end of the spine of the scapula, near to the vertebral column.

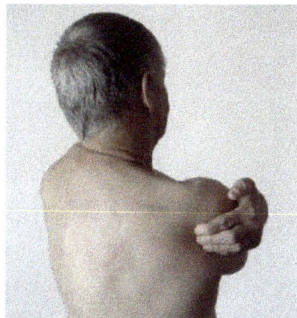

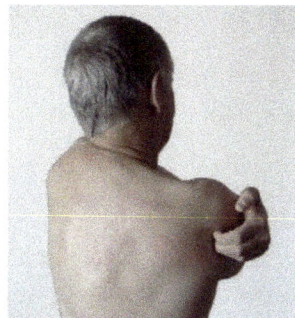

- Slide your fingertips across the muscle and towards the tip of your shoulder using a rake like action, following a line just under the spine of the scapula while simultaneously taking your right upper limb further to the left across the front of the body and around your rib cage.
- Work down the arm along parallel strips until the muscle attaches on the deltoid tubercle.
- Keep perpendicular to the muscle fibres by changing from moving in a more horizontal direction to a more upward direction.
- The muscle is wide at the top and tapers to a narrow tendon, and so the distance for kneading the muscle becomes less as you go down the arm.

Biceps brachii and Brachialis

Massaging biceps can be useful when there is pain from a muscle strain, perhaps because of atrophy, weakness or shortness or from a forceful or unexpected overload of the muscle. It can also help when there is a strain of the tendon, tendinitis or tendinopathy. Repetitive forces and poor posture can cause the tendon of the long head of biceps to become irritated, inflamed and undergo degenerative changes. Biceps pain and tightness can occur when there is a rotator cuff problem or another shoulder condition.

Massaging brachialis can be useful if the muscle is strained by repetitive or forceful contraction such as during heavy physical labour, weightlifting, rope climbing, rock climbing or forceful pull ups and curls.

Biceps brachii has two heads. The short head of biceps arises on the apex of the coracoid process of the scapula.

The long head of biceps arises from a bony tubercle just above the shoulder joint cavity of the scapular. At the top of the shoulder the tendon of the long head passes over the intertubercular sulcus, a groove in the humerus between two bony protuberances, the greater and lesser tuberosities.

The two muscles from each head join as a tendon that attaches onto the back of the radial tuberosity of the radius and a fibrous part, the bicipital aponeurosis, which merges with the deep fascia of the forearm. The biceps tendon twists before attaching on the radial tuberosity.

Biceps brachii flexes and supinates the forearm at the elbow and is a weak flexor of the arm at the shoulder.

Brachialis arises down the front of the lower half of the shaft of the humerus. It narrows to a thick broad tendon which attaches at the top and front of the ulna.

The muscle lies deep to biceps and may split into two or more parts or fuse with biceps and other muscles.

Brachialis is the main flexor of the forearm at the elbow joint, flexing it in all positions.

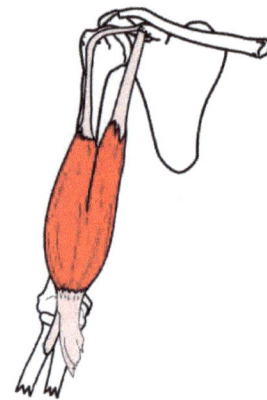

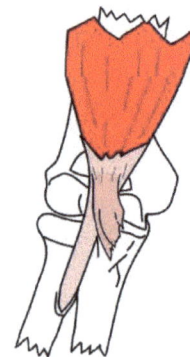

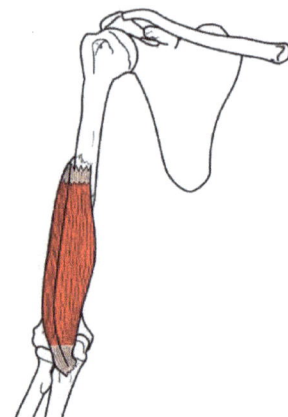

2.2a Kneading biceps brachii and brachialis using the tips of your fingers and thumb

- Stand, sit on a chair or kneel on the floor.
- Flex your right elbow about 90 degrees and rotate your forearm outwards so your palm faces upwards.
- If you are sitting, then rest the back of your right hand on your right thigh.

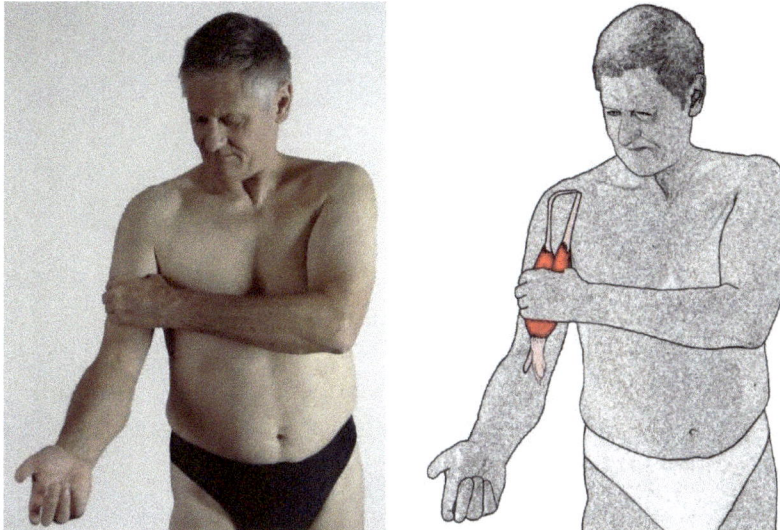

- Grasp your right biceps between the fingers and thumb of your left hand.
- Place your thumb on the inside of the arm and your fingers on the outside.
- Push into the muscle with your thumb and pull with your fingers using a twisting action of the wrist while simultaneously extending your forearm at the elbow, but do not fully straighten your elbow.

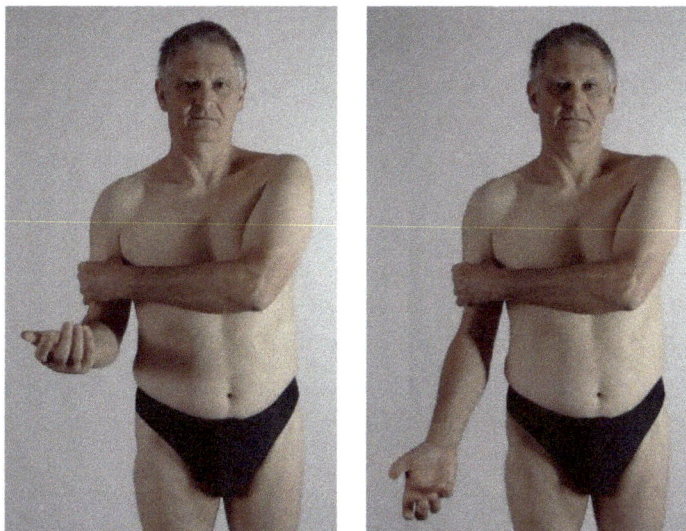

- Use a push pull squeezing action with fingers and thumb.
- Do not slide the fingers or thumb over the skin or pinch the skin.
- Push your thumb outwards and away from your body, and pull your fingers inwards and towards your body, while rotating your forearm outwards to increasing leverage.

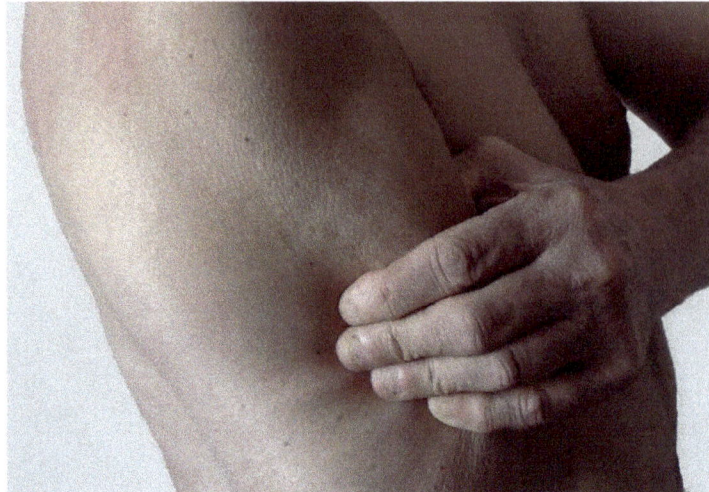

- Start from where the biceps emerge from under deltoid at the front and top of the arm and work down the arm as far as the biceps tendon at the front of the elbow.
- Brachialis is deep to the biceps and so to knead this muscle you must either push through biceps or push under it and over the bone, while keeping biceps relaxed.

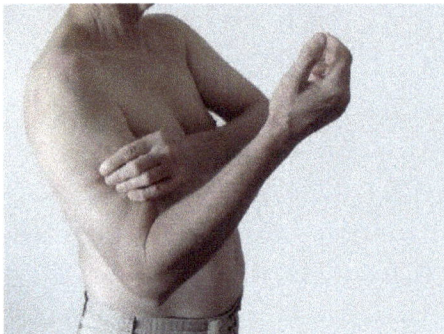

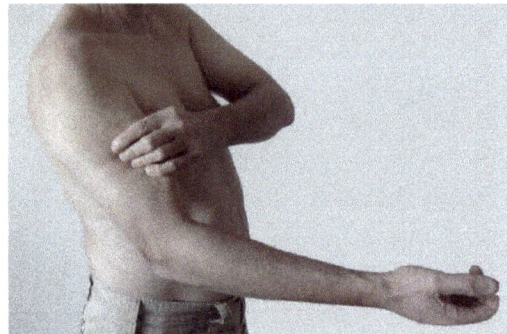

- Work down the inside of your arm, pushing the tip of your thumb as far as you can across the shaft of the humerus and under the biceps and then work down the outside of your arm, pulling with your fingertips.

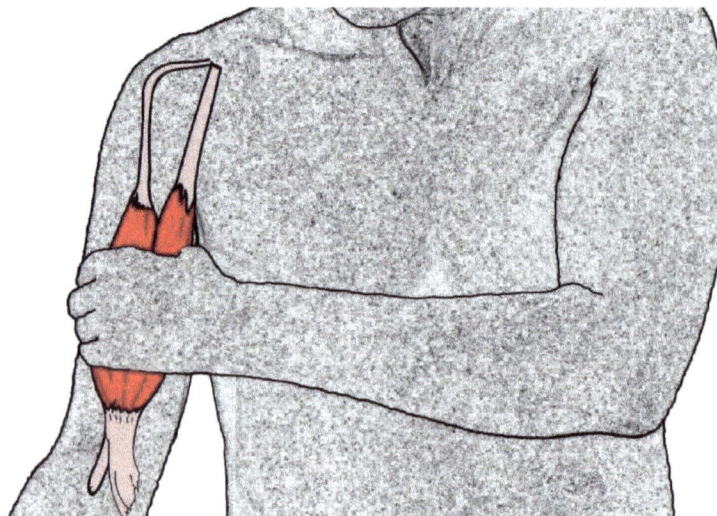

2.2b Kneading biceps and triceps brachii standing or seated with your hand under your thigh and using your fingertips and the tip of your thumb

- Sit on a chair, lift your right thigh, reach under the inside of your thigh with your right hand and grasp the muscles at the back of your thigh.
- Return your thigh and hand to the chair so that your fingers are wedged between your thigh and the chair, and your palm is upwards.
- Roll your right arm inwards so your shoulder and elbow face forwards.

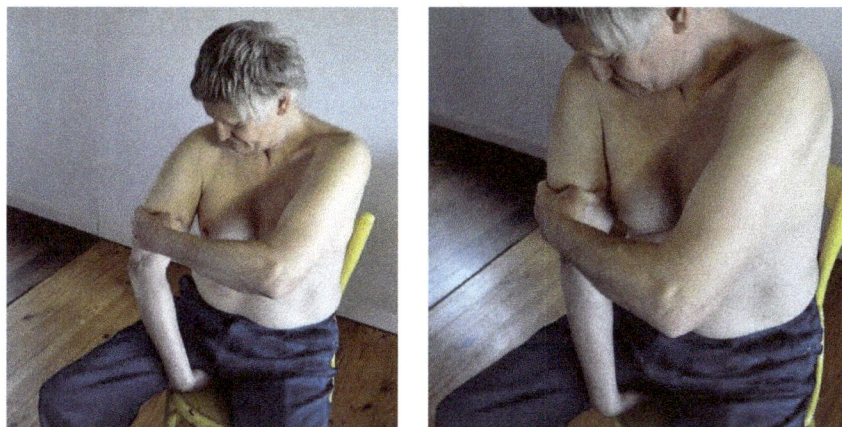

- An alternative to the seated techniques is the standing technique and most of the remaining bullet points apply to both of them.
- Reach in front of your body and around your right arm with your left hand and hook your fingers around the back of your triceps muscle.
- Lift your left elbow, rotate your forearm inwards and turn your wrist so that your thumb points backwards towards your body.
- Place the tip of your thumb on the outside of your biceps muscle, taking care not to lose contact with the triceps.

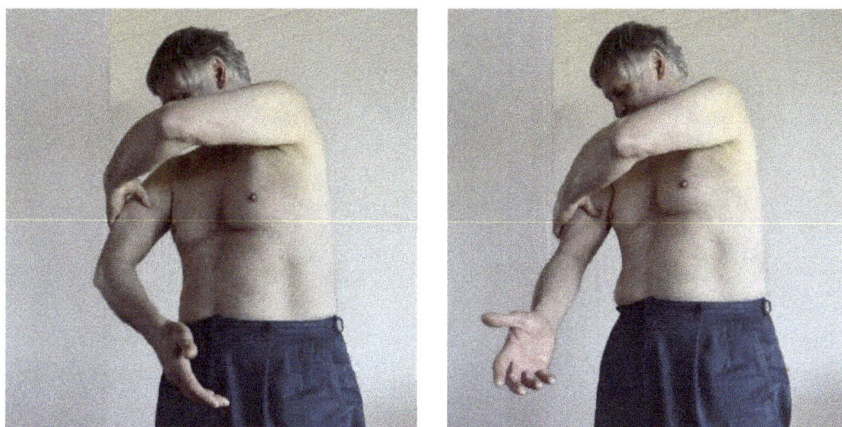

- Push against your biceps with the tip of your thumb and pull on the triceps with your fingertips while simultaneously extending (straightening) your right elbow and outwardly rotating your arm.
- Rotation acts as a counterforce against your finger and thumb pressure.
- Extending your right elbow means bringing your arm closer to your side.
- Start at the top of the arm where the biceps and triceps emerge from under deltoid and move down to their attachments at the elbow.

Triceps brachii

Massaging triceps can be useful when there is pain from a muscle strain, partial tendon strain or tendinopathy where overuse or repetitive activities lead to degenerative changes in one of the tendons. The pain and swelling are usually experienced at the triceps insertion on the elbow. As the muscle helps stabilise the shoulder joint it should be massaged when there is a rotator cuff problem.

Triceps brachii has three heads. The long head arises just under the shoulder joint. The lateral head arises from a flattened tendon which attaches on a ridge on the outside and back of the shaft of the humerus and from fascia arising on muscle and bone. The medial or deep head arises from the back surface of the shaft of the humerus and from fascia arising on muscle and bone.

A common tendon inserts on the upper olecranon at the back of the elbow and onto deep fascia in the forearm.

Triceps brachii straightens the arm at the elbow joint by extending the forearm.

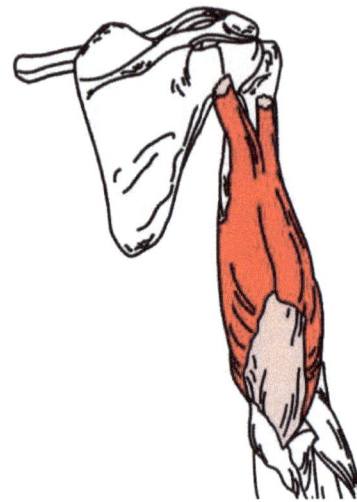

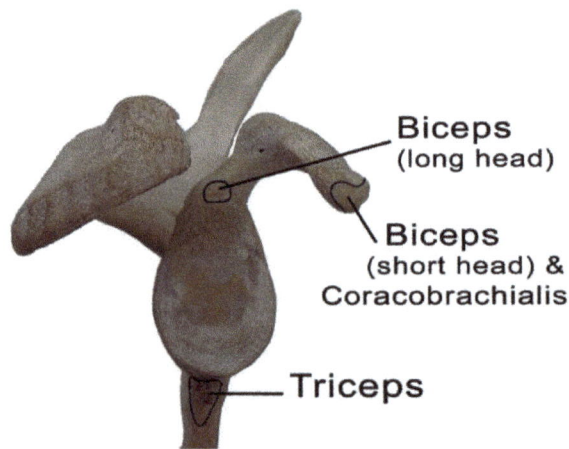

Biceps
(long head)

Biceps
(short head) &
Coracobrachialis

Triceps

Scapula - lateral view

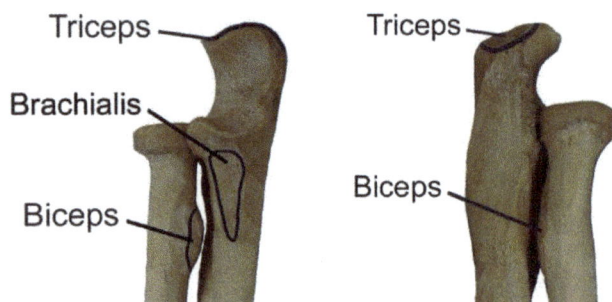

Triceps

Brachialis

Biceps

Triceps

Biceps

Radius and Ulna - anterior view (left) posterior (right)

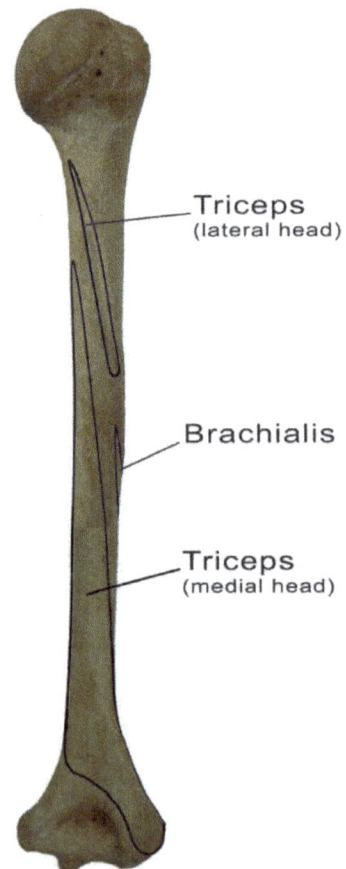

Triceps
(lateral head)

Brachialis

Triceps
(medial head)

Humerus - posterior view

2.3a Kneading triceps brachii using the tips of your fingers and thumb

- Stand, sit on a chair or kneel on the floor.
- Flex your right elbow to about 120 degrees flexion, then move your arm away from your side until your hand and wrist are behind the upper part of your head.

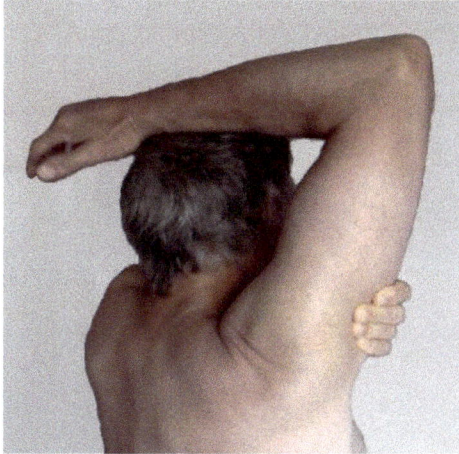

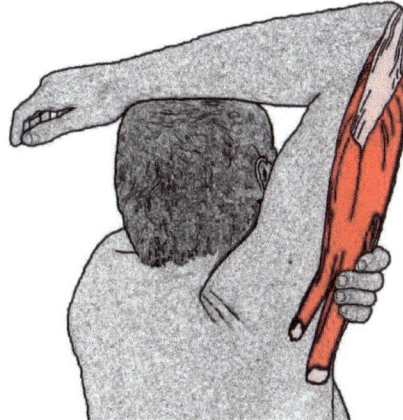

- Reach across the front of your body with your left hand and grasp your right triceps between the pads of your fingers and thumb.
- Place your fingertips on the outside of the muscle and your thumb on the inside.

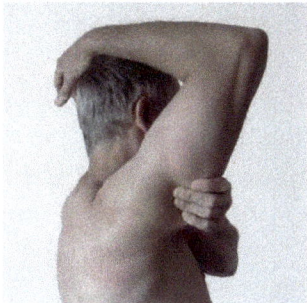

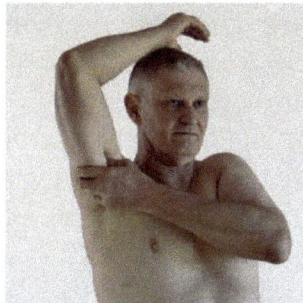

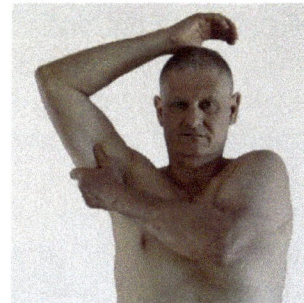

Start of kneading cycle

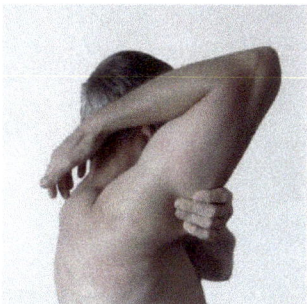

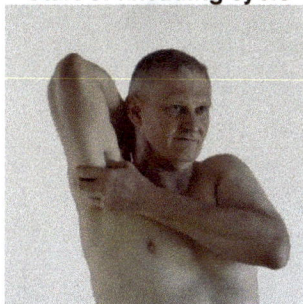

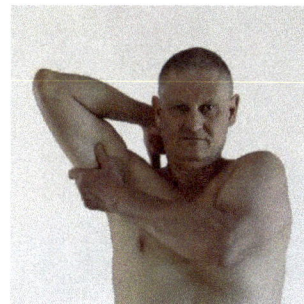

End of kneading cycle

- Knead the triceps with a push-pull action of your fingers and thumb and a twisting action of your wrist while simultaneously increasing elbow flexion by allowing your forearm to drop behind your neck.
- Work from where the long head of triceps attaches near the arm pit to the common tendon attachment on the olecranon process.

2.3b Kneading triceps using your fingertips with one hand fixed under your thigh

- Sit in a chair, lift your right thigh, reach under the inside of it with your right hand and grasp the back of your thigh with your hand.
- Return your thigh to the chair so the back of your fingers are in contact with the chair, your palm faces upwards and your hand wraps around the back of your thigh.

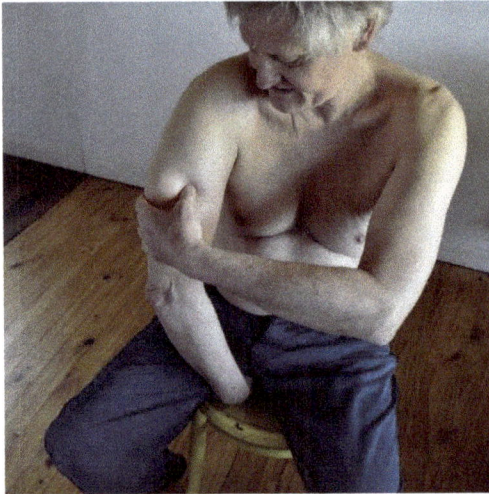

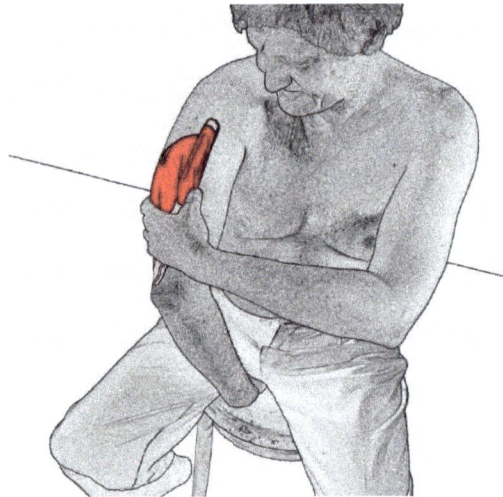

- To make the triceps more accessible roll your right shoulder forwards and turn your arm inwards so that your elbow points more forwards.
- Reach in front and around your right arm with your left hand and grasp your triceps between your fingers and thumb.
- Pull across your triceps muscle with your fingertips and push with your thumb and use a twisting action with the wrist.
- Alternatively use a squeezing action with your fingers and heal of hand.
- Simultaneous with your hand actions, flex your right elbow by taking your elbow more backwards, downwards and to the right with a pivoting movement around your right wrist.

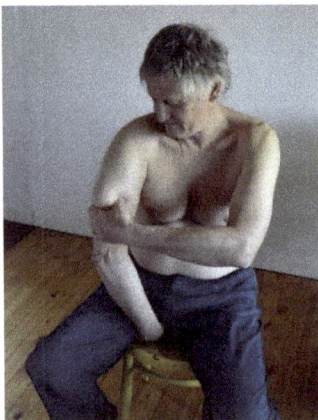

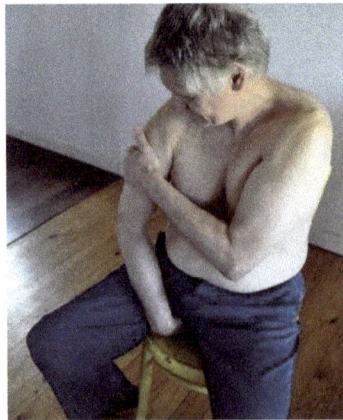

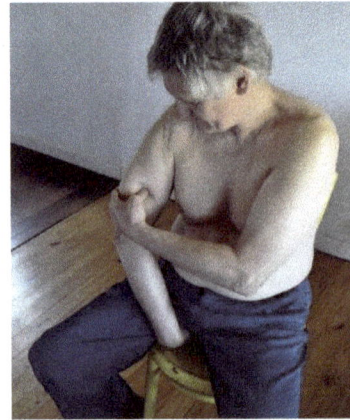

- Move your right arm as a counterforce against your left hand.
- Work from the long head in your armpit and down your arm to the elbow.
- The lateral head is on the outside of the arm, more towards the top of the arm and the medial head is on the inside of the arm, nearer the elbow.

Latissimus dorsi and teres major

Massaging latissimus dorsi can be useful when the muscle is short or when there is pain from a strain. The pain may be in the back, behind the shoulders or in the arm pit. There may also be tingling in the arm and fingers.

A strain or tear in latissimus dorsi is rare and occurs in sports that involve throwing, pulling and reaching overhead. Overuse, poor posture, faulty sport or exercise technique, inadequate stretching and not warming up before exercising can also contribute to latissimus dorsi strains.

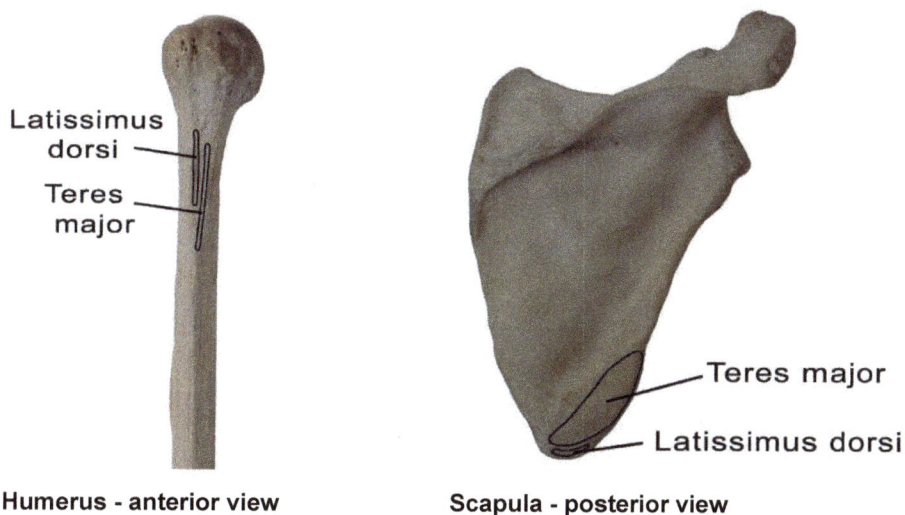

Latissimus dorsi

Teres major

Teres major

Latissimus dorsi

Humerus - anterior view   **Scapula - posterior view**

Latissimus dorsi is a triangular muscle which arises on thoracolumbar fascia, sacrum, iliac crest and spinous processes of all lumbar vertebrae and thoracic T6 to T12. The muscle arises directly from ribs 9 to 12, a small area on the iliac crest and the inferior angle of the scapula. Between T6 and T12 it lies under trapezius.

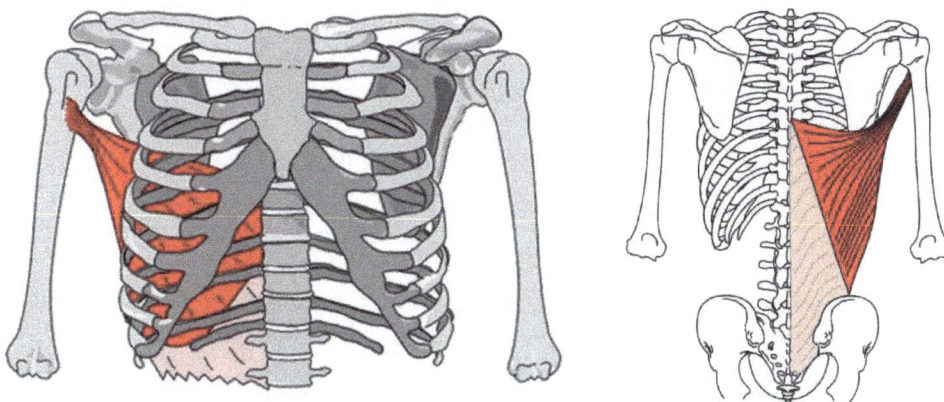

Latissimus dorsi - anterior view (left) and posterior view (right)

Latissimus dorsi runs upwards and outwards, passes over the lower part of teres major then twist around it so that its front part faces backwards and presses against teres major. Together the two muscles form the posterior axillary fold. The latissimus dorsi tendon attaches onto a lower part intertubercular sulcus of the humerus. Because of its twisting action the highest midline fibres form the lowest tendon attachment and the lowest midline fibres form the highest tendon attachment on the humerus.

Teres major injuries are rare but when they occur are usually the result of vigorous throwing or reaching actions. The pain is usually localised at the side of the scapula or deep under the arm pit. Massage and rest are usually effective in fixing this injury.

Teres major arises as muscle from the outside and back surface of the scapula and near the inferior angle at the bottom and from fascia attached to other muscles.

The flat tendon attaches on an area of bone at the front of the shoulder and on the lip of the intertubercular sulcus.

The muscle acts with latissimus dorsi to bring the arm to the side of the body (adduction), backwards (extension) and to rotate the arm inwards (medial rotation).

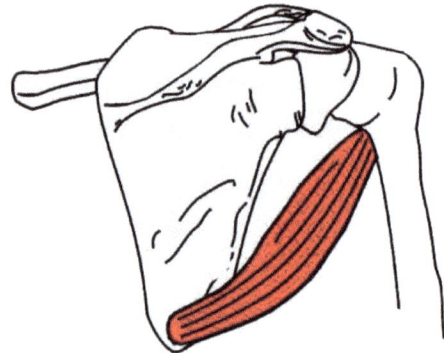

2.4a Kneading latissimus dorsi, teres major and teres minor using your fingertips and tip of your thumb

- Stand, sit straight on a chair or kneel on the floor.
- Lift your right arm and place your right hand on your head.
- Reach across the front and right side of your body with your left hand and place your fingers on the bone pointing downwards at the bottom of your scapula, the inferior angle.

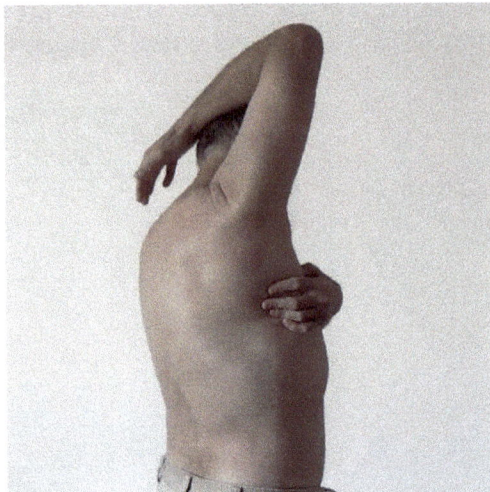

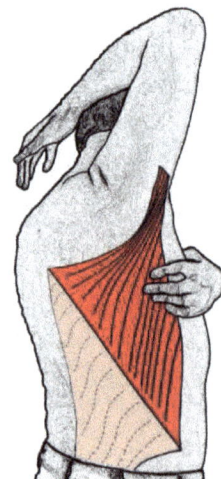

- Now reach further behind the scapula and towards the spine.
- Flex your fingers and hook your fingertips over the upper border of latissimus dorsi which swings from T6 in the thoracic spine, across the back of the rib cage and lower scapula.
- To keep your hooked fingertips perpendicular to the latissimus dorsi fibres move downwards, then outward along the rib angles, and then forwards across the rib cage and just under the inferior angle.

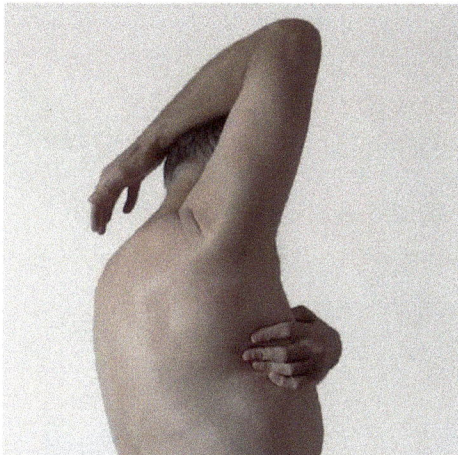

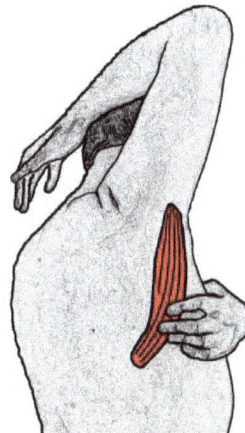

- As you slide your fingertips over the muscle move your arm further towards your head.
- From the inferior angle latissimus dorsi is joined by teres major fibres and they project up the side of the scapula to the back of the arm pit.
- Slide your fingertips forwards across the bottom of the scapula and across the ribs to about the mid-point of the rib cage.
- Work progressively along short parallel strips over the back and side of the scapula and then drop down to the ribs - use a rake like action.

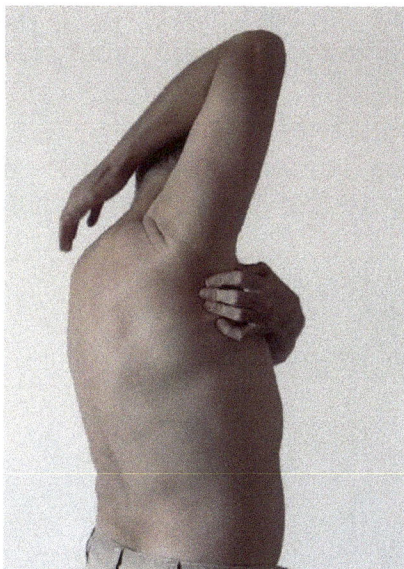

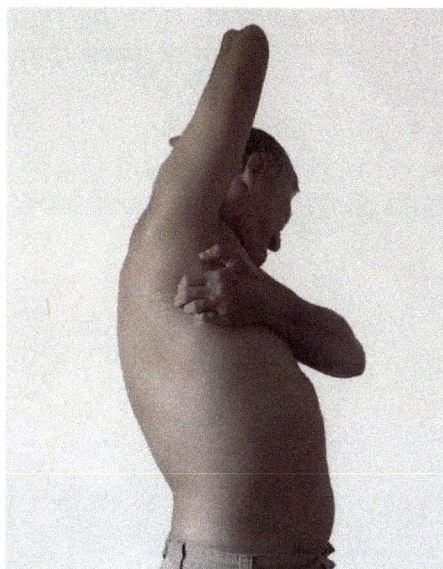

- Latissimus dorsi and teres major are joined by teres minor about halfway up the outer border of the scapula.
- Continue with the sliding action of the fingertips but press harder as the muscle fold becomes thicker towards the back of the arm pit.
- Grasp the thicker muscle fold between your fingers and thumb and knead them with a twisting action - but take care not to press your thumb hard into the arm pit where there are sensitive tissues.
- To localise on teres minor, return your right arm to the side of your body and increase inward rotation of your right arm as you knead the muscle.

2.4b Kneading teres major, teres minor, and the upper fibres of latissimus dorsi using the wadi or two balls in a net

- Lie on your right side with your right hip and knee flexed about 90 degrees and your left leg flexed a bit less so that it is resting behind the right leg.
- Flex your right arm and place your hand just behind your head.
- Place the palm of your left hand on the floor in front of your body.

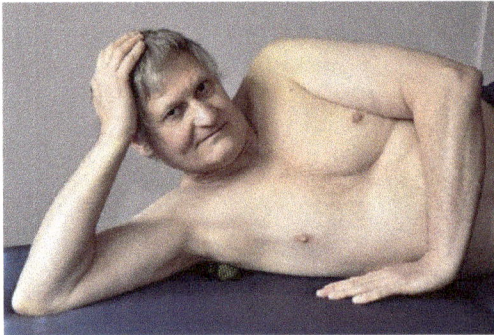

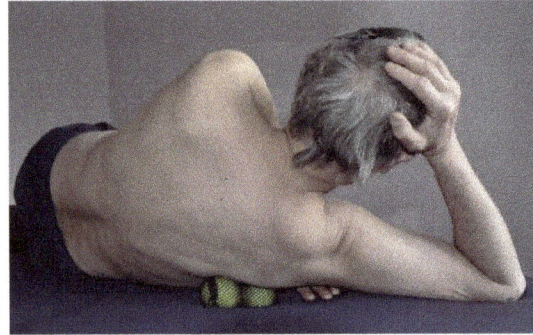

- Use your left hand for controlling balance and moving the wadi or balls.
- Lift your upper body off the floor and place the wadi/balls against the outside edge of the scapula, just at the bottom, so one wheel/ball is in front of the scapula and the other is behind.
- Return the wadi/balls and the right side of your trunk to the floor, relax and allow the domes or balls to push into the muscles either side of the scapula.
- The scapula sits in valley between the domes or balls.
- Take a deep breath in and then exhale and relax and allow the wadi or balls to push further into the muscles - let the weight of your body do the work.

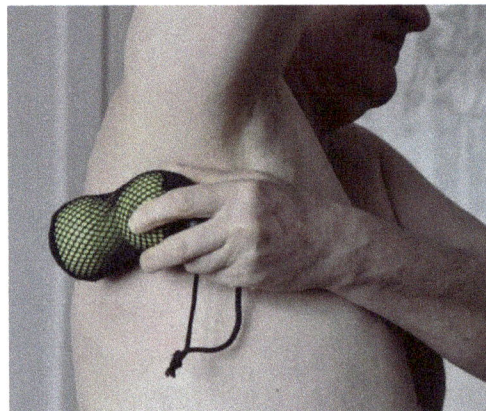

- Rotate your trunk forwards or backwards to adjust your body's centre of gravity and weight over the wadi/balls and pressure on the muscle.
- Repeat the technique from the inferior angle at the bottom of the scapular to the top, following a line along the outside of the scapula to the back of the arm pit where latissimus dorsi, teres major and teres minor form a thick fold.
- Avoid this technique if you have a rotator cuff problem.

Serratus anterior

Massaging serratus anterior can be useful when there is pain in the arm, shoulder or chest, tightness in the chest or difficulty breathing.

Trauma to the muscle or the long thoracic nerve in the lower cervical spine, can cause muscle weakness and the inability to lift the arm. It can also result in scapula winging, where the medial border of the scapula sticks out at an angle on the rib cage. Massage can help muscle tightness from a chronic rotator cuff problem.

Serratus anterior arises from the outer surface and upper border of ribs 1 to 8 and from fascia covering the intercostal muscles. It runs back and around the rib cage as a muscular sheet, passing under the scapula to attach along the entire length of the inner border of the scapula, including two triangular areas at the top and bottom of the front of the scapula.

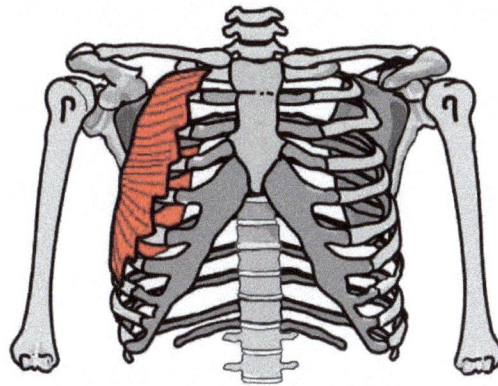

Fibres arising from ribs 1 and 2 attach on the upper area of the scapula and fibres from ribs 3 and 4 attach along the inner border of the scapula and they produce outward movement or protraction of the scapula.

Fibres arising from ribs 5 to 8 attach on the lower area of the scapula near the inferior angle and they produce upward rotation of the scapula, so the shoulder joint faces more vertically. The muscle steadies the scapular during arm movements and assists with pushing, reaching and taking the arm above the head.

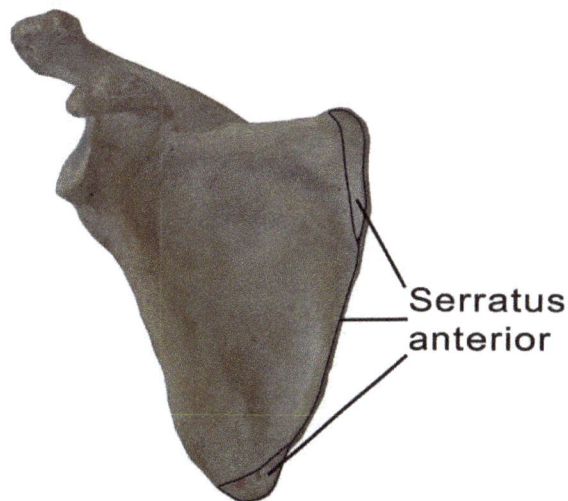

Serratus anterior

2.5a Kneading serratus anterior using your fingertips

- Stand, sit straight on a chair or kneel on the floor.
- The lower fibres of serratus anterior arise on the inferior angle, which is the sharp bone pointing downwards at the bottom of the scapula.
- The lower fibres fan out from here to attach on ribs 5, 6, 7 and 8.
- Reach across the front and right side of your rib cage with your left hand and place your fingertips on the inferior angle.

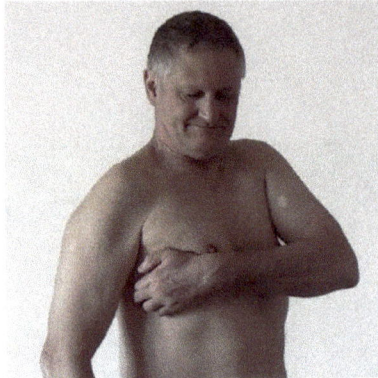

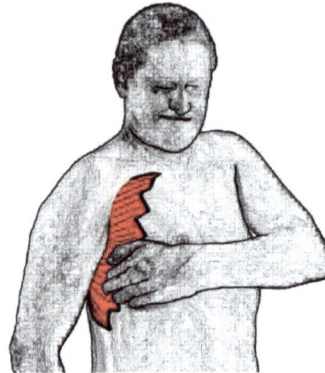

- Flex your fingers and hook your fingertips over the very lowest fibres of serratus anterior, which run forwards and slightly downwards to rib 8.
- Using a rake like action move your fingertips downwards, forwards and then upwards in an arc around the inferior angle of the scapula.
- Start close to the inferior angle, but then make progressively wider arcs around bottom of the scapula and then up the outside.
- Slide your hooked fingertips across the ribs, muscles and overlying skin.
- As you move your fingertips across the muscle pull your right shoulder down (depression) and move your scapula towards the spine (retraction).

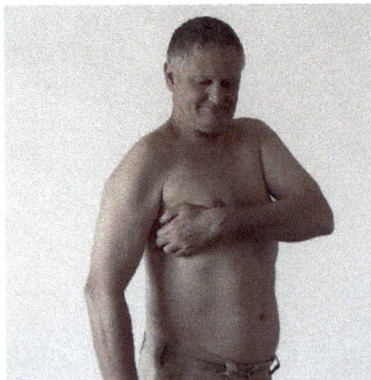

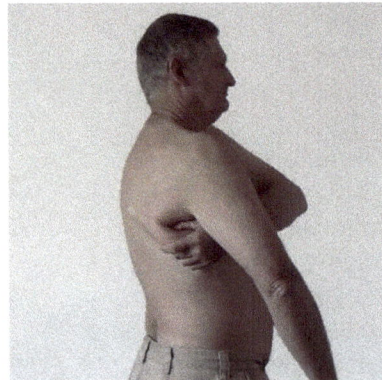

- Now move your fingertips to the outside of your scapula.
- Slide your fingertips up the right side of your rib cage, staying close to the outside edge of the scapula until your reach the arm pit - this area is sensitive so go more lightly here.
- Move your shoulder down and back as you slide your fingertips.
- Repeat the movement along two or three other vertical strips of the rib cage, staying parallel with the outer border of the scapula.
- Keep perpendicular to the upper fibres of serratus anterior by moving upwards and sliding over each rib with your rake-like action.

2.5b Kneading serratus anterior using the wadi or two balls in a net

- Lie on your right side with your right hip and knee flexed about 90 degrees and your left leg flexed a bit less so that it is resting behind the right leg.
- Flex your right arm and place your hand just behind your head.
- Place the palm of your left hand on the floor in front of your body.
- Use your left hand for controlling balance and moving the balls.
- Lift your upper body off the floor and place the wadi/balls against the outside edge of the scapula, just at the bottom, so one wheel/ball is in front of the scapula and the other is behind.

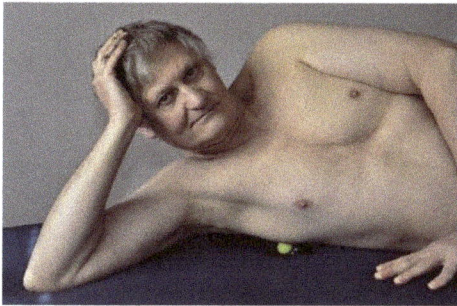

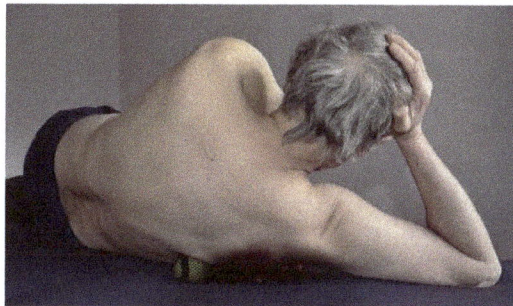

- Return the wadi/balls and the right side of your trunk to the floor, relax and let the domes or balls push into the muscles either side of the scapula.
- The scapula sits in valley between the domes or balls.
- Take a deep breath and then exhale and relax and allow the wadi or balls to push further into the muscles - let the weight of your body do the work.
- Rotate your trunk forwards or backwards to adjust your body's centre of gravity and weight over the wadi/balls and pressure on the muscle.
- Rotate your trunk forwards to increase pressure on serratus anterior.

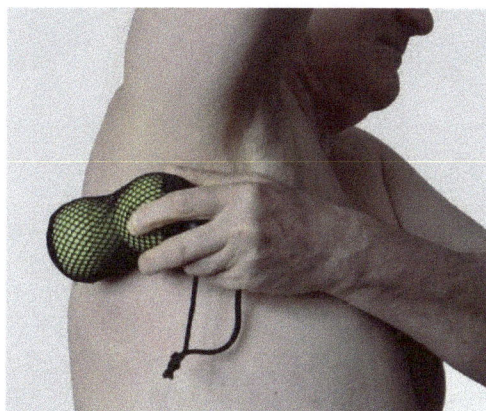

- Repeat the technique all the way up to the side of the rib cage and into the arm pit where the upper fibres of serratus anterior attach.
- Avoid this technique if you have a rotator cuff problem.

Pectoralis major and pectoralis minor

Massaging pectoralis major and pectoralis minor can be useful for pain from a strain to the muscles or their tendons, tendinitis and tendinopathy. It can help when poor posture results in muscle shortness, which can restrict breathing and shoulder movement, and affect circulation and nerve function in the upper limb.

A pectoralis major strain is more common than a minor and usually occurs at the musculotendinous junction from overloading during bench presses or weightlifting. It can occur in the muscle as a result of a direct blow to the front of the chest during contact sports. A strain in pectoralis major or minor may result in pain in the front of the chest or shoulder, difficulty breathing, muscle weakness and restricted movement, especially when lifting the arm. Tendinitis is more common in pectoralis major and results in pain and swelling over the tendon.

Pectoralis major is a thick triangular muscle that forms the front of the arm pit. Its upper part, the clavicular fibres, arises from the inner half of the clavicle. Its lower part, the sternocostal fibres, arises from the front of the sternum, costal cartilages of ribs 2 to 6 and the fascia covering the external oblique muscle of the abdomen.

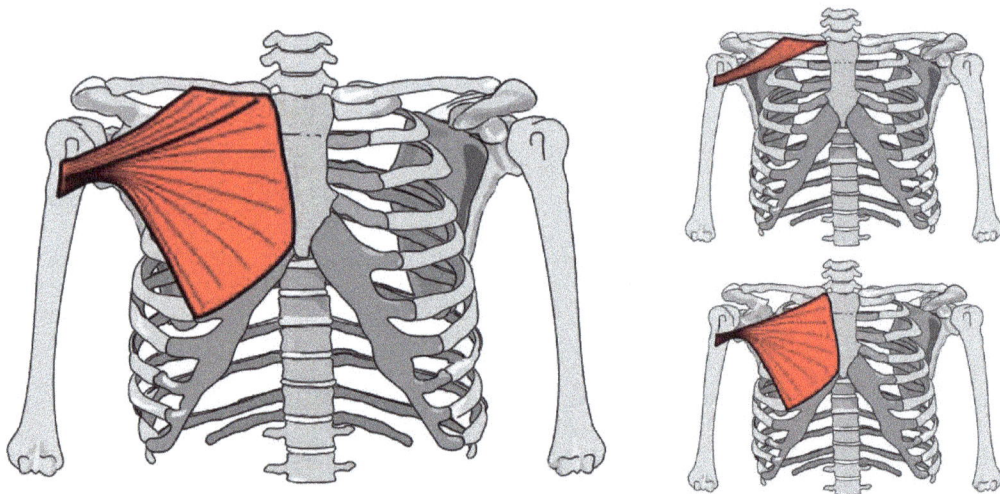

Pectoralis major - clavicular and sternal costal fibres

The two heads unite on a narrow flat tendon about 5 cm wide, which passes under deltoid to insert on the outer lip of the intertubercular sulcus of the humerus. The tendon has two layers, and the outer layer comes from the upper muscle and the inner layer comes from the lower and in front of the sternum. The sternal and abdominal fibres twist so that the lowest fibres attach highest on the arm and the highest fibres attach lowest.

From a position of extension, the clavicular fibres produce flexion of the humerus. In addition, they produce medial rotation and horizontal flexion of the humerus. From a position of flexion, the sternocostal fibres produce extension of the humerus. In addition, they produce adduction, medial rotation and horizontal flexion of the humerus. When the upper limb is fixed above the head the muscle pulls the torso upwards and forwards as in climbing. The muscle may be involved in forced inhalation.

2.6a Kneading the clavicular fibres of pectoralis major using the side of your thumb or your fingertips

- Stand facing a post or the corner of a wall.
- Place the palm of your right hand against the post or wall.
- Take a short step forward and allow your right arm to drop back behind your body.
- Rotate your spine to the left and allow your right arm to rotate outwards at the shoulder.
- Keep your right arm near the side of your body and allow your elbow to flex a little.
- Hook your fingers under the bottom of pectoralis major and place the side of your left thumb under your clavicle, near the sternum.

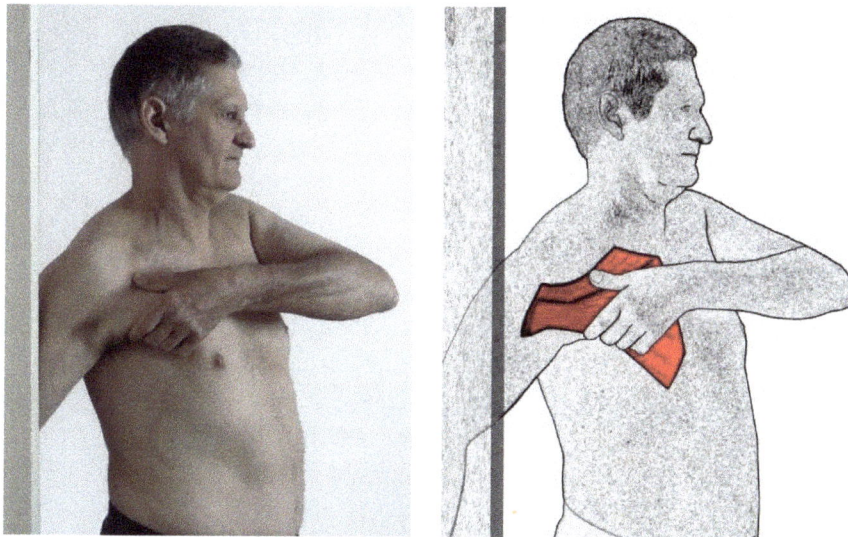

- Slide your thumb across the muscle which attaches along the bottom of the clavicle while simultaneously leaning your body further forwards to increase the backward movement and outward rotation of your arm.
- Stop where the muscle attachment about halfway along the clavicle.
- Now change direction and slide your thumb obliquely downwards and towards your sternum while leaning forwards and rotating your body.
- This part of the muscle is only a few centimetres wide so do not move your thumb too far.
- Repeat this over short parallel strips until your reach the tendon in front of the arm.

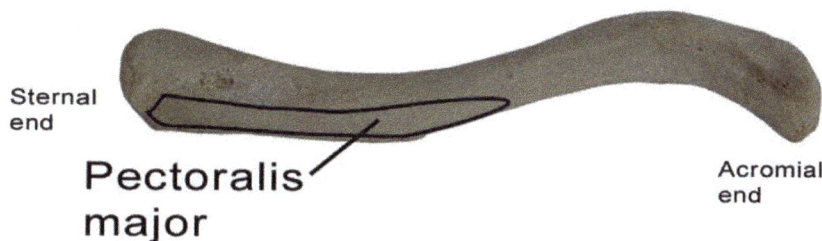

Sternal end

Pectoralis major

Acromial end

Clavicle viewed from below

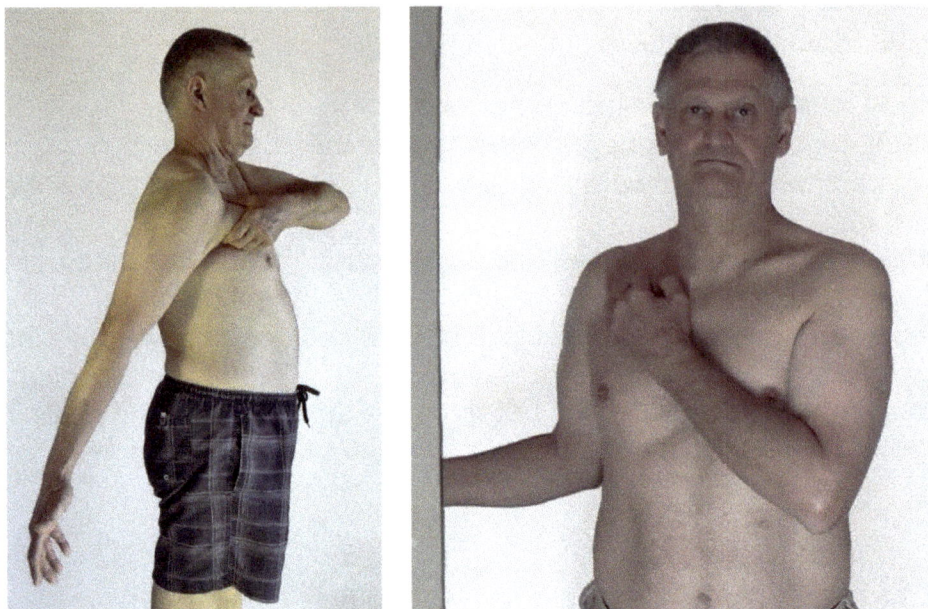

- There are several other options with this technique:

  - Use your fingers as a counterforce against your thumb and knead the sternal fibres of pectoralis major as well as the clavicular fibre.
  - Use your fingertips instead of your thumb and slide them in a downwards direction across the clavicular fibres of pectoralis major, just like with the thumb.
  - Flex your right forearm 90 degrees at the elbow, place your palm on the post or wall and rotate your body so your arm turns outwards at the shoulder, and then knead the muscle with your fingertips or thumb as you increase the rotation.
  - Actively move your arm backwards and/or rotate it instead of using a post or wall.

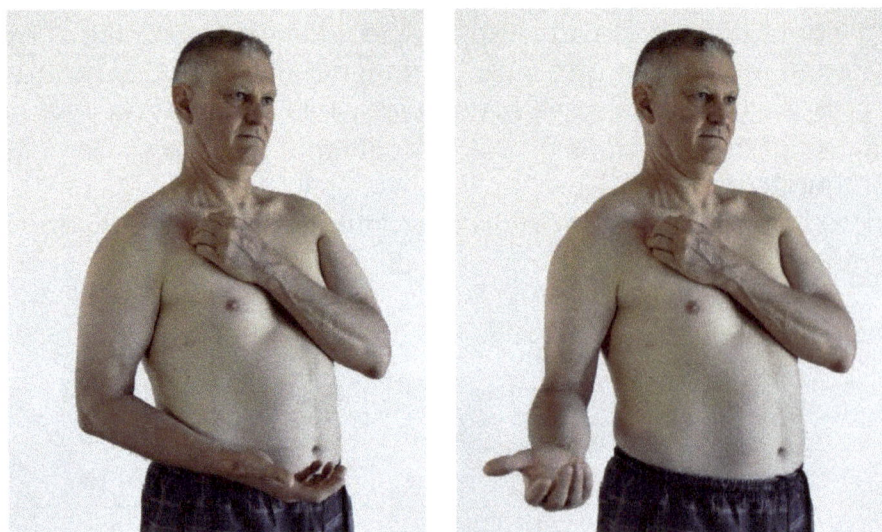

2.6b Kneading the sternal fibres of pectoralis major using the tip of your thumb or your fingertips

- Stand facing the corner of a wall.
- Flex your right forearm 90 degrees at the elbow, then take your arm 90 degrees away from your body and then outwardly rotate it.
- Place the palm of your right hand, forearm and elbow against the wall.
- Your hand is level with the top of your head, your forearm vertical and your arm horizontal so your elbow is about level with your shoulder.

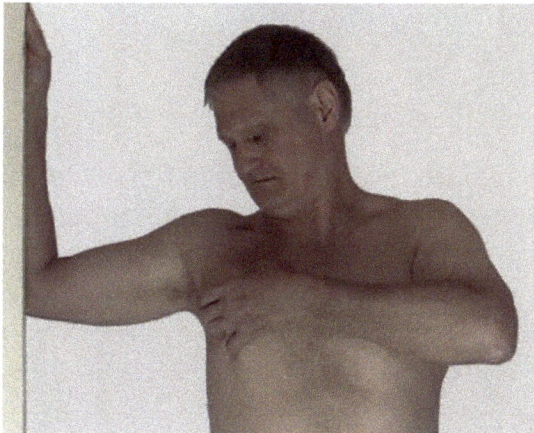

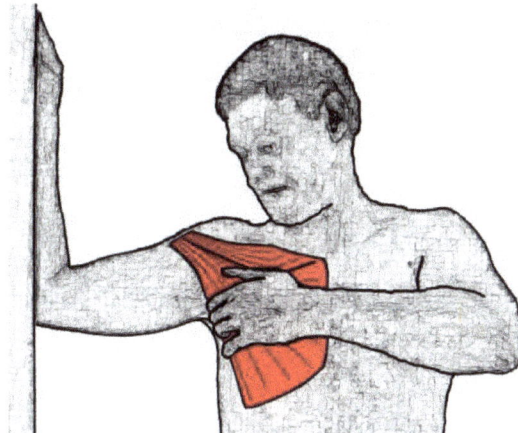

- Lean forwards so your arm rotates outwards a bit and rotate your spine to the left so your arm moves horizontally backwards - do not stretch the muscle too hard.
- Reach across the front of your body with your left hand and grasp your pectoralis major muscle between your fingers and thumb.
- Start where the muscle attaches on the sternum.
- Curl your fingers around the bottom of the muscle and place the side of your thumb on the top of the muscle, or as far as you can easily reach.

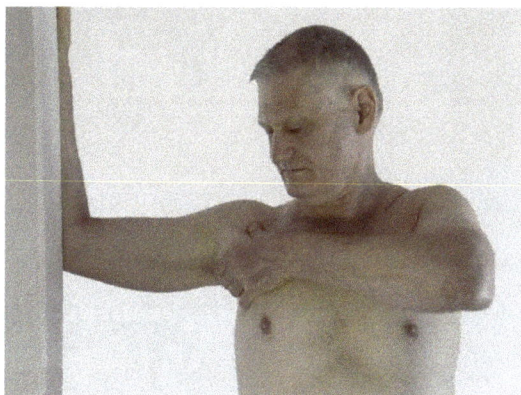

- Knead the muscle by pushing downwards with your thumb and pulling upwards with your hooked fingers, combining the finger and thumb actions with a twisting of the wrist.
- Lean forwards and rotate your body to the left as you knead the muscle.
- Repeat these actions further along the muscle, which gets progressively narrower towards the arm pit, before attaching on an 8 cm wide tendon in front of the arm.

- Work your fingertips high up and deep into the armpit but do not press hard against the ribs and the sensitive structures here.

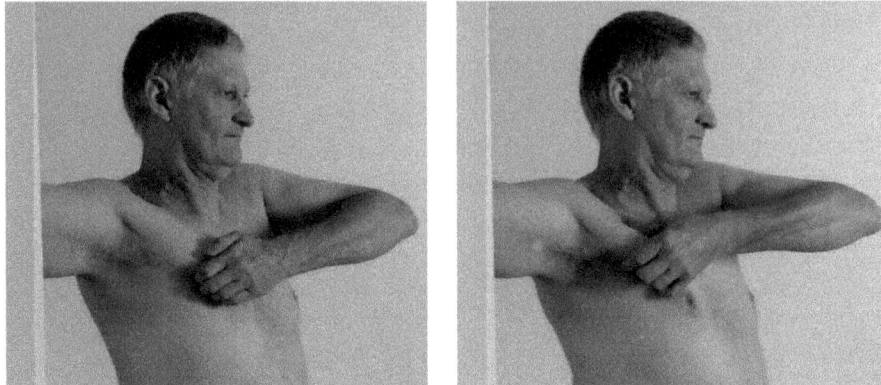

- Place your thumb in the depression just under the end of the clavicle.
- Work across these outer fibres, where the muscle is at its narrowest.
- The fibres of pectoralis major change direction along their length and to keep your thumb perpendicular to the fibres you must follow a downwards and outwards arc.

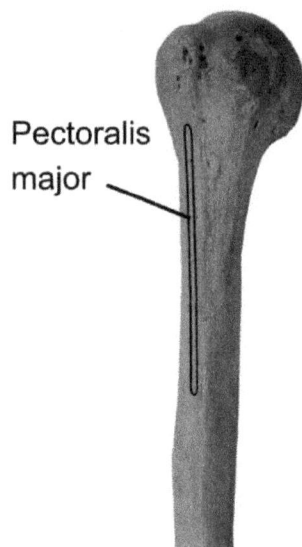

Pectoralis major

Humerus - anterior view

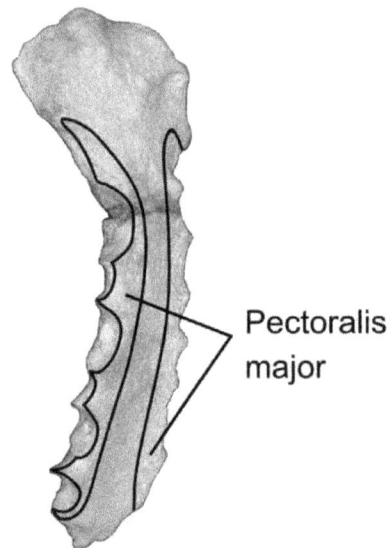

Pectoralis major

Sternum - anterior view

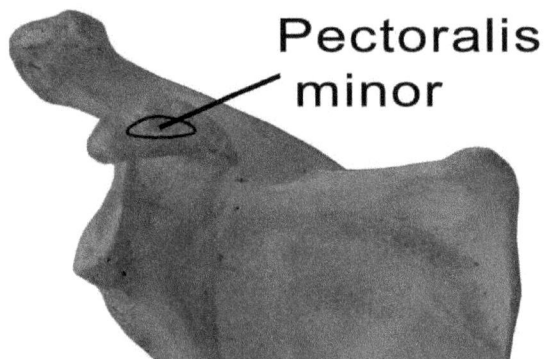

Pectoralis minor

Scapula - anterior view

Pectoralis minor is a thin muscle beneath pectoralis major. It arises from the upper and outer surface of ribs 3, 4 and 5, near the front of the rib cage and from fascia covering the external intercostal muscles. The fibres run upwards and outwards to attach onto the upper surface of the coracoid process of the scapula.

The muscle produces depression, protraction, forward tilt and downward rotation of the scapula and assists with stabilization of the shoulder. When the scapula is fixed, it lifts the rib cage and assists with inhalation.

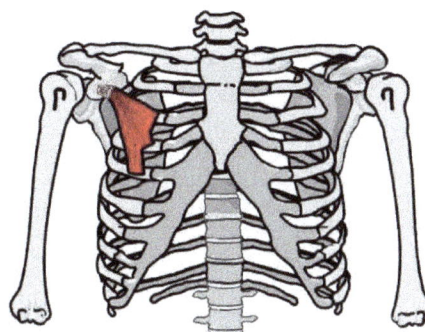

2.6c Kneading pectoralis minor using the tip of your thumb and your fingertips over a rolled-up towel

- Sit on the floor.
- Place a rolled-up towel across your thoracic spine and lower half of your scapula.
- Holding the rolled-up towel in place bring your body and the towel to the floor so you are lying over it.
- If you have placed the towel correctly across the lower half of the scapula, then it will tip backwards in the lying position.
- Flex your right arm and forearm so your right hand rests behind your head.

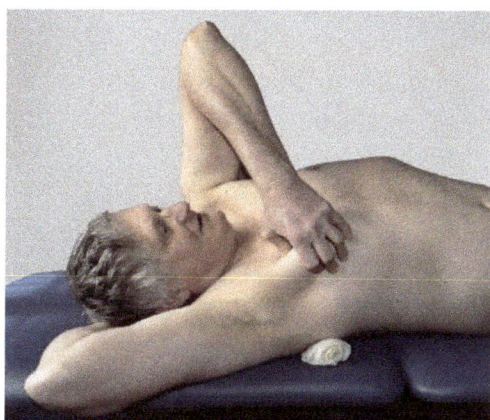

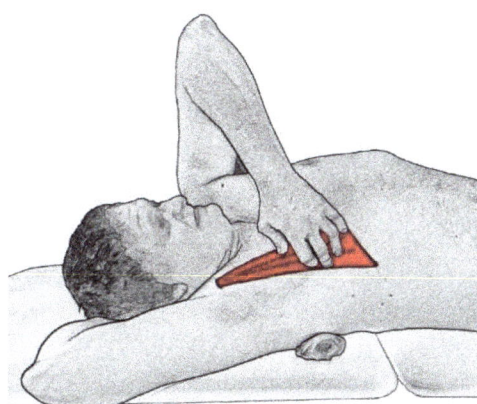

- Adjust your right shoulder and make your scapula tilt backward to the floor.
- Adjust the rolled-up towel so that it pins the inferior angle against the rib cage.
- Reach across the front of your body with your left hand and hook your fingers around the outside of pectoralis major.
- Find the halfway point of the clavicle and place the tip of your thumb just under the clavicle here, which is just above rib 3 and the top of the inner border of pectoralis minor.

- Take a deep breath in and then exhale and push the tip of your thumb outwards and slightly downwards, over the rib cage and push your fingertips inwards and upwards, again by moving over the rib cage and over the outer fibres of pectoralis minor.
- Combine this with greater scapula elevation and backward tilt with your right shoulder.
- Push through pectoralis major with your thumb to reach pectoralis minor.
- Reposition your thumb one rib lower to rib 4 and repeat these actions and then do them again on the fibres attaching on rib 5, the lowest rib attachment for this muscle.
- The muscle fans out in a downward and inwards direction and you will need consider this and its attachments on ribs 3, 4 and 5.

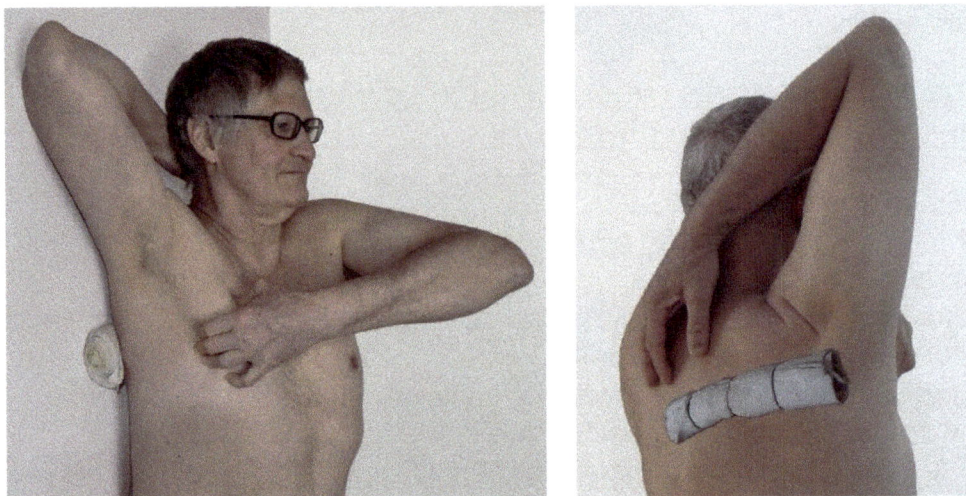

- This technique can be done standing with the rolled-up towel sandwiched between the back of your scapula and the wall.
- The image above and on the right is digitally manipulated to show the correct placement of the rolled-up towel against the lower half of your scapula.
- This technique can also be done seated with the rolled-up towel sandwiched between the back of your scapula and the back of the chair - take care not to fall backwards.
- Instead of combining thumb and fingers, this technique can be done by focusing on just pushing with your thumb or just pulling with your fingers.
- To treat the outermost fibres of pectoralis minor, pull your hooked fingers under pectoralis major and over the rib cage.
- To treat the innermost and middle fibres of pectoralis minor, push the tip of your thumb through pectoralis major.

THE ELBOW, FOREARM AND WRIST

Wrist and finger flexor muscles of the anterior forearm

Massaging the wrist and finger flexor muscles and common flexor tendon on the inside of the elbow, can be useful when there is pain from a muscle strain, partial tendon strain, ligament sprain, bursitis or repetitive strain injury (RSI).

Muscle strains are usually the result of sudden loading of unprepared muscles, over-stretching of muscles or a direct blow to the forearm. Short tight forearm muscles lead to painful and restricted hand and wrist movement. Massage on the medial epicondyle, the bony knob on the inside of the elbow, can be useful when there is a golfers' elbow, which is a strain of the common flexor tendon. Golfer's elbow is usually the result of overuse, overloading or repetition. Symptoms include a dull ache on or near the epicondyle when at rest, pain with hand or wrist movement, weakness, especially when grasping objects and referred pain into the forearm or wrist.

Massage over the joint line just below the bony knob can be useful when there is pain from a medial collateral ligament sprain. Medial collateral ligament sprains occur from a single force directed to the outside of the elbow or from repetitive forces such as overhead throwing. The inside of the elbow may be swollen, tender, bruised, stiff and painful.

Bursitis from repetitive activities, pressure or injury can occur at several locations around the elbow. RSI can develop as a result of fatigue in weak or tired muscles, from a previous injury or from the prolonged use of a computer keyboard or musical instrument.

The following muscles share common features - they mostly arise on a common flexor tendon at the inside of the elbow, merge with fascia that surrounds other muscles within and in front of the forearm and they are bundled together inside and at the front of the forearm.

Wrist flexor muscles of the forearm

Palmaris longus arises on the medial epicondyle of the humerus. It lies between flexor carpi radialis and flexor carpi ulnaris. Its long tendon bisects the wrist, runs under a strap-like structure in front of the wrist, the flexor retinaculum and attaches onto the palmar aponeurosis. It produces wrist flexion, and it tenses the palmar fascia.

Flexor carpi ulnaris arises on the medial epicondyle of the humerus and has a larger head which arises on the ulna and fascia within the forearm. It primarily attaches on the pisiform bone in front of the wrist and then goes on to attach on other bones and tissues in the wrist and hand. The muscle produces wrist flexion and adduction, and stabilisation of the wrist during movements of the thumb and little finger.

Flexor carpi radialis arises on the medial epicondyle. Its long tendon attaches onto the base of the second and third metacarpal. It is palpable. It produces wrist flexion and abduction.

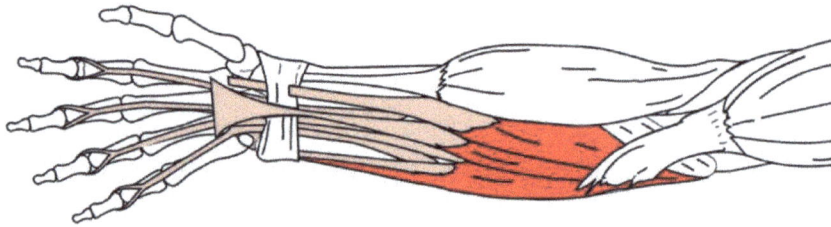

Finger flexor muscles of the forearm

Flexor pollicis longus arises over a broad area in front of the shaft of the radius. The tendon passes under the flexor retinaculum and attaches on the base of last digit of the thumb. The muscle produces flexion of the thumb. It assists with adduction of the thumb and flexion of the wrist.

Flexor digitorum profundus arises on a broad area in front of the ulna. The muscle gives rise to four tendons, which diverge after passing under the flexor retinaculum and then attach on the base of the last digits of the fingers. The muscle produces flexion of the fingers and wrist.

Flexor digitorum superficialis has two heads. One head arises from the medial epicondyle of the humerus and a small area of bone at the top, front and inside of the ulna. The other head arises as a thin sheet, from an oblique line running down the front of the radius. The muscle gives rise to four tendons, which diverge after passing under the flexor retinaculum and then insert onto either side of the middle digits of all four fingers. The muscle produces fast and resisted finger flexion.

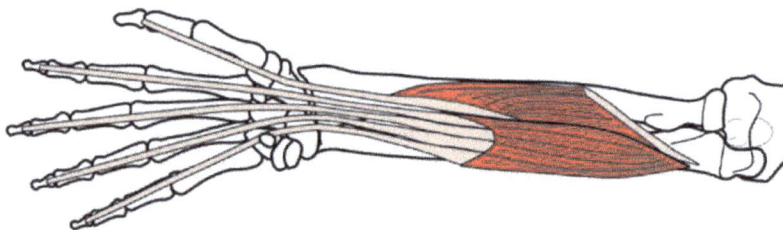

Pronator teres has two heads. The humeral head arises from just above the medial epicondyle of the humerus and from fascia between other muscles. The smaller and deeper ulna head arises from just in front of the elbow. The muscle runs diagonally across the front of the forearm and attaches on a flat tendon attaching about halfway down the outside of the radius. Pronator teres produces pronation of the forearm and is a weak flexor of the forearm.

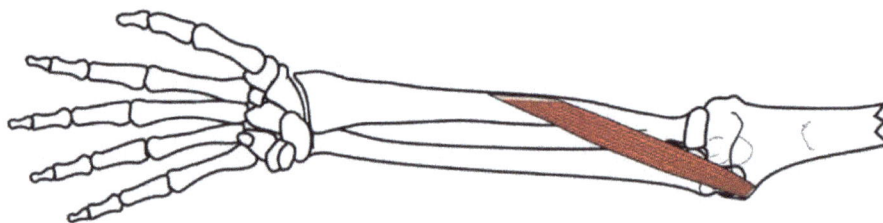

Anterior forearm muscles including wrist and finger flexors

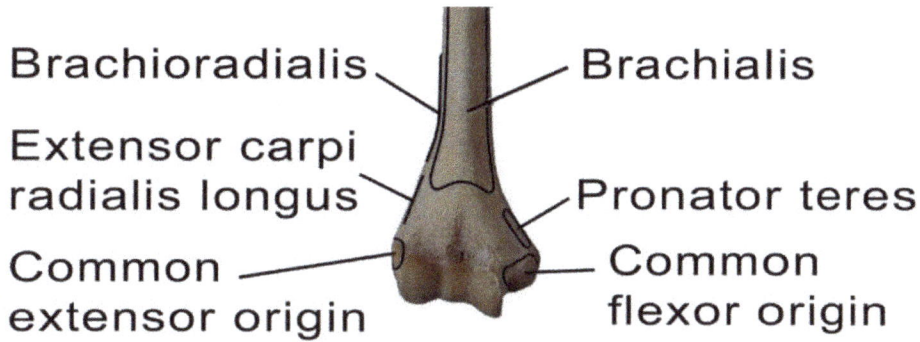

Brachioradialis

Brachialis

Extensor carpi
radialis longus

Pronator teres

Common
extensor origin

Common
flexor origin

Distal humerus and muscle attachments - anterior view

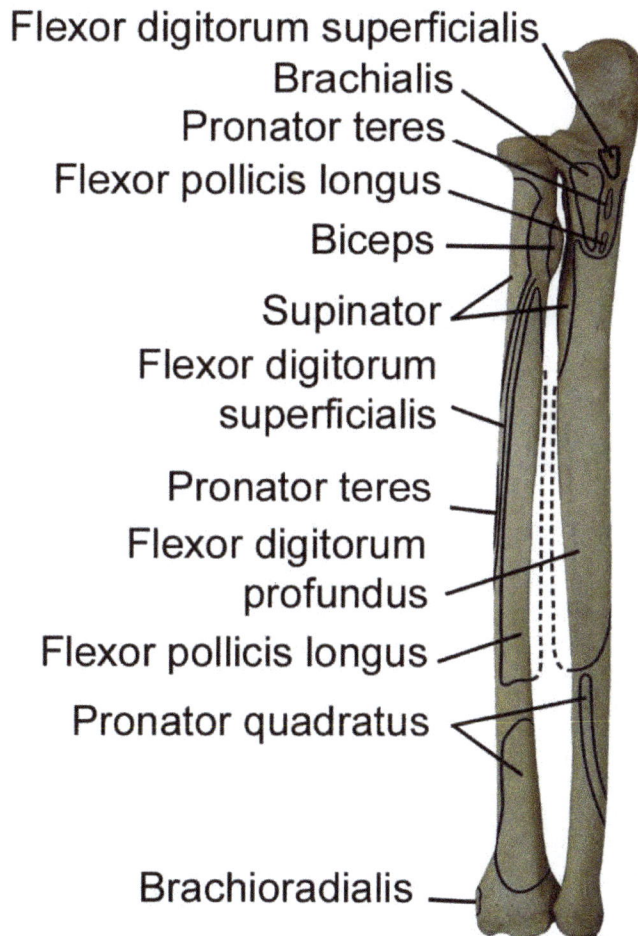

Flexor digitorum superficialis

Brachialis

Pronator teres

Flexor pollicis longus

Biceps

Supinator

Flexor digitorum
superficialis

Pronator teres

Flexor digitorum
profundus

Flexor pollicis longus

Pronator quadratus

Brachioradialis

Radius and ulna and muscle attachments - anterior view

2.7a Kneading the wrist and finger flexor muscles of your forearm using the tip of your thumb seated

The next three techniques are best for the outer or more lateral flexor muscles, such as flexor carpi radialis, the middle flexor muscles and the deeper muscles.

- Sit on a chair with your right elbow flexed and forearm pointing away.
- Rest the back of your lower right forearm on your right thigh.
- Reach across the front of your body with your left hand and grasp your right forearm between the fingers and thumb of your left hand.
- Place your fingertips behind your forearm and the pad of your thumb in front, pressed against the outer border of your flexor muscles, which run down the front and inside of your forearm.

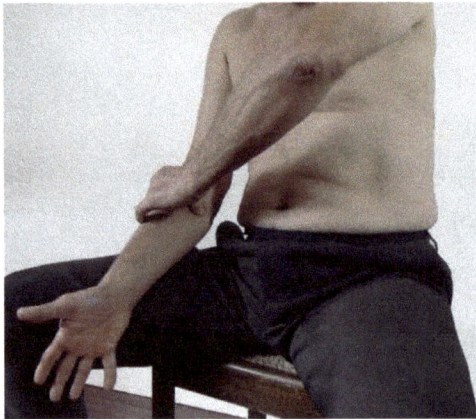

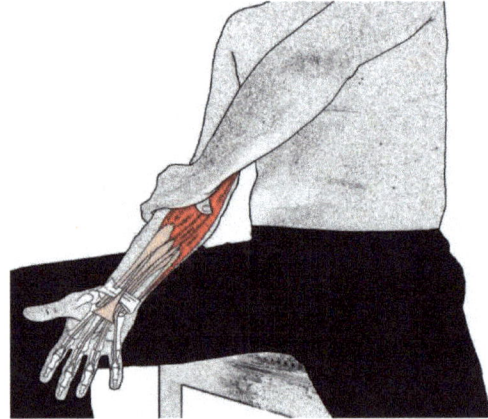

- Point your thumb down and back towards the right side of your body.
- Push across your flexor muscles with your left thumb while simultaneously extending your right hand at the wrist and forearm at the elbow.
- Straightening your forearm produces a counterforce against the force of your thumb and taking your hand backwards stretches the flexor muscles.
- Start at the common flexor tendon at the elbow and work down the muscles until you reach their tendons near the wrist.
- Knead down the lateral flexor muscles and then the middle muscles.
- Press firmly to reach the deeper finger flexor muscles and pronator teres.

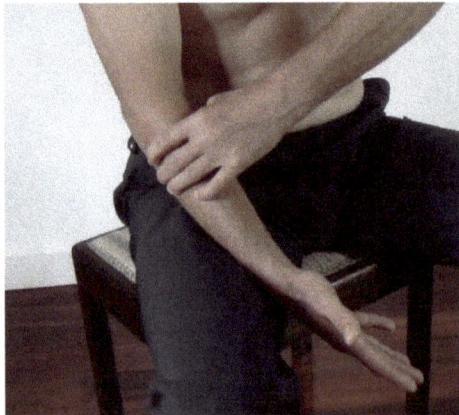

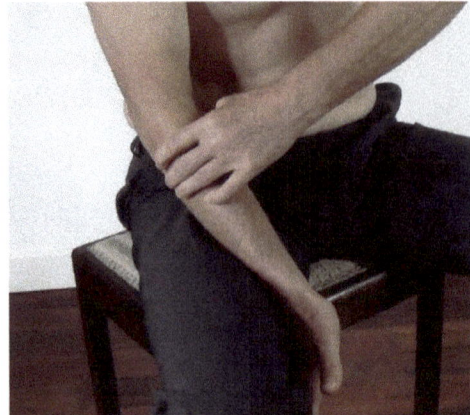

2.7b Kneading the wrist and finger flexor muscles of the forearm using your thumb standing

- Stand over a table and place your hand, palm down on the table so your fingers point away.
- Flex or extend your knees to adjust your posture and for optimal control over the technique.
- Reach across the front of your body and forearm with your left hand and grasp your right forearm between the fingers and thumb of your left hand.

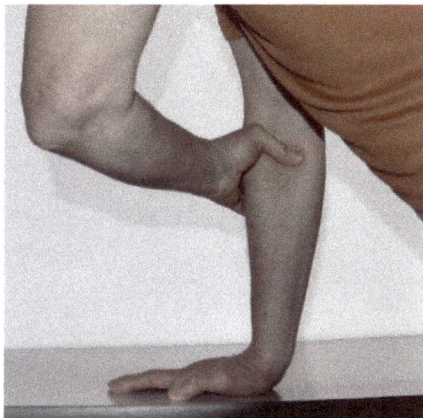

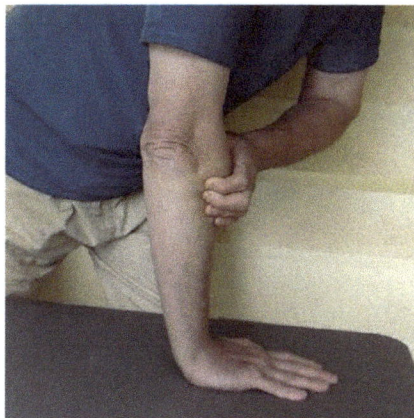

- Place your fingertips on the outside of your forearm and the pad of your thumb on the inside of your forearm, so your fingers and thumb are either side of your extensor muscles.
- Start near your elbow and press your thumb against the outer border of your flexor muscles, which run down the inside of your forearm.
- Push across the muscles with your thumb while simultaneously externally rotating your arm at the shoulder and extending your forearm at the elbow as a counterforce against your thumb.

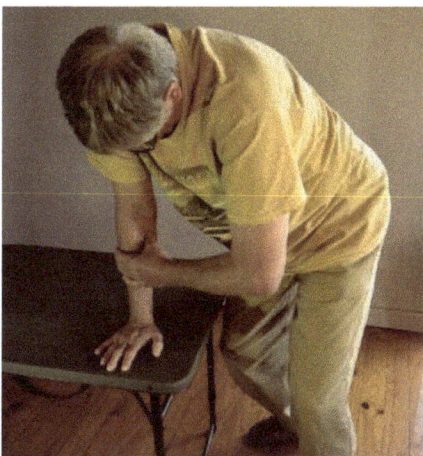

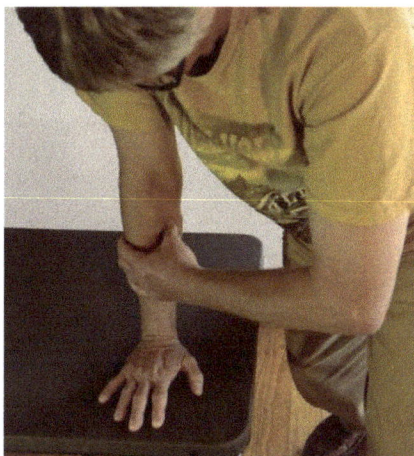

- The tip of your thumb should point backwards and to the right.
- Fix your hand on the table and keep your elbow loose.
- Keep your right shoulder over your right hand and your arm vertical.
- Work down the forearm from the medial epicondyle where the muscles arise to where they become tendons near the front of the wrist.

2.7c Kneading the wrist and finger flexor muscles of the forearm using the tip or pad of your thumb

- Stand straight.
- Flex your right forearm about 90 degrees and then supinate your forearm by rotating it outwards so your palm is turned upwards.

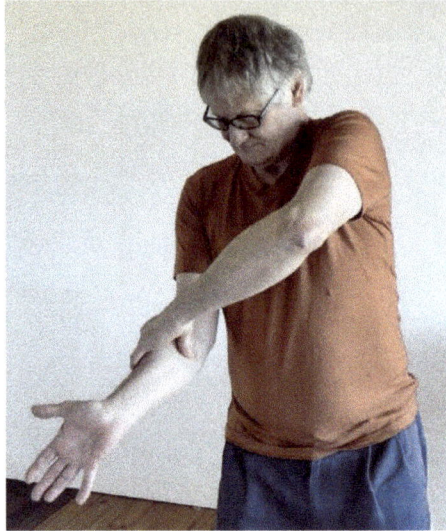

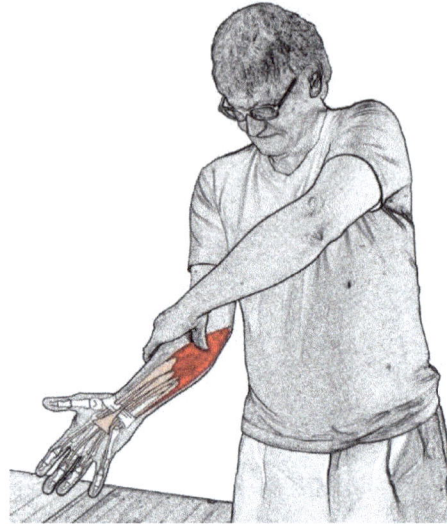

- Reach across the front of your body with your left hand and grasp your forearm between the pads of your fingers and the pad of your thumb.
- Place the pads of your fingers on the outside and back of your forearm.

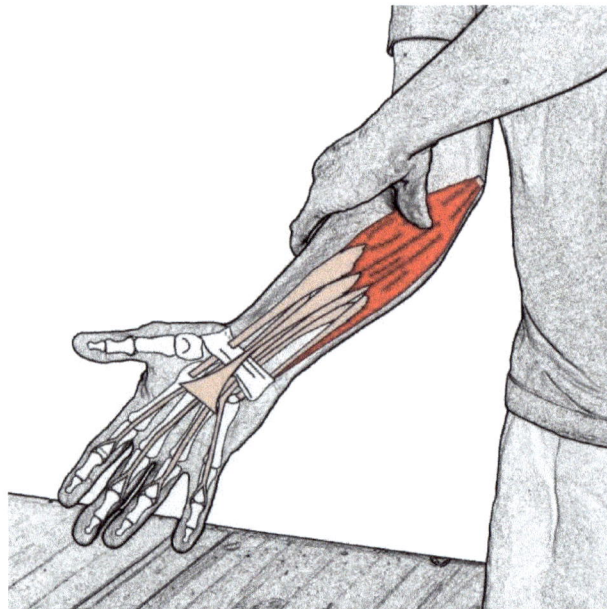

- Place the tip of your thumb against the flexor muscles running down the inside and front of your forearm.
- Start with the tip of your thumb just below the medial epicondyle, the bump on the inside of your elbow where most of the flexor muscles emerge.

- Your thumb points downwards, backwards and to the right.
- Press the tip of your left thumb into and across the muscles while simultaneously extending your right hand at the wrist and extending your right forearm at the elbow.

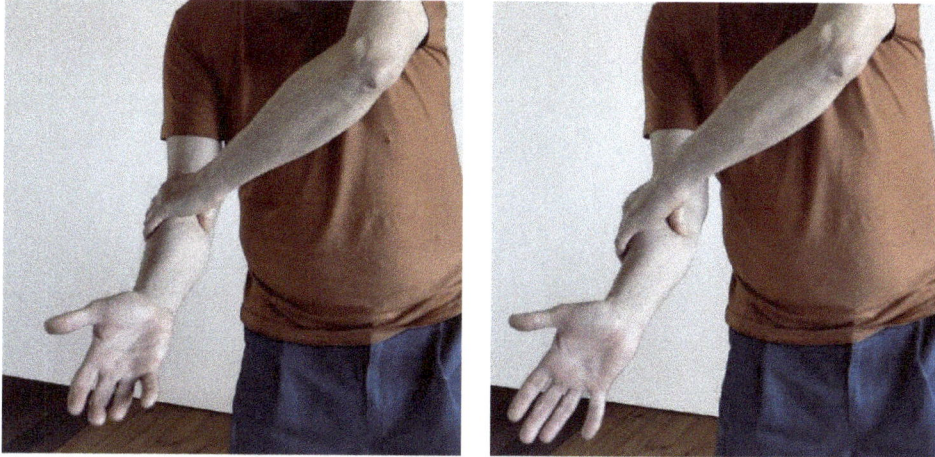

- Straightening your forearm provides a counterforce against the pressure of your thumb and taking your hand backwards stretches the muscles.
- Do not take your right elbow to the fully straight 'locked' position.
- Work down the forearm from the inside of your elbow to where the muscles become tendons near the wrist.
- This technique is like the one done sitting with the back of your right wrist on your right thigh.

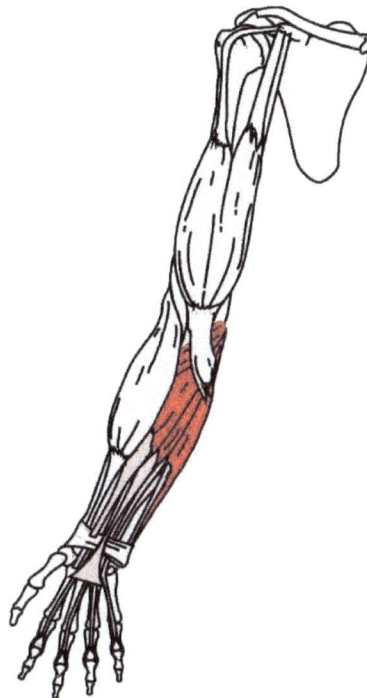

Upper limb muscles - anterior view

2.7d Kneading the wrist and finger flexor muscles of the forearm using the tip of your thumb

The next couple of techniques are best for the inner or more medial flexor muscles, such as flexor carpi ulnaris.

- This is best done standing but can be done seated.
- Flex your right forearm about 120 degrees and then rotate it outwards so your palm is turned towards your right shoulder.

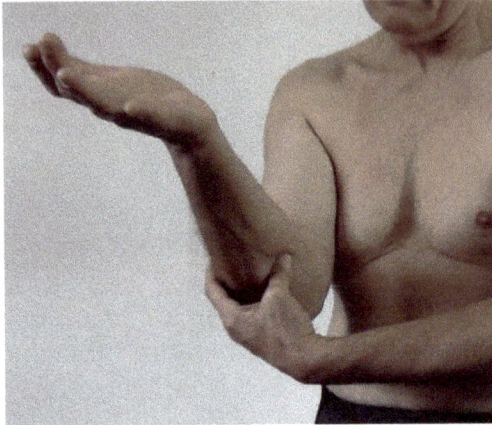

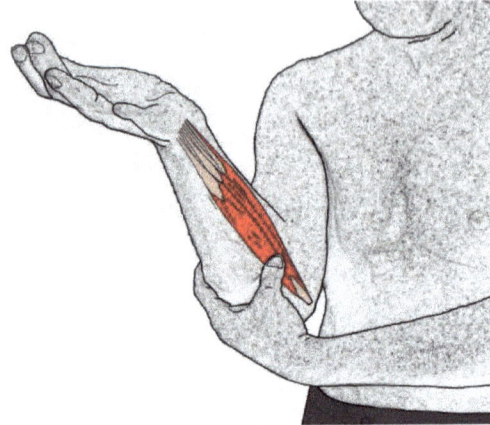

- Reach across the front of your body with your left hand and grasp your upper forearm near the elbow, between the pads of your fingers and the pad of your thumb.
- Turn your arms inwards and roll your shoulders forwards.

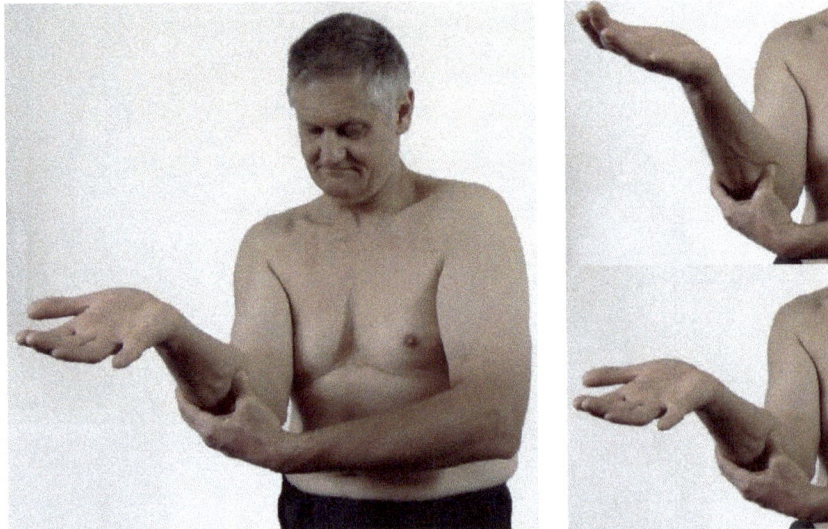

- Place the tip of your thumb between the sharp edge of the ulna bone passing down the inside of your forearm and the inner border of the flexor muscles beside it.
- Lift your left elbow and flex your left wrist so that your left thumb points backwards and to your right side of your body and into the flexor muscles.

- Push your thumb into the muscles while simultaneously extending your right hand at the wrist, pronating your right forearm and extending your right forearm at the elbow.
- Taking your right wrist backwards stretches the flexor muscles while straightening your right forearm and turning it inwards produces a counterforce against the pressure of your thumb.

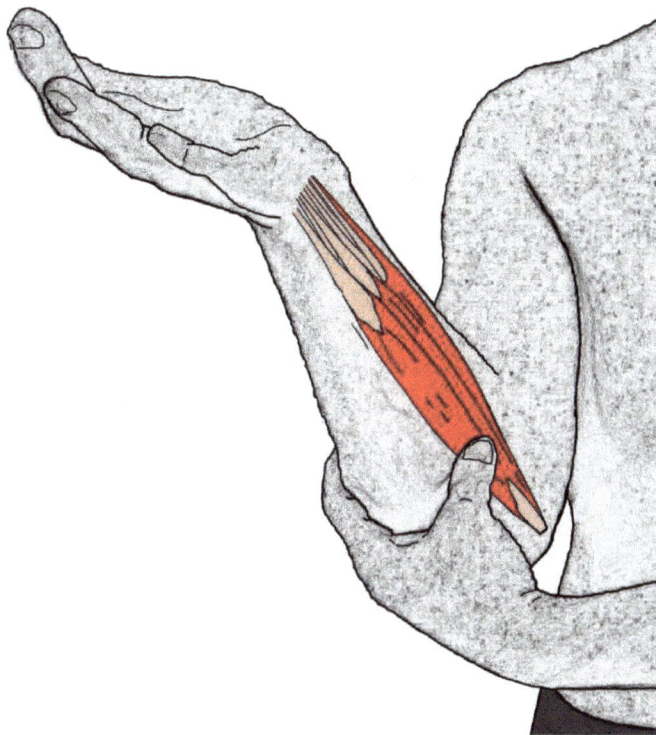

- Keep the pads of your fingers anchored to the back and outside of your forearm and pull with your fingers to help get easier thumb pressure.
- Work along short parallel strips from the inside of your elbow, down the back and inside of your forearm until the muscles become tendons near the wrist.

2.7e Kneading the wrist and finger flexor muscles of the forearm pulling with your hooked thumb standing

- Stand over a table and place your hand, palm down on the table so your fingers point away.
- Flex or extend your knees to adjust your posture and for optimal control over the technique.
- Reach across the front of your body and forearm with your left hand and grasp your right forearm between the fingers and thumb of your left hand.
- Place the pads of your fingers on the extensor muscles running down the outside of your forearm and wrap your thumb around your flexor muscles running down the inside of your forearm.

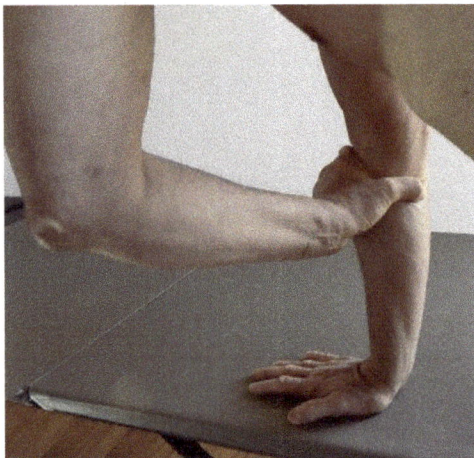

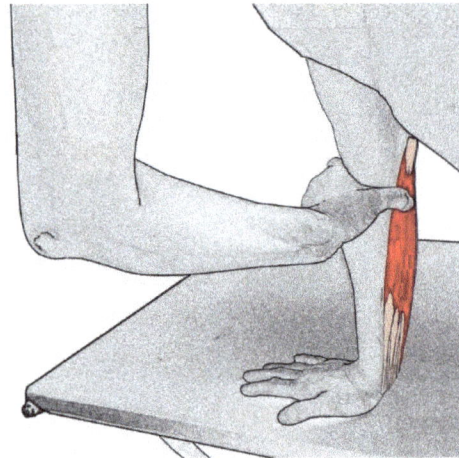

- Start on the muscles at the top of your forearm, near your elbow.
- Hook your thumb around the inside and back of your forearm so the tip of your thumb touches the ulnar bone, and the pd of your thumb is against the medial wrist and finger flexor muscles, specifically flexor carpi ulnaris.
- Keep your fingertips hooked behind the extensor muscles at the back and outside of your forearm.
- Pull your fixed hooked thumb into the muscles while simultaneously internally rotating your right arm at the shoulder and flexing your elbow as counterforces against your thumb pressure.

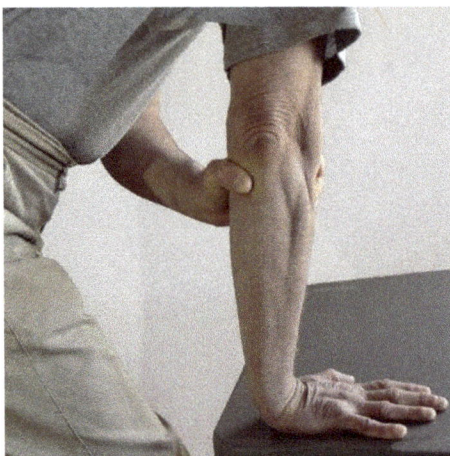

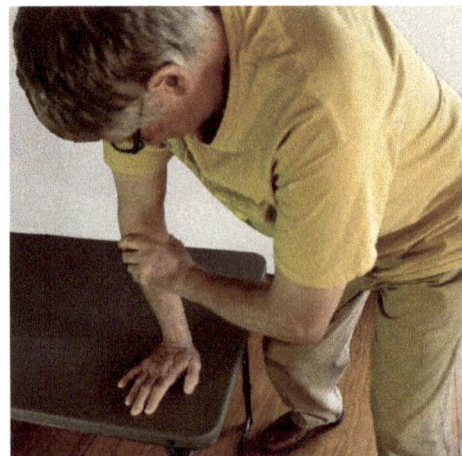

- Increase the pulling action of your left arm by taking your left elbow forwards and keep your thumb in a fixed hooked position.
- The tip of your thumb should point to the right and away from your body.
- Do not lock your elbow in the fully straight position.
- Keep your hand fixed on the table.
- Keep your right shoulder over your right hand and your arm vertical
- Work down the forearm from the elbow to where the muscles become tendons in the wrist.
- The pulling action is not as strong as the pushing action of the previous technique, but it may be easier for people with inflexible shoulders.

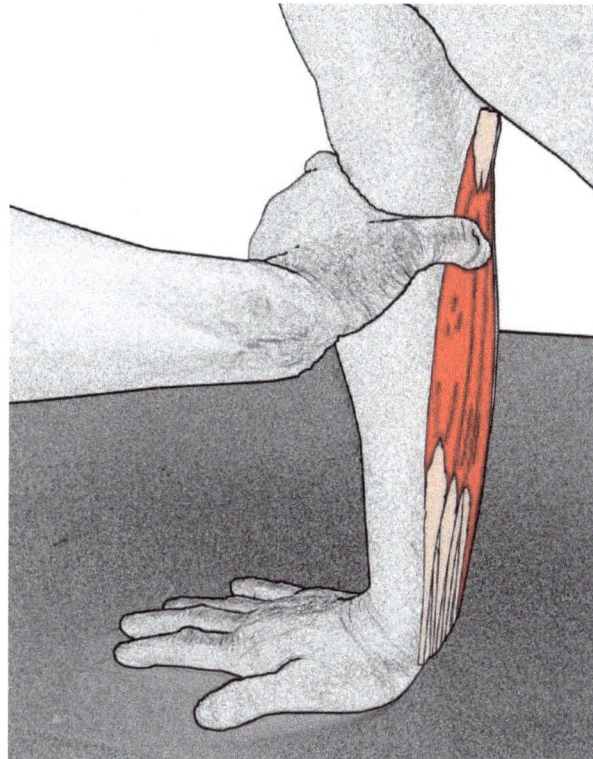

2.7f Transverse friction over the medial collateral ligament and flexor tendon of the medial elbow (golfer's elbow) using the tip of your thumb

- Stand straight or sit in a chair.
- Flex your right arm about 20 degrees and forearm about 90 degrees and then rotate your forearm outwards so your palm is up.

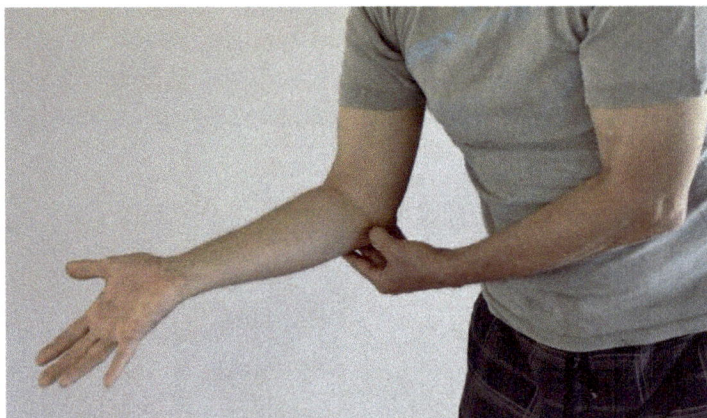

- Reach across the front of your body with your left hand and grasp the back of your right elbow between your fingers and thumb.
- Your fingers wrap around the back and outside of your elbow and the tip of your thumb rests against the bony bump (medial epicondyle) on the inside of your elbow.

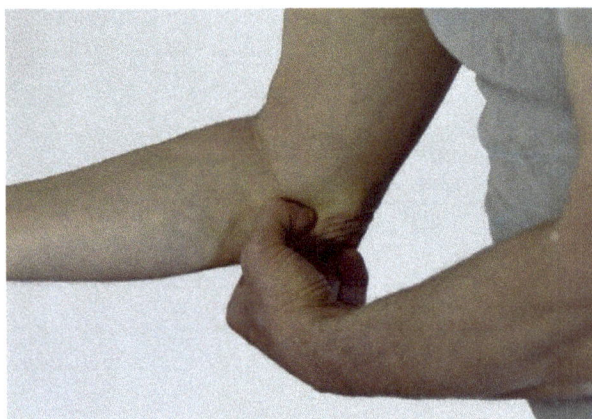

- The common tendon to the wrist flexor muscles of your forearm arises on this bump and the muscles run down the inside and front of your forearm.
- Golfer's elbow is a strain of this tendon which is usually painful to touch.
- Slide your thumb off the bump, towards your hand and onto the tendon.
- Apply transverse friction across the tendon with the tip of your thumb.
- Move along parallel strips from the bone to the start of the muscle.
- The medial collateral ligament lies beneath flexor tendon and just behind it and runs from the humerus to the ulna, on the inside of the elbow.
- The technique for the treatment of this ligament is similar to the one just described for golfer's elbow but since the ligament is deeper, you will need to press harder.
- Apply transverse friction here with the tip of your thumb.

Brachioradialis and the wrist and finger extensor muscles of the posterior forearm

Massaging brachioradialis and the wrist and finger extensor muscles of the posterior forearm can be useful when there is forearm and wrist pain from a muscle strain, bursitis or repetitive strain injury (RSI). Massaging the common extensor tendon and the lateral collateral ligament, both on the outside of the elbow, can be useful when there is pain from a partial tendon strain or a ligament sprain. Pain can also arise from tendinitis or tenosynovitis of the extensor tendons at the back of the wrist.

The extensor muscles may be strained by over-stretching, overloading, overuse or repetitive use such as with a computer. There may be restricted hand and wrist movement and the muscles usually feel short, tight and fibrous. An extensor tendon strain, also known as a tennis elbow, is a type of tendinitis. There may be swelling over the tendon and difficulty moving the wrist and thumb.

Posterior forearm muscles including wrist and finger extensors

Brachioradialis arises on a ridge of bone at the end and outside of the humerus and fascia between muscles. The muscle ends in the middle of the forearm as a long flat tendon which attaches at the end and outside of the radius. The muscle is close to the surface and is easily observed down the outside of the forearm with resisted elbow flexion. The muscle is a forearm flexor and helps to stabilise the elbow during rapid flexion.

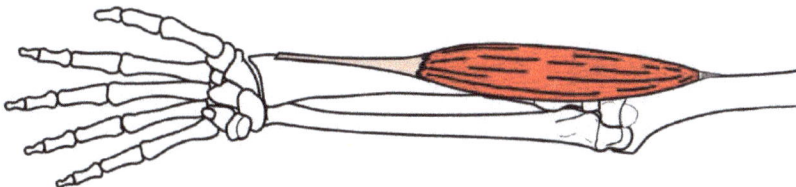

Wrist and finger extensor muscles of the forearm

Extensor carpi ulnaris arises on the lateral epicondyle of the humerus. It attaches onto the base of the fifth metacarpal bone of the hand. The muscle produces wrist extension and adduction and wrist stabilisation when grasping objects.

Extensor carpi radialis longus arises on a ridge of bone at the end of the humerus, on the lateral epicondyle and from fascia between muscles. It attaches onto the base of the second metacarpal at the back of the wrist. The muscle produces wrist extension and abduction and wrist stabilisation when grasping objects.

Extensor carpi radialis brevis arises on the lateral epicondyle of the humerus by the common extensor tendon, from fascia between muscles and from a ligament on the outside of the elbow. It attaches onto the base of the third metacarpal bone at the back of the wrist. The muscle produces wrist extension and abduction and wrist stabilisation when grasping objects.

Extensor digitorum arises on the lateral epicondyle of the humerus by the common extensor tendon and from fascia between and covering muscles. It attaches onto the base of the second and third phalanges of all fingers. The muscle produces extension of hand and fingers.

Extensor indicis arises from the back of the ulna and fascia between the ulna and radius. The tendon of extensor indicis passes behind the wrist and attach onto the index finger.

Extensor digiti minimi arises from the common extensor tendon and from fascia between muscles, and its tendon attaches onto the back of the first phalanx of the little finger.

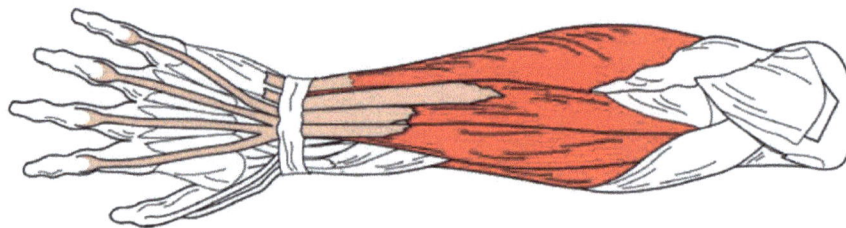

Thumb and finger extensors

Abductor pollicis longus arises on the lateral posterior ulna, interosseous membrane and posterior radius and attaches to the lateral side of the base of the first metacarpal bone.

Extensor pollicis longus arises from the back of the ulna and from fascia between the ulna and radius. Its tendon attaches on the base of the last phalanx of the thumb.

Extensor pollicis brevis arises on the back of the radius and fascia between the ulna and radius. It attaches on the base of the first phalanx of the thumb.

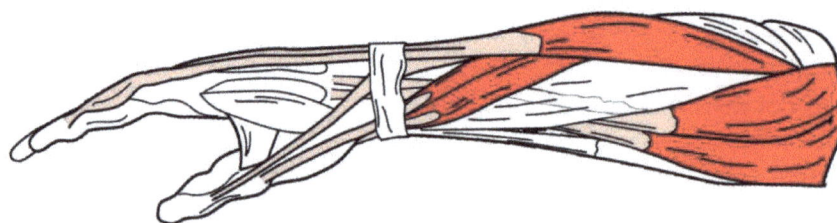

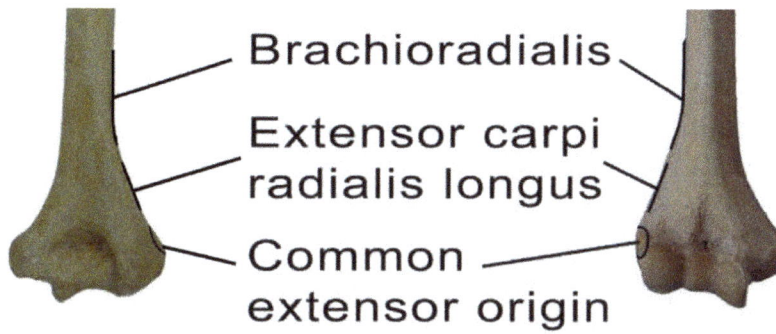

Distal humerus - posterior view (left) & anterior view (right)

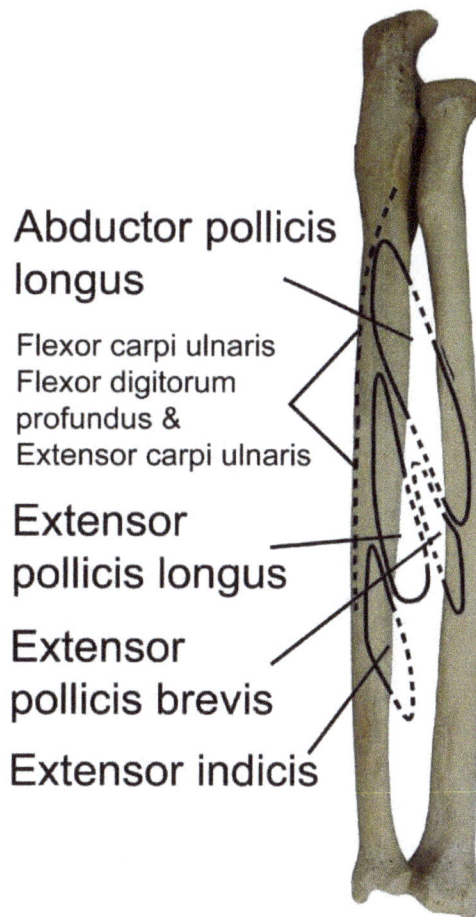

Abductor pollicis longus

Flexor carpi ulnaris
Flexor digitorum profundus &
Extensor carpi ulnaris

Extensor pollicis longus

Extensor pollicis brevis

Extensor indicis

Radius and ulna and muscle attachments - posterior view

The following six kneading techniques are either done sitting with the hand under the thigh, standing with the back of the hand on a table or standing with the hand free and in each of them the thumb either pushes outwards against the lateral fibres or inwards against the medial fibres.

2.8a Kneading brachioradialis and the wrist and finger extensor muscles of your forearm using your fingertips and the tip of your thumb, with your hand fixed under your thigh

This technique delivers the strongest thumb pressure to extensor carpi radialis and brachioradialis but can work for any of the forearm extensors.

- Sit in a chair and then lift your left thigh, reach under it with your right hand and grasp the back of your thigh.
- Relax your hand and return your hand and thigh to the chair so your thigh rests on your fingers and anchors your hand to the chair.

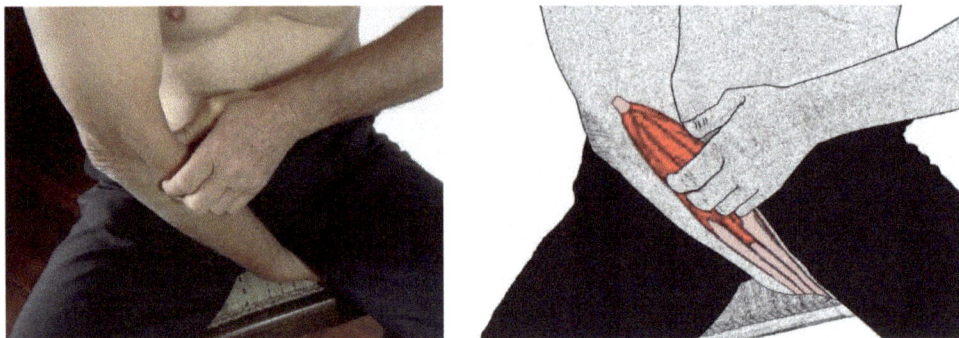

- The back of your fingers are in contact with the seat of the chair, your palm faces upwards, and your right elbow is partially flexed.
- Reach in front and around the outside of your right forearm with your left hand and grasp your forearm extensor muscles between your fingers and thumb.
- Place your fingertips behind your extensor muscles and brachioradialis and your thumb in front - down the outside and back of your forearm.

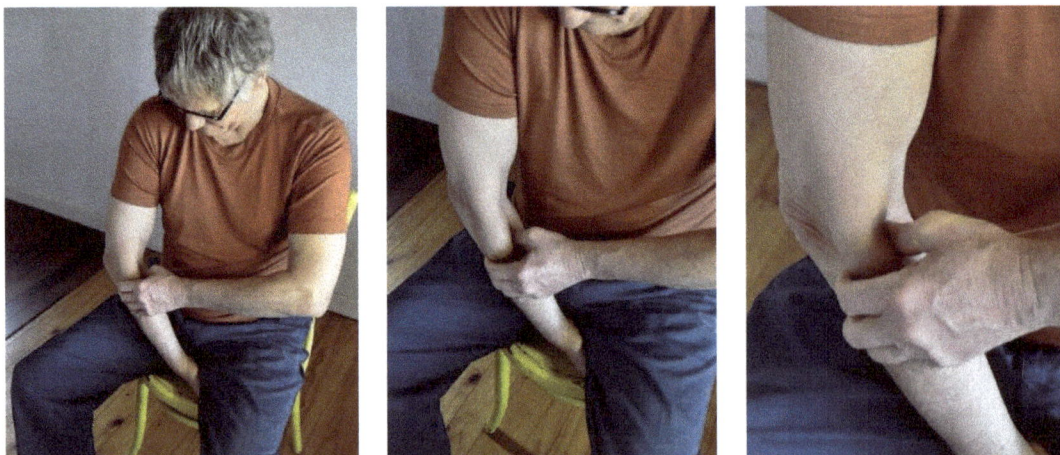

- Push on your forearm extensor muscles with the tip or pad of your thumb and pull on them with the pads of your fingers while simultaneously straightening your right elbow and flexing your wrist.
- Use the movement as a counterforce against the pressure of your thumb.
- Use a squeezing and twisting action with your wrist, fingers and thumb.
- Start at the muscle origin at your elbow and finish when the muscles become tendons, towards the end of your forearm.

2.8b Kneading brachioradialis and the wrist and finger extensor muscles of your forearm using the tip or pad of your thumb, with your hand fixed under your thigh

This technique delivers the strongest thumb pressure to extensor carpi ulnaris, the extensor muscles to the fingers, long muscles to the thumb and posterior and lateral fibres of brachioradialis.

- Sit in a chair.
- Lift your right thigh, reach around the inside and back of your thigh with your right hand and grasp the back of your thigh.
- Relax your hand and return your thigh to the chair so it rests on your fingers and anchors your hand to the chair.
- The back of your fingers are in contact with the chair, your palm faces upwards, and your fingers point backwards and to your right.
- Allow your right elbow to flex.

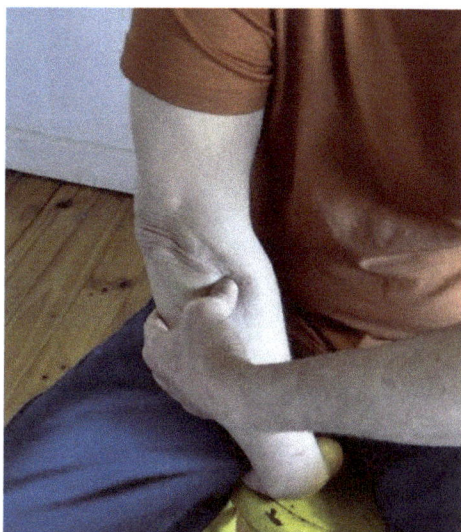

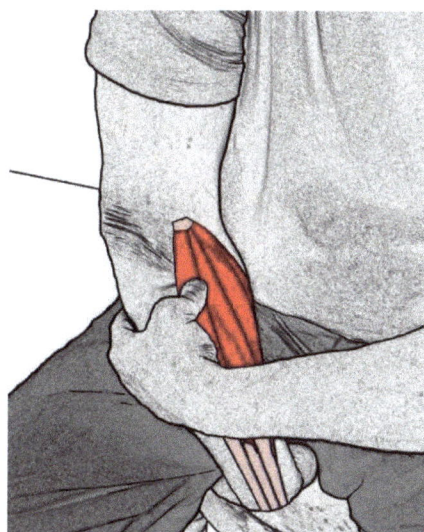

- Reach across the front of your body and the front and outside of your right forearm with your left hand and grasp the back of your right forearm with the fingers and thumb of your left hand.
- Hook the pads of the fingers of your left hand around the upper forearm muscles situated near the elbow.
- Lift both elbows so your arms rotate inwards, and your shoulders become more rounded.
- Flex your left wrist and curl your hand around the back of your forearm so your thumb points backwards towards your body.
- Place the tip of your thumb on the outside of your forearm extensor muscles but keep your fingers anchored around the back of your forearm.
- Push into the extensor muscles with the tip or pad of your thumb while simultaneously straightening your right elbow and turning your forearm outwards as a counterforce to the push of your thumb.

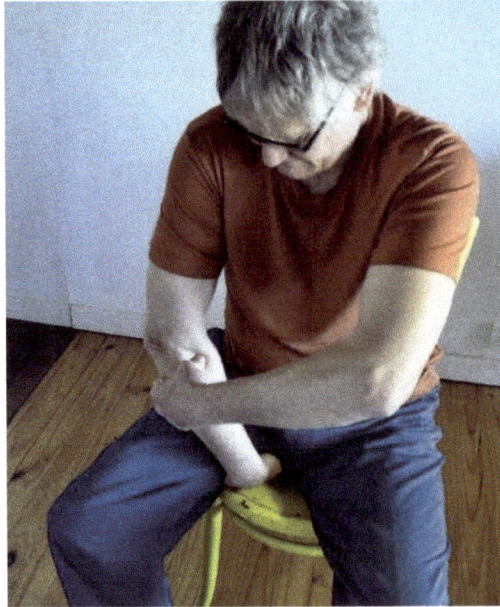

- Straightening your right elbow also produces wrist flexion which stretches the extensor muscles.
- Allow your left hand, and right elbow and forearm to come closer towards your body.
- Start where the muscles emerge from the common extensor tendon near the bump on the outside of your elbow (lateral epicondyle) and work down the forearm until the muscles become tendons near your wrist.

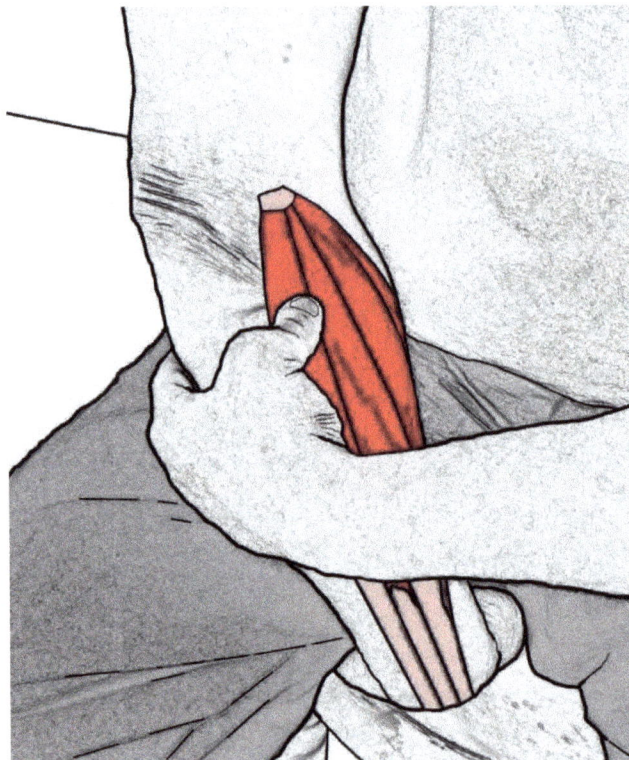

2.8c Kneading the anterior and medial fibres of brachioradialis and wrist and finger extensor muscles of your forearm using your thumb and fingertips with the back of the fingers of one hand resting on a table

This technique delivers the strongest thumb pressure to extensor carpi radialis and brachioradialis but can work for any of the forearm extensors.

- Stand over a table, flex your right forearm about 90 degrees at the elbow and then rotate your arm inwards at the shoulder until your right hand contacts your abdomen.
- Reach across the front of your body and the outside of your right forearm with your left hand and grasp your forearm near the elbow between the pads of your fingers and thumb.

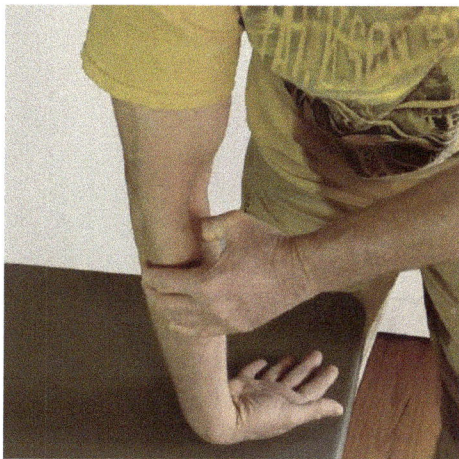

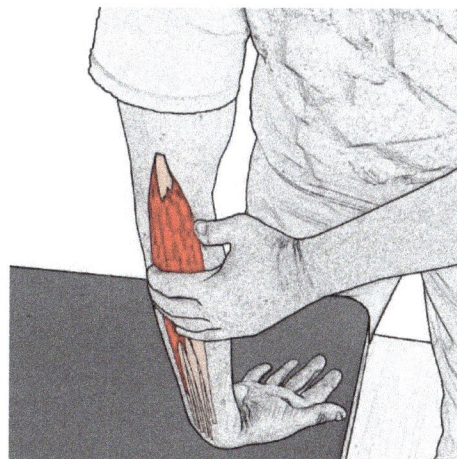

- Place your fingertips on the outside and back of your forearm and the tip or pad of your thumb on the inside and front of the muscles running down the outside of your forearm.
- Make sure the tip of your thumb is on the outside of the thick biceps tendon passing across the front of the pit of your elbow.

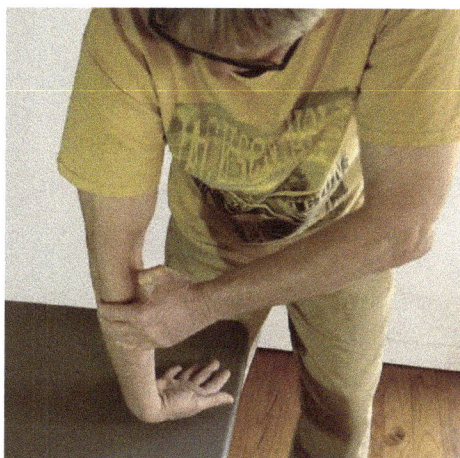

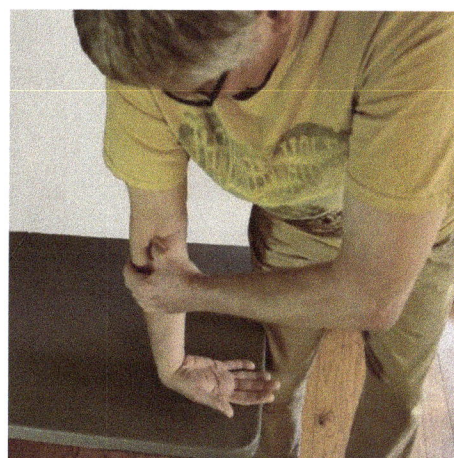

- Allow your right forearm to extend a few degrees and then flex your right wrist and place the back of your fingers on the table.

- Your right wrist and fingers are in a relaxed, partially flexed position and your fingers point towards your left hip.
- Point the tip of your left thumb forwards and outwards to your right.
- The muscles at the front of your forearm face the front and right side of your body.
- Grasp brachioradialis and the extensor muscles at the back of your forearm between the pads of your fingers and the tip or pad of your thumb.
- Push the tip or pad of your thumb into the muscles and pull against the muscles with your fingers while simultaneously bending your knees to increase wrist flexion.

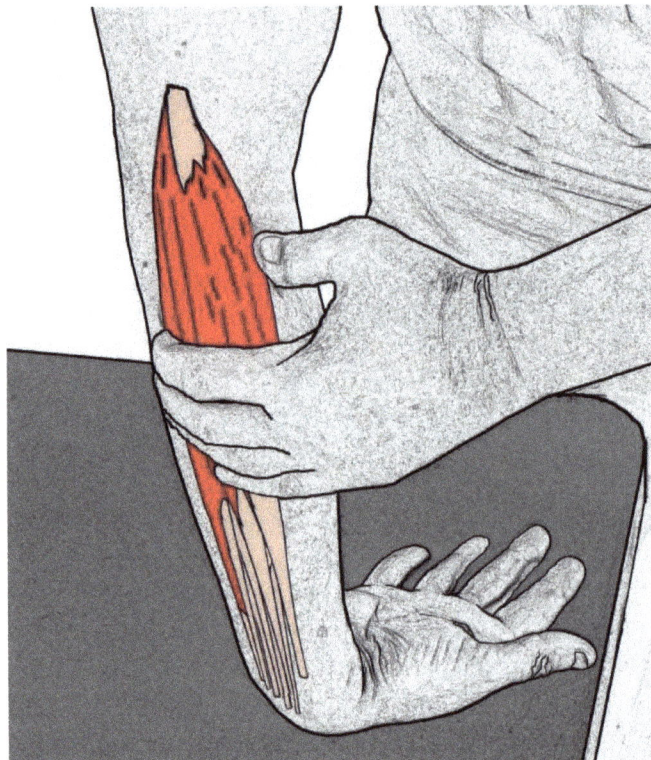

- Keep your right elbow straight but not locked.
- Use a squeezing action of the wrist, fingers and thumb.
- Keep the pads of your fingers on the muscles at the back of your forearm.
- Start at the lateral epicondyle, the bump on the outside of the elbow where the muscles arise, and work down your forearm until the muscles become tendons near the wrist.
- Use thumb pressure to knead the muscles at the front of your forearm and fingertip pressure to knead the muscles at the back of your forearm.

2.8d Kneading the wrist and finger extensor muscles of the forearm and brachioradialis using the tip of your thumb with the back of the fingers of one hand resting on a table

This technique delivers the strongest thumb pressure to extensor carpi ulnaris, the extensor muscles to the fingers, long muscles to the thumb and posterior and lateral fibres of brachioradialis.

- Stand over a table, flex your right forearm about 90 degrees at the elbow and then rotate your arm inwards at the shoulder until your right hand contacts your abdomen.
- Reach across the front of your body and right forearm with your left hand and grasp the back of your right elbow between the pads of your fingers and thumb.

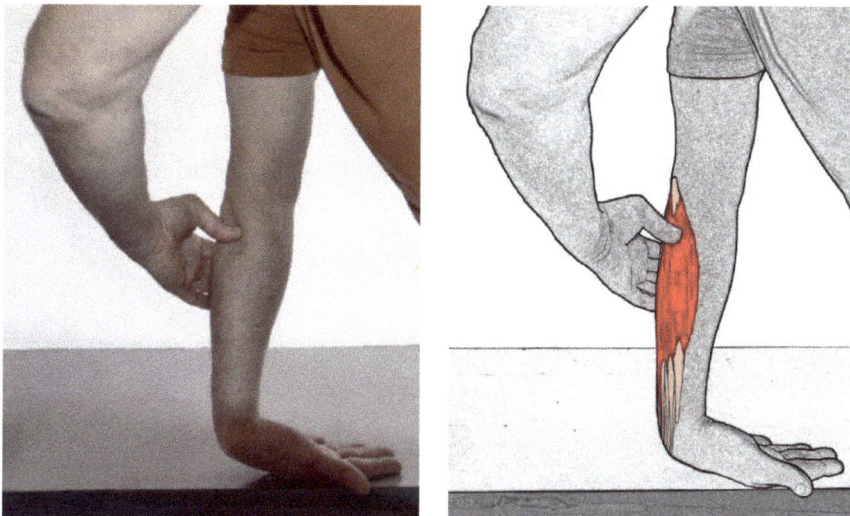

- Slide your hand down your forearm so your fingertips rest on the flexor muscles running down the inside of your forearm.
- Extend your right forearm a few degrees and then flex your wrist and place the back of your fingers on the table.
- Internally rotate your right arm so that your fingers point towards your right hip but keep your wrist and fingers in a relaxed, partially flexed position.
- Flex or extend your knees to adjust your posture and for optimal control over the technique.
- Flex and internally rotate your left arm at the shoulder by lifting your left elbow and then flex your left wrist and thumb so your thumb points backwards towards your body.
- Place the tip of your thumb against the muscles arising from the large bump, the lateral epicondyle, at the back and outside of your elbow.
- Keep your fingers anchored behind your forearm so they can be used to generate greater force with the thumb.
- Push the tip of your thumb into the muscles while simultaneously bending your knees to increase wrist flexion.

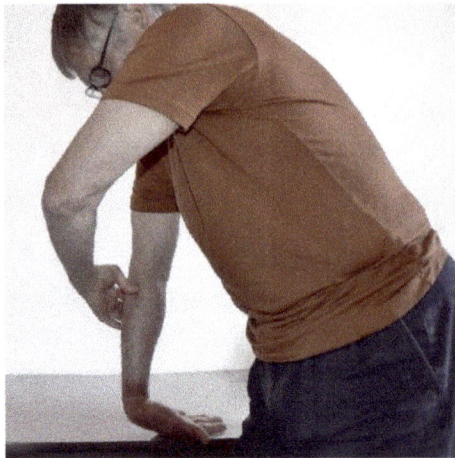

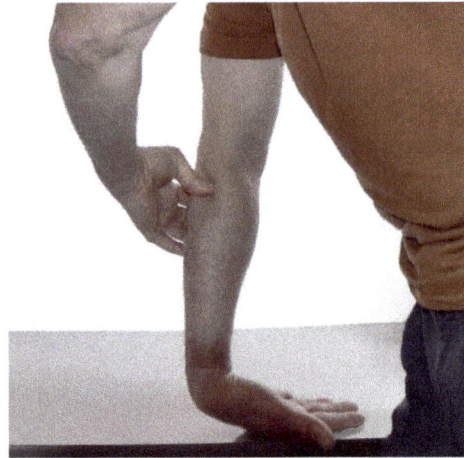

- Work down the muscles close to the shaft of the ulnar bone - this requires good flexibility of your left wrist.
- Then return the tip of your thumb to the lateral epicondyle and work down the muscles passing down the middle of the back of the forearm.
- Then work down the brachioradialis, the fleshy muscle arising just above the elbow and ending on the outside of the forearm, near your wrist.

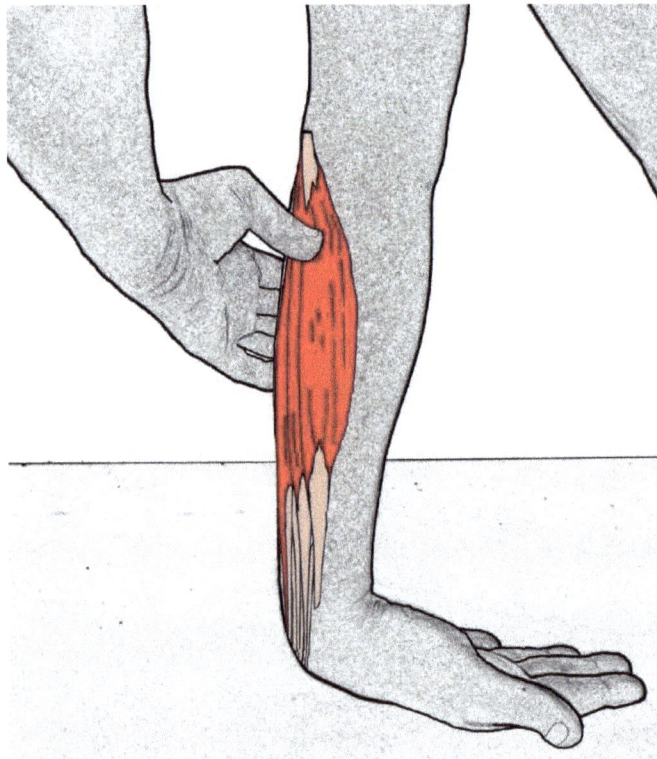

2.8e Kneading brachioradialis and the wrist and finger extensor muscles of the forearm using the tips of your fingers and thumb standing

This technique delivers the strongest thumb pressure to extensor carpi radialis and brachioradialis but can work for any of the forearm extensors.

- Reach across the front of your body with your left hand and grasp your forearm near the elbow between the pads of your fingers and thumb.
- Place the tip of your thumb in the crease in front of your elbow, just to the outside of the biceps tendon so the pad of your thumb rests in front of brachioradialis.

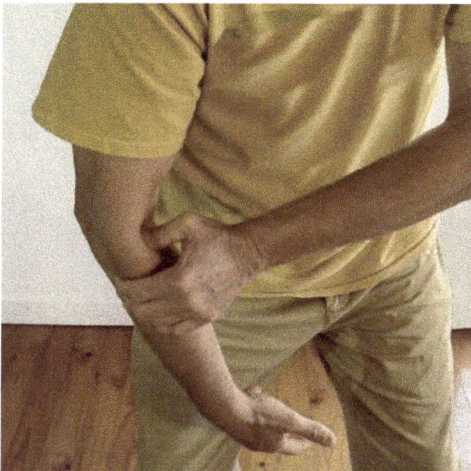

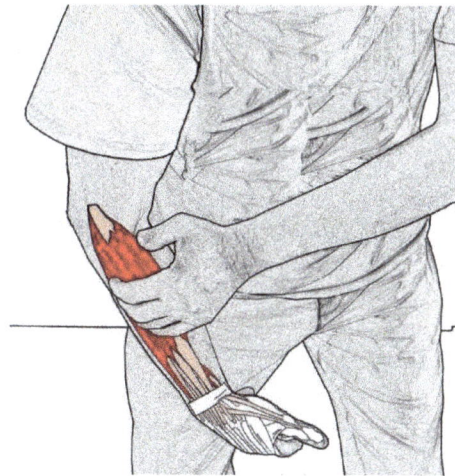

- Place your fingertips behind brachioradialis and the extensor muscles running down the outside and back of your forearm.
- Brachioradialis is the large fleshy muscle arising above the outside of your elbow and running down the outside and back of your forearm.
- The tip of your left thumb points outwards to your right.

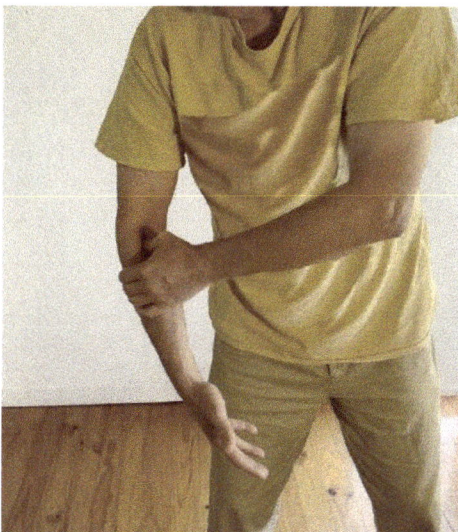

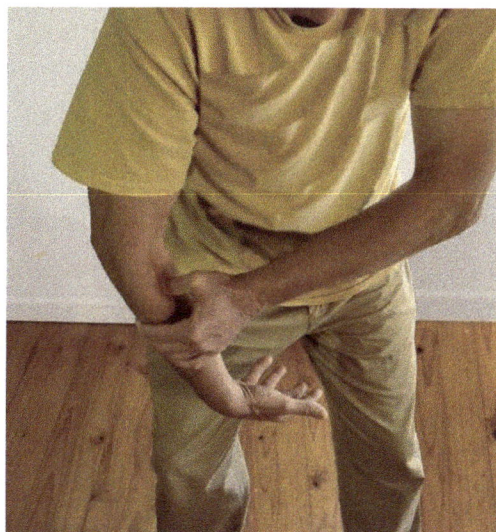

- Push on brachioradialis with the tip or pad of your thumb and pull on brachioradialis or one of the forearm extensor muscles with the pads of your fingers while simultaneously straightening your right elbow and flexing your wrist.

- Use a squeezing action with the fingers and thumb of your left hand, an outwards twisting action with your left wrist and drop your left elbow a bit to increase leverage.
- Start where the muscles arise on the lateral epicondyle, the bump on the outside of the elbow, and work down the forearm to the wrist.
- The thumb kneads the anterior and medial fibres of brachioradialis whereas the tips of the hooked fingers knead the wrist and finger extensor muscles and posterior and lateral fibres of brachioradialis.

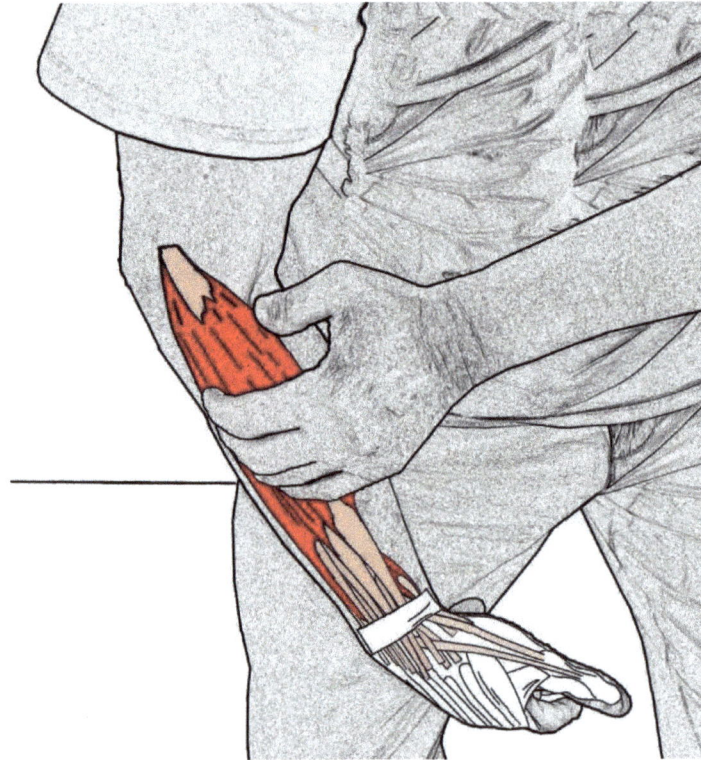

- Use the pads of your fingers for a general kneading of the muscles and use hooked fingertips to target specific muscles.
- With the tips of your hooked fingertips work down the back of the forearm to the wrist along three parallel lines - first along a line near the shaft of the ulnar bone, then along a line down the middle of the forearm and finally along a line down the outside of brachioradialis.

2.8f Kneading brachioradialis and the wrist and finger extensor muscles of the forearm using the tip or pad of your thumb standing

This technique delivers the strongest thumb pressure to extensor carpi ulnaris, the extensor muscles to the fingers, the long muscles to the thumb and the posterior and lateral fibres of brachioradialis.

- Stand straight and flex your right forearm about 90 degrees at the elbow and then internally rotate your right arm at the shoulder.
- Flex your left forearm at the elbow and then flex and internally rotate your left arm at the shoulder.

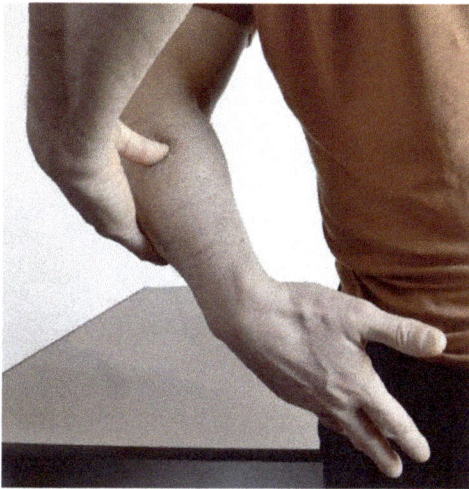

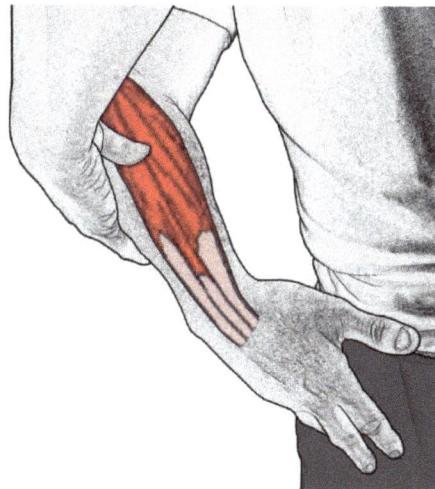

- Reach across the front of your body and over and around the outside of your right forearm with your left hand and grasp your right forearm near the elbow between the pads of your fingers and thumb.
- The pads of your fingers rest on the flexor muscles running down the front of your forearm and the tip of your thumb rests on the extensor muscles running down the back of your forearm.

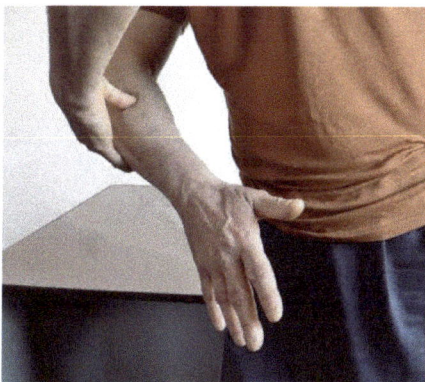

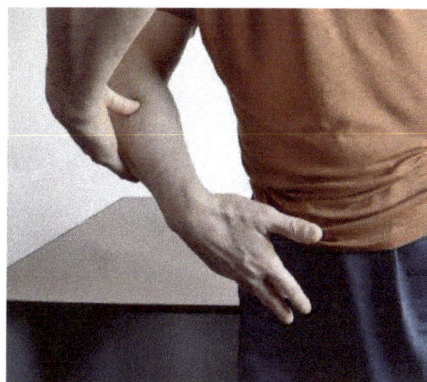

- Lift your left elbow and flex your left wrist and thumb so your thumb is pointing backwards towards your body.
- Place the tip of your thumb against the muscles arising from the large bump, the lateral epicondyle, at the back and outside of your elbow.
- Keep your fingers anchored on the flexor muscles on the far side of your forearm so they can be used to generate greater force with your thumb.

- Push your thumb into the forearm extensor muscles while simultaneously extending your right elbow and rotating your forearm outwards, both acting as counterforces to the pressure of your thumb.

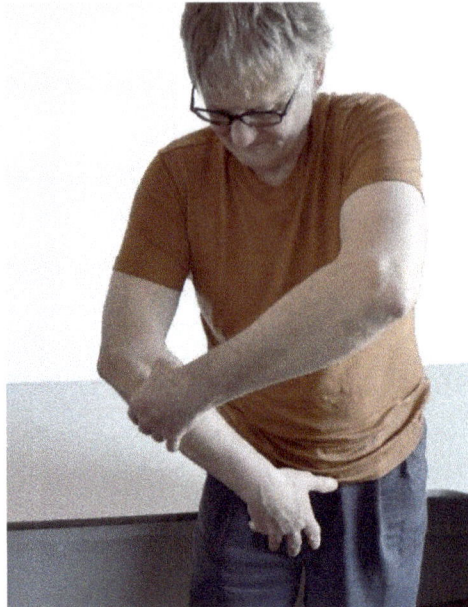

- Add right wrist flexion during the kneading technique to stretch the extensor muscles.
- Lift your left elbow higher to increase the pressure with your thumb.
- Work down the muscles close to the shaft of the ulnar bone then return to the lateral epicondyle and work down the muscles passing down the middle of the back of the forearm, and finally work down the brachioradialis, the fleshy muscle arising just above the elbow and ending on the outside of the forearm, near the wrist.

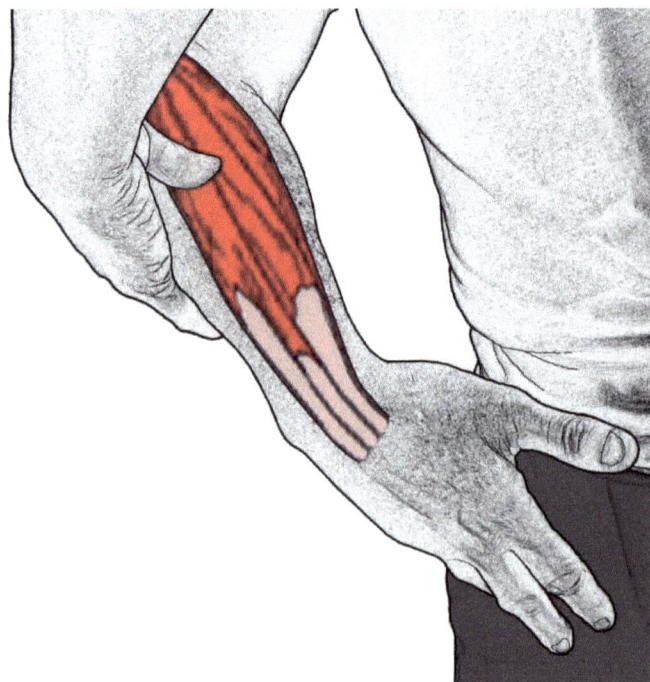

2.8g Transverse friction over the lateral collateral ligament and extensor tendon of the lateral elbow (tennis elbow) using the tip of your index finger

- Sit on a chair with your feet planted on the floor.
- Flex your right elbow and place your hand under your right thigh with your palm facing upwards and into your thigh.
- Grasp your right elbow between the fingers and thumb of your left hand.
- Your fingers wrap around the back of your forearm and the pad of your thumb rests against your biceps tendon in front of your elbow.
- Tennis elbow is a strain of the common extensor tendon which arises on the lateral epicondyle, the bony bump on the outside of the elbow, and merges with muscles on the outside and back of your forearm.

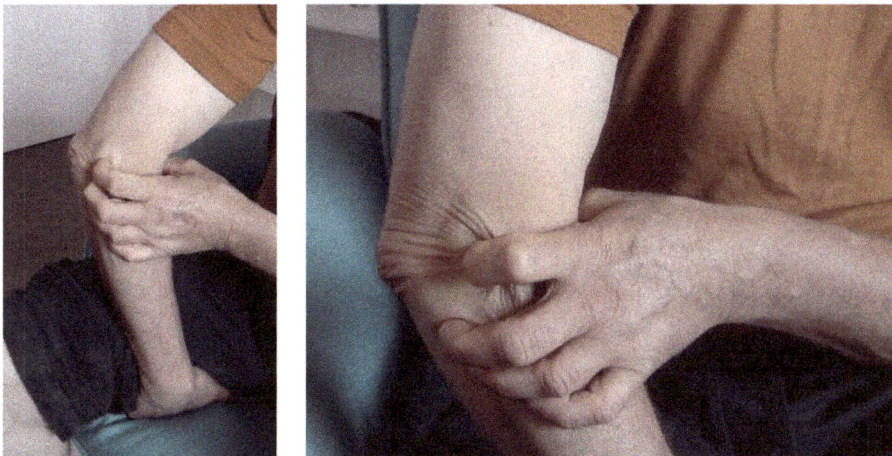

- Place the tip of your index finger on the bump and then slide off it and onto the tendon.
- Apply transverse friction on the tendon with the tip of your index finger.
- Move along parallel strips from the bone to start of the muscles.
- Points of tenderness may indicate the location of the strain.
- The lateral collateral ligament lies beneath extensor tendon and runs from the humerus to the radius, on the outside of the elbow.
- The technique for the treatment of this ligament is similar to the one just described for tennis elbow but since the ligament is deeper, you will need to press harder.
- Apply transverse friction on the ligament with the tip of your index finger.

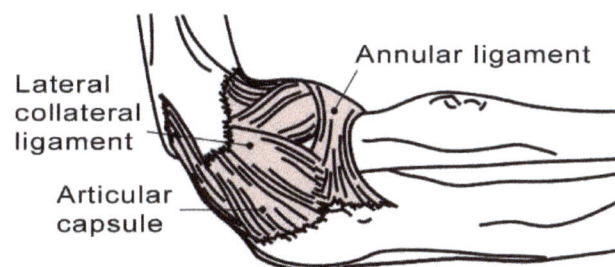

Lateral ligaments of the elbow

THE WRIST AND HAND

Massaging the wrist and hand can be useful when there is pain from a strain or cramping in one of the muscles, a strain in one of the tendons, tendinitis or tendinopathy, tenosynovitis in the tendon sheaths enclosing the tendons to the thumb and fingers, a ligament sprain, osteoarthritis or rheumatoid arthritis.

Tendinitis and tenosynovitis can occur in the wrist as a result of a single injury or from repetitive activities. Symptoms include pain, swelling and tenderness of the tendon and reduced strength and movement in the hand. The most common type of tenosynovitis affects the extensor and abductor tendons to the thumb.

Writer's cramps can occur in the hand as a result of repeated hand and finger movements such as in writing, typing and using tools. Muscle strains in the hands and ligament sprains in the wrist can occur as a result of falls, strong forces in work and sport and weight-bearing by the hands during gymnastics.

Osteoarthritis can occur in the hand as a result of trauma or heavy use. It usually develops in the base of the thumb or at the end or middle joint of a finger. Rheumatoid arthritis can develop in the hands and results in pain, swelling, weakness and stiffness in the fingers and hand.

Muscles of the hand

There are two types of muscles to the hand, the long finger muscles, which arise from the arm and forearm and the short muscles to the thumb and fingers, which arise from the carpal bones of the wrist and a fibrous tissue in front of the wrist called the flexor retinaculum. The long finger muscles are covered in the previous chapter.

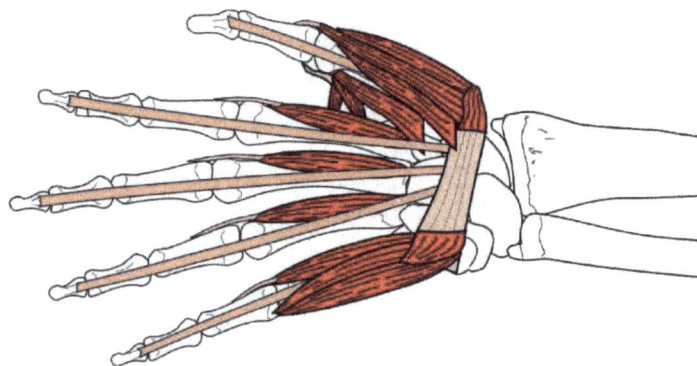

Short finger flexor muscles: thenar, hypothenar, interossei muscles and flexor digitorum profundus tendons

The short muscles of the thumb form the soft pad at the base of the thumb called the thenar eminence and the short muscle of the little finger form the soft pad at the base of the little finger called the hypothenar eminence. The thenar muscles move the thumb and include **abductor pollicis brevis** (closest to the surface), **opponens pollicis** (the outer muscle), **flexor pollicis brevis** a (deep muscle) and **adductor pollicis** (the deepest muscle). The hypothenar muscles move the little finger and include **abductor digiti minimi, opponens digiti minimi** and **flexor digiti minimi.**

2.9a Kneading the palmar aponeurosis of the hand using the tip of your thumb standing

- Stand straight or sit on a chair with your hips and knees flexed and your feet planted on the floor.
- Flex your right forearm about 90 degrees and then turn it outwards so your palm faces upwards.

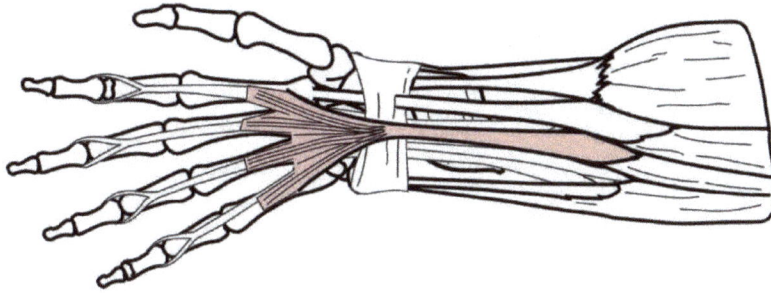

Palmar aponeurosis - anterior view

- Turn your right arm inwards until the side of your forearm touches the side of your body.
- Reach across the front of your body with your left hand and grasp your right hand between the fingers and thumb of your left hand.
- The fingers of your left hand are behind the back of your right hand.

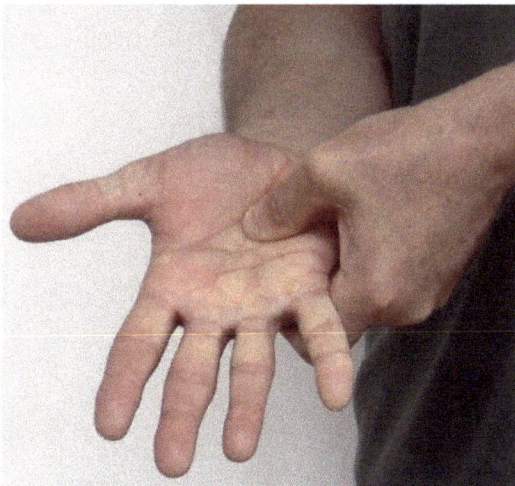

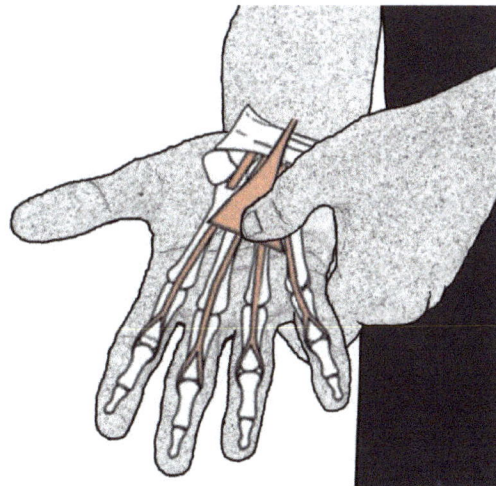

- Place the tip of your left thumb in the middle of the palm of your hand, between your thenar and hypothenar muscles.
- Push the tip of your thumb into the palm of your right hand while simultaneously bending your wrist and fingers backwards.
- Systematically work across the palm of your hand, from your wrist to the base of your fingers.

2.9b Kneading the thenar muscles of the hand using the tip of your thumb standing

- Stand straight or sit on a chair with your hips and knees flexed and your feet planted on the floor.
- Flex your right forearm about 90 degrees and then turn it outwards so your palm faces upwards.
- Rotate your right arm inwards so the side of your hand and forearm are against your abdomen.

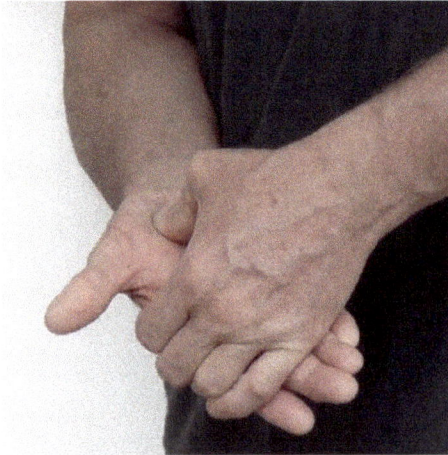

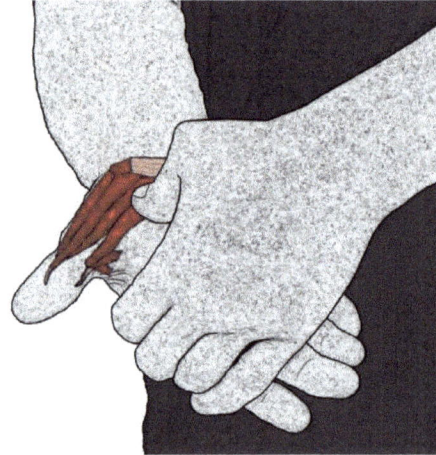

- Reach across the front of your body with your left hand and grasp your right hand between your fingers and thumb.
- Place the pads of your fingers on the back of your wrist and index finger.
- Place the tip of your thumb against your inner thenar muscles which arise near the middle and front of your wrist.
- Move your right thumb backwards and outwards (extension) until there is a mild stretch on the thenar muscles.

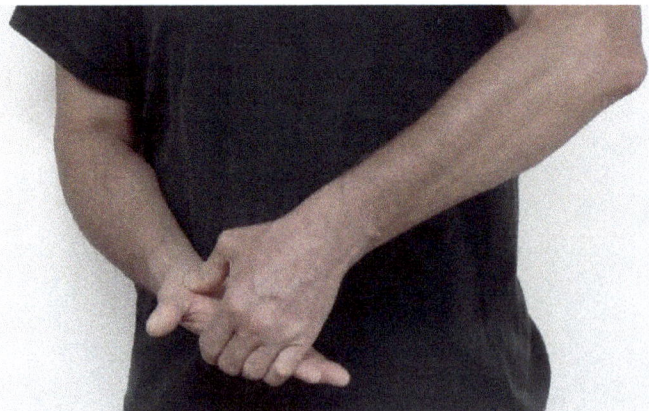

- Push the tip of your left thumb into the thenar muscles while simultaneously taking your right thumb even further backwards.
- Work down your inner thenar muscles following a line from the middle of your wrist to the base of your index finger.
- To treat the middle and deep thenar muscles reposition your thumb where they arise, towards the outside and front of your wrist.
- Work down these muscles following a line from your wrist to the web area of your thumb.

- The lines fan out as you move from the wrist to the thumb.
- Continue to push the tip of your left thumb into the muscles while taking your right thumb backwards and outwards.
- To treat the outer thenar muscles change your hand positions.
- Move your right thumb forwards and inwards (flexion) until the inside of your thumb rests against the front of the index finger of your right hand.
- Do not flex it so hard the muscles are too tight for kneading.

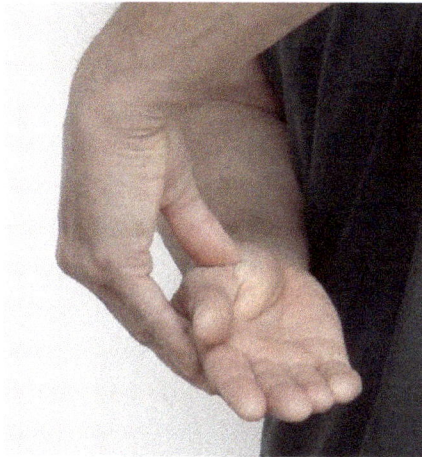

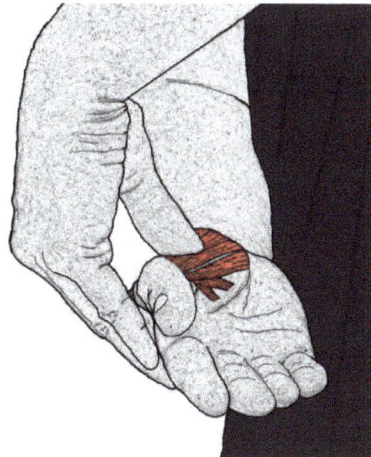

- Flex and then internally rotate your left arm at the shoulder by lifting your left elbow and then flex your left hand at the wrist so your thumb points back towards your body.
- Reach around the outside and back of your right hand and place the fingers of your left hand against the back of your right hand.
- Place the tip of your left thumb on the point where the outer thenar muscles arise from the bones at the front and outside of your wrist.
- Push the tip of your left thumb into the outer thenar muscles while simultaneously taking your right thumb even further into flexion.
- Work down your outer thenar muscles following a line from the outside and front of your wrist down the edge of the long bone of the thumb to the base of the first digit of your thumb.
- To treat the middle thenar muscles reposition your thumb where these muscles arise more towards the middle and front of your wrist.
- Work down these muscles following a line from your wrist to the base of the first digit of your thumb.

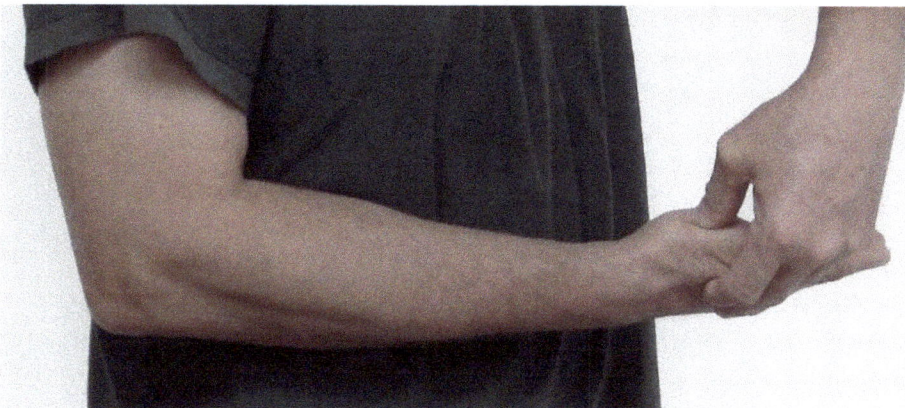

2.9c Kneading the hypothenar muscles of the hand using the tip of your thumb standing

- Stand straight or sit on a chair with your hips and knees flexed and your feet planted on the floor.
- Flex your right forearm about 90 degrees and then turn it outwards so your palm faces upwards.
- Rotate your right arm at the shoulder so that your hand and forearm are straight out in front of you.

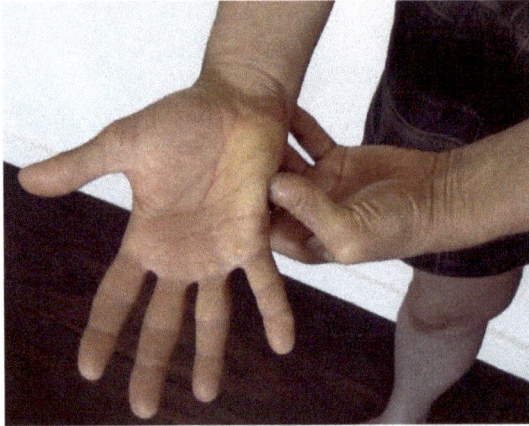

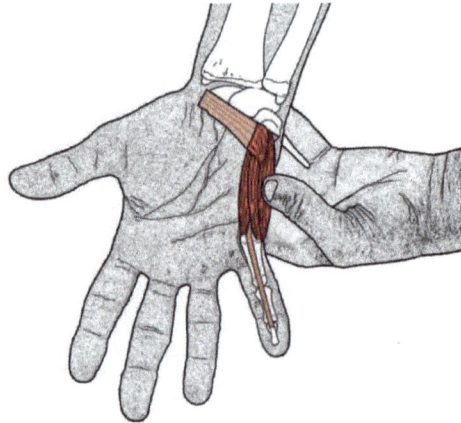

- Reach across the front of your body with your left hand and grasp your right hand between your fingers and thumb. Place the fingers of your left hand around the back of your right wrist.
- Place the tip of your left thumb on the side of the small round pisiform bone at the front and inside of your wrist and then slide off the bone towards the little finger and onto the origin of the medial hypothenar muscles.

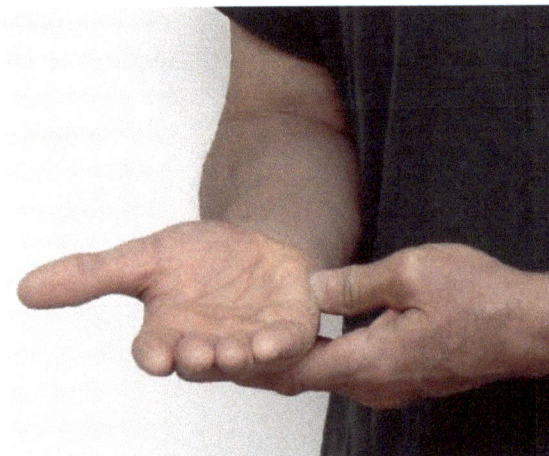

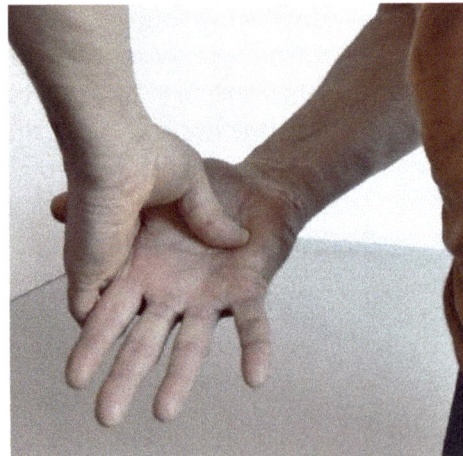

- Push the tip of your left thumb into the hypothenar muscles while simultaneously spreading your fingers.
- Work down the medial hypothenar muscles to the first digit of your little finger following a line down the side of the long metatarsal bone of your little finger.

- Return to the pisiform bone and place the tip of your thumb on the front of the pisiform bone and then slide off the bone towards the little finger and onto the origin of the middle hypothenar muscles.
- Work down the middle hypothenar muscles following a line from the pisiform bone down the muscles to the first digit of your little finger.
- To treat the lateral hypothenar muscles, you need to reposition your hand.
- Turn your right forearm until your palm faces left.

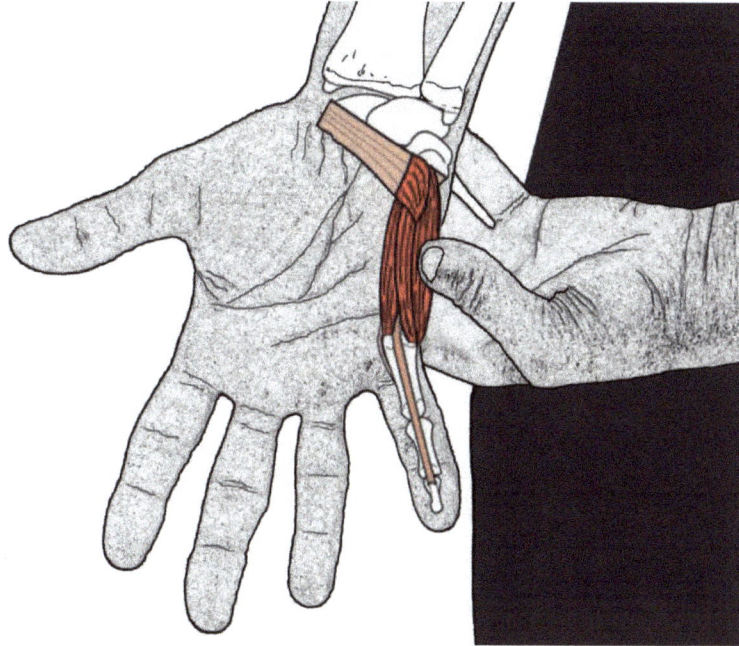

- Reach over and around the back of your right hand with your left hand and place your fingers against the back of your hand.
- Place the tip of your left thumb on where your lateral hypothenar muscles arise on the front of your wrist.
- Push the tip of your left thumb into the lateral hypothenar muscles while simultaneously spreading your fingers.
- Rotate your forearm outwards as a counterforce against your thumb pressure.
- Work down the lateral hypothenar muscles to the base of your little finger.

2.9d Transverse friction over the tendon sheaths of extensor pollicis brevis and abductor pollicis longus using the tip of your thumb

- Stand straight or sit on a chair with your hips and knees flexed and your feet planted on the floor.
- Flex your right forearm 90 degrees and rotate your arm 45 degrees inwards so your palm faces towards your abdomen.

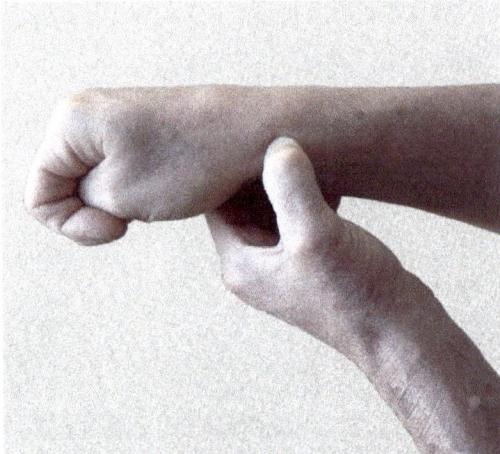

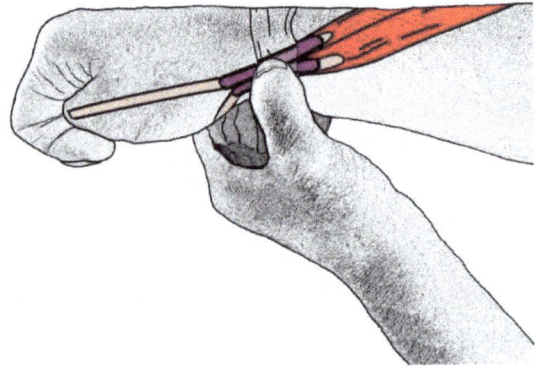

- Reach across the front of your body with your left hand and grasp your right wrist between your fingertips and the tip of your thumb.
- Your fingers are below your wrist facing upwards and your thumb is above your wrist facing downwards.
- To find the two tendons of extensor pollicis brevis and abductor pollicis longus lift your right thumb upward and generate the hollowed out 'anatomical snuff box' at the side of the wrist.

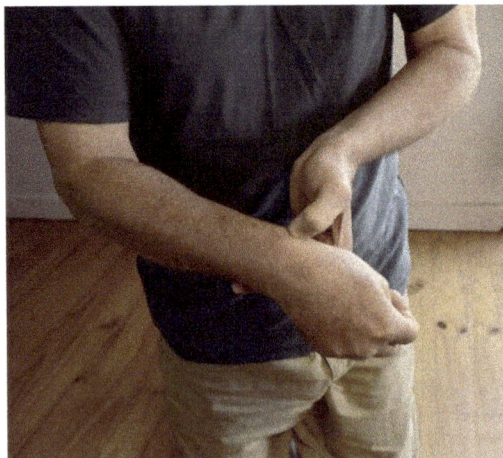

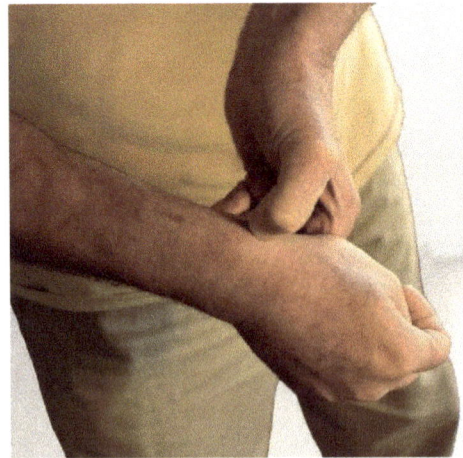

- The tendons run down the side of the wrist and form the boundary of the snuff box that is closest to the front of your wrist.
- Place the tip of your thumb against each of the tendons and search for any areas of tenderness.
- You will be able to identify the tendon-sheath tenosynovitis because the area will be tender.

- Flex your right thumb until it sits against the palm of your hand and then close your fingers around your thumb and make a loose fist.
- Tilt your hand downward towards the floor (wrist adduction) to mildly stretch the muscles and take up some slack on the sheath and skin.

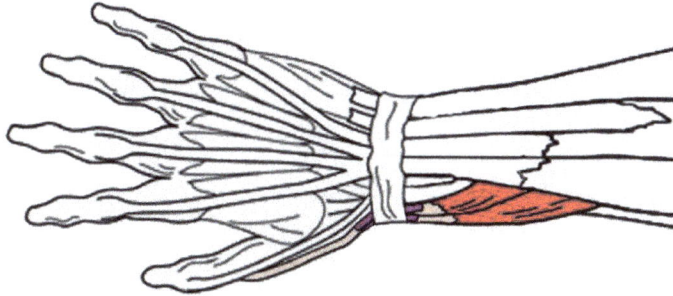

- Push the tip of your left thumb across the tendon sheath for 15 seconds.
- After completing transverse friction on one area move the tip of your thumb to a new location further down the sheath.
- Cover the whole tendon-sheath from where it starts at the bottom of the forearm to just past the wrist.
- After completing the transverse friction apply ice over the tendon for about ten minutes.

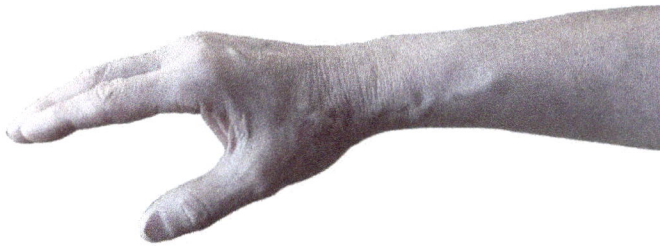

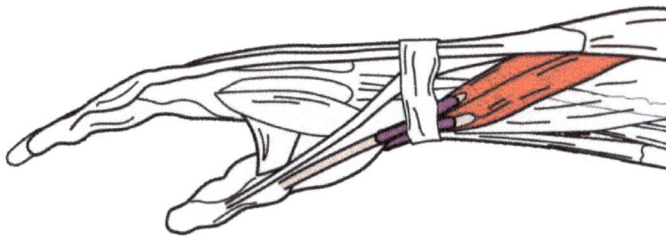

Extensor pollicis brevis and abductor pollicis longus tendon sheaths

Part C The lower limbs

THE HIP

Massaging the hip muscles can be useful for hip, buttock, groin and back pain caused by muscle spasms, ligament sprains, muscle and tendon strains, bursitis, and damage or loss of hip joint cartilage. Hip pain can result from repetitive loading, overuse and injury or be referred from the knee, ankle or lower back.

Massaging the hip muscles can help piriformis syndrome, where the muscle, located deep in the buttock, goes into spasm, causing buttock pain and irritating the sciatic nerve; trochanteric bursitis, where friction between the hip bone and the strap like iliotibial band, on the outside of the thigh, irritates the bursa and causes hip pain; a mild tear of the inguinal ligament or abdominal muscles attaching to it, causing groin pain; and hip pain and stiffness from osteoarthritis.

Muscles of the posterior and lateral hips

Gluteus maximus arises on the back and side of the ilium, sacrum and coccyx, on fascia attached to the erector spinae and gluteus medius, and on the sacrospinous and sacrotuberous ligaments. The upper part of the muscle attaches on the iliotibial tract and the deeper fibres of the lower part of the muscle attaches on the gluteal tuberosity at the back of the femur.

Gluteus maximus is a hip extensor and external rotator, and its upper fibres participate in hip abduction. It adds tension to the iliotibial tract and helps balance the femur on the tibia when the quadriceps are relaxed. It is important in climbing and coming up from flexion.

Gluteus medius arises on the crest of the outer ilium and from the deep fascia that covers it. It attaches on an outer part of the greater trochanter by a flat tendon. It can be felt all around the outside of the pelvis except where is covered by gluteus maximus at the back.

Gluteus medius is mainly a hip abductor but anterior fibres rotate the hip inwards, and posterior fibres weakly rotate it outwards. It is important in walking and supporting the weight bearing leg.

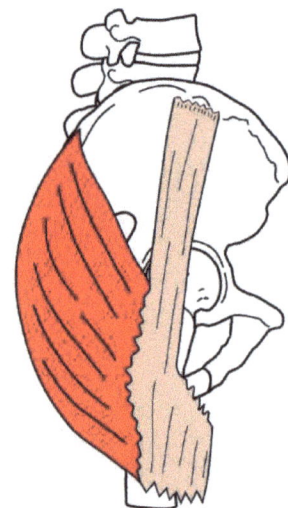

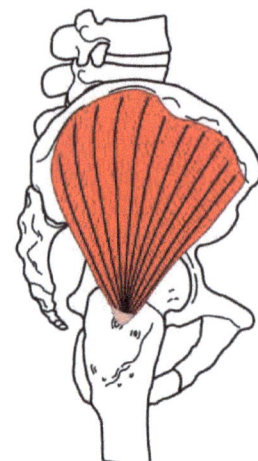

Gluteus minimus arises on the outer ilium towards the front. It attaches on the outside and front of the greater trochanter. Most of the muscle is under gluteus medius.

The muscle rotates the hip inwards and abducts the hip. With gluteus medius it counters the tendency of the pelvis to drop when the foot is lifted off the ground, such as in walking.

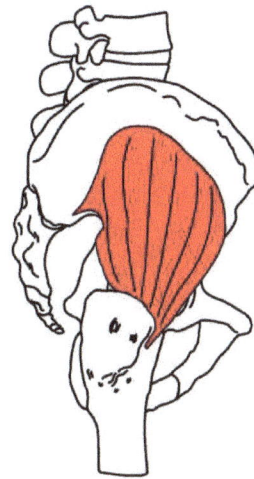

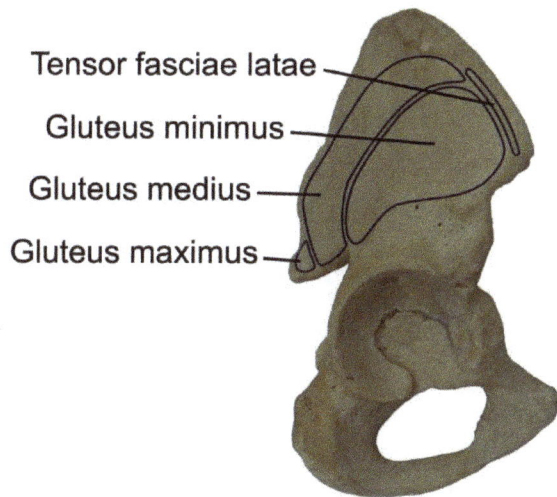

Tensor fasciae latae
Gluteus minimus
Gluteus medius
Gluteus maximus

Pelvis - side view

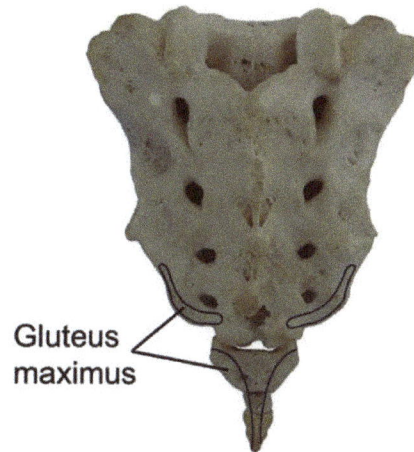

Gluteus maximus

Sacrum - posterior view

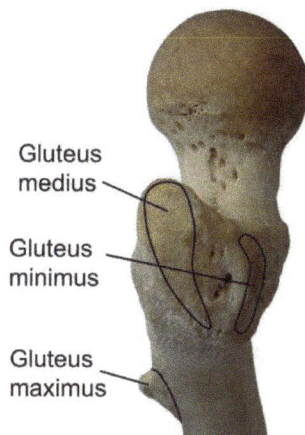

Gluteus medius
Gluteus minimus
Gluteus maximus

Upper femur - side view

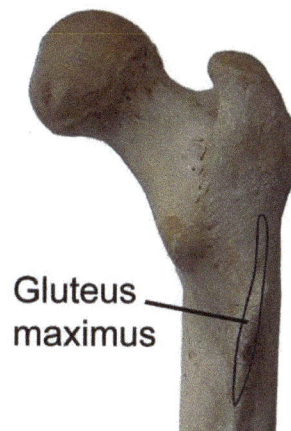

Gluteus maximus

Upper femur posterior view

133

Tensor fasciae latae arises on the iliac spine, iliac crest and on deep fascia and attaches about one third of the way down the iliotibial tract. The iliotibial tract inserts onto the condyle of the tibia on the outside of the knee. The muscle is palpable.

The muscle extends the knee and abducts and internally rotates the hip. In the erect position it stabilises the pelvis on the head of the femur and the condyles of the femur on the tibia and helps control posture.

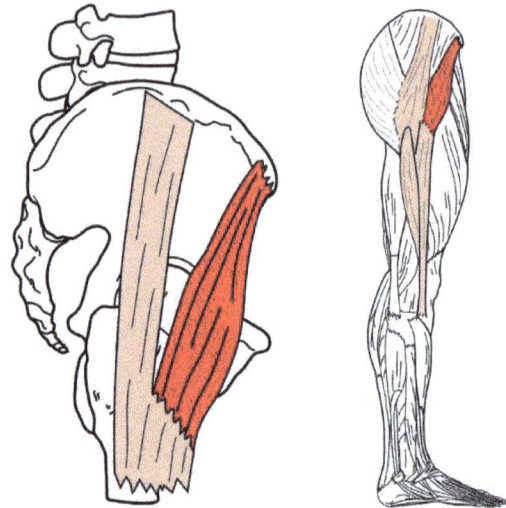

The **Iliotibial band or tract** is the thickened part of the outside of the **fascia lata,** the deep fascia of the thigh, which surrounds the thigh like a stocking and runs the length of the thigh.

The **hip external rotator muscles** are behind the hip joint and under the gluteal muscles.

They include piriformis, gamellus superior, gamellus inferior, obturator internus, obturator externus and quadratus femoris.

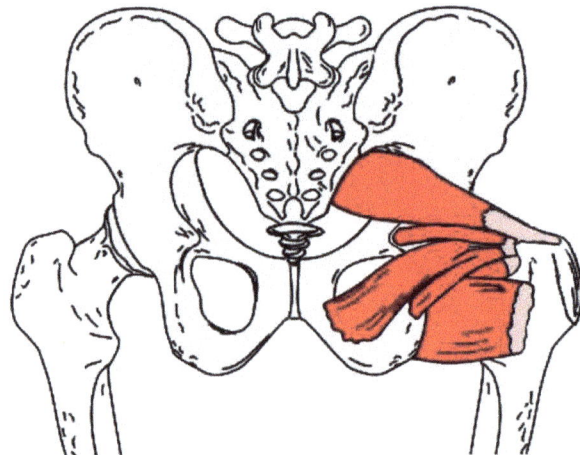

Pelvis and proximal femur - posterior view

Piriformis arises at the front of the sacrum and on a small area on the ilium and attaches on the top of the greater trochanter. The **gamellus superior** arises at the back of the pelvis and attaches on the inside of the greater trochanter. **Obturator internus** arises from the inside of the pelvis and the bottom of the pubic bone and attaches onto the inside of the greater trochanter. These muscles externally rotate the extended thigh and abduct the flexed thigh.

Obturator externus arises from a broad area on the outside of the lower pelvis and attaches on a depression on the inside of the greater trochanter of the femur. The **quadratus femoris** arises from the top and outside of the sit bone and attaches onto the back of the femur, just under the greater trochanter. These muscles produce external rotation of the thigh.

Piriformis
Gamellus superior
Obturator externus
Quadratus femoris

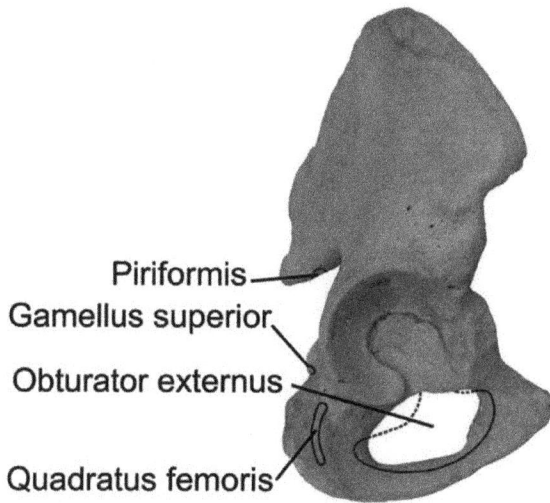

Ilium - lateral view

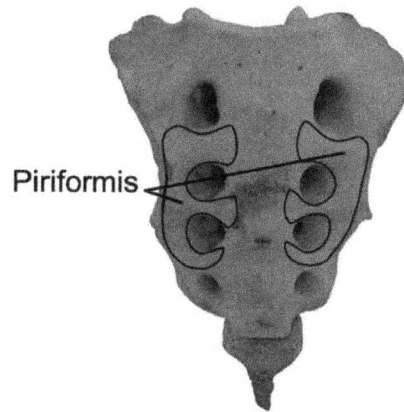

Piriformis

Sacrum - anterior view

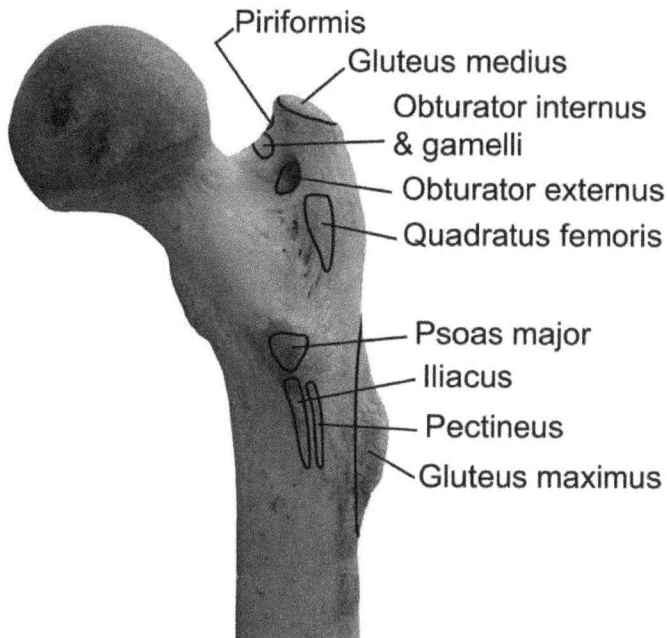

Piriformis
Gluteus medius
Obturator internus
& gamelli
Obturator externus
Quadratus femoris

Psoas major
Iliacus
Pectineus
Gluteus maximus

Proximal femur - posterior view

The inguinal ligament is a band of fibrous tissue that runs from the anterior superior iliac spine of the ilium to the pubic tubercle on the pubic bone. It attaches on abdominal fascia and the lower border of the external oblique muscle, and it merges with fascia that surrounds the thigh.

135

3.0a Kneading gluteus maximus and medius and the hip external rotator muscles using the wadi on its side

- Lie on your back, on a carpet or mat on the floor.
- Flex both hips and knees and then lift your pelvis off the floor.
- Grasp the wadi between the thumb and index finger of your right hand and place the apex of one dome against the muscles at the top and outside of your right sacroiliac joint.
- These are the upper fibres of gluteus maximus and the posterior fibres of gluteus medius.
- Lower your pelvis and the wadi to the floor.
- The wadi is on its side with the apex of one dome on the floor and the other pressed against the muscle.

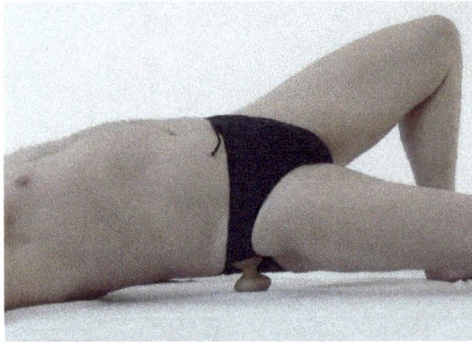

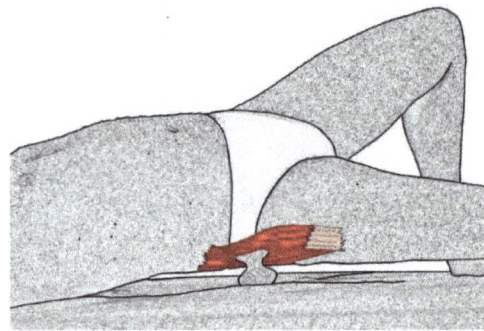

- Straighten your right knee.
- Lift the left side of your pelvis so it is tilted a few degrees to the right.
- Move your left knee to the right so your pelvis and the muscle are balanced directly over the wadi.
- Take a deep breath in, then exhale and relax the muscle while simultaneously moving your left knee to the right to take more of your body weight over the wadi and increase the pressure on the muscle.
- Focus on letting go of the muscle if it tenses up with the initial pressure.
- Relax and let the weight of your pelvis do the work.

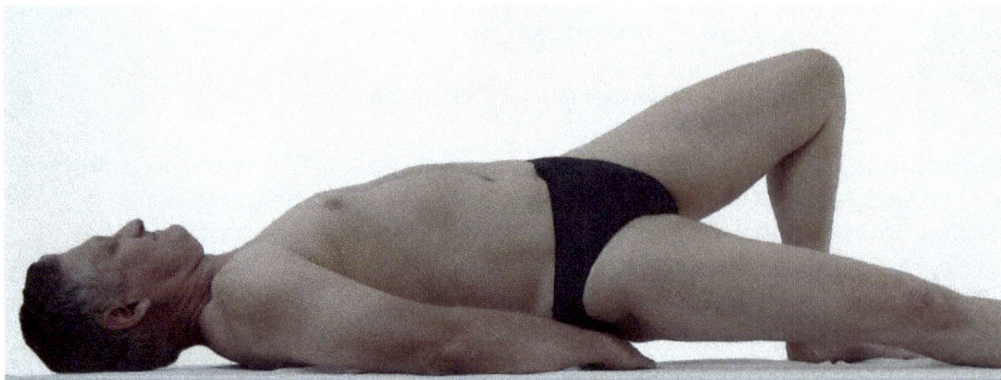

- After a couple of breaths lift your pelvis off the floor and reposition the wadi on an area of muscle further down the back and side of your pelvis.
- Follow a line down the outside of the sacroiliac joint and side of the sacrum to the bottom or the sacrum then reposition the wadi at the top of the pelvis again but about one centimetre further out from the sacrum.

- Move the wadi along a second line roughly parallel with the first, down muscles at the side of the pelvis and stop before the sit bone.
- These are gluteus maximus and medius and the deeper hip external rotator muscles.
- Stay behind the hip joint and shaft of the femur.
- When you work down lines that are further away from the sacrum adjust the tilt of your pelvis and the position of your left knee, so your weight stays directly over the wadi.

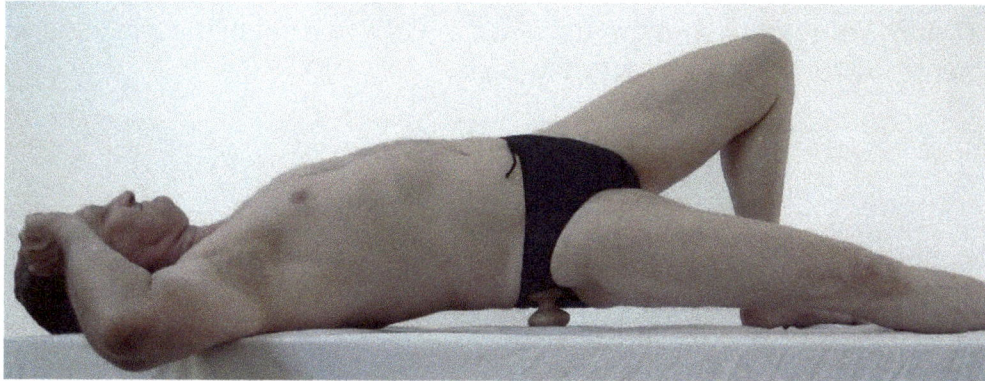

- Your pelvis may need to tilt up to about 45 degrees to treat some muscles.
- Your head, right shoulder, rib cage, calf and foot, and the sole of your left foot stay in contact with the floor throughout the technique.
- People who are thin or have gluteus maximus atrophy should take care not to put too much weight over the wadi because the sciatic nerve passes directly below the muscles, and it can be irritated.

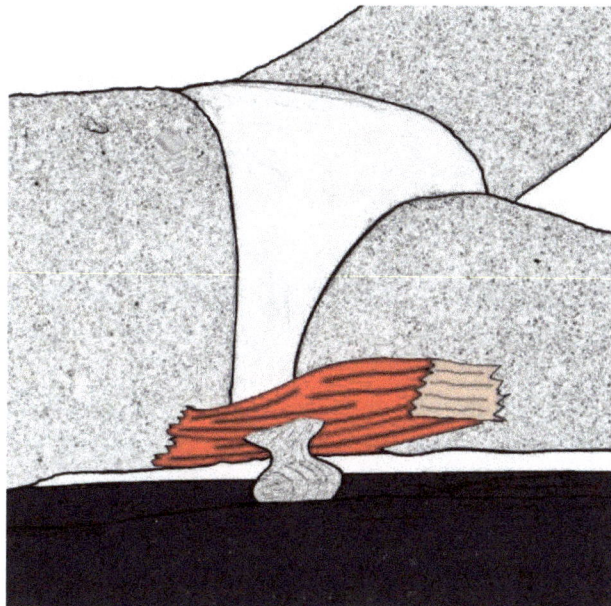

3.0b Kneading gluteus maximus, medius and minimus, the posterior fibres of tensor fasciae latae and the hip external rotator muscles using two balls in a net or the wadi or a tightly rolled-up towel

- Lie on your back, on a carpet or mat on the floor.
- Flex both hips and knees and then lift your pelvis off the floor.
- Grasp the two balls in your right hand and place them against the muscles at the top and outside of your pelvis.
- Align the balls in a head-to-toe direction behind your right sacroiliac joint.
- Return your pelvis and the balls to the floor and relax the muscles as you slowly lower your body over the balls.

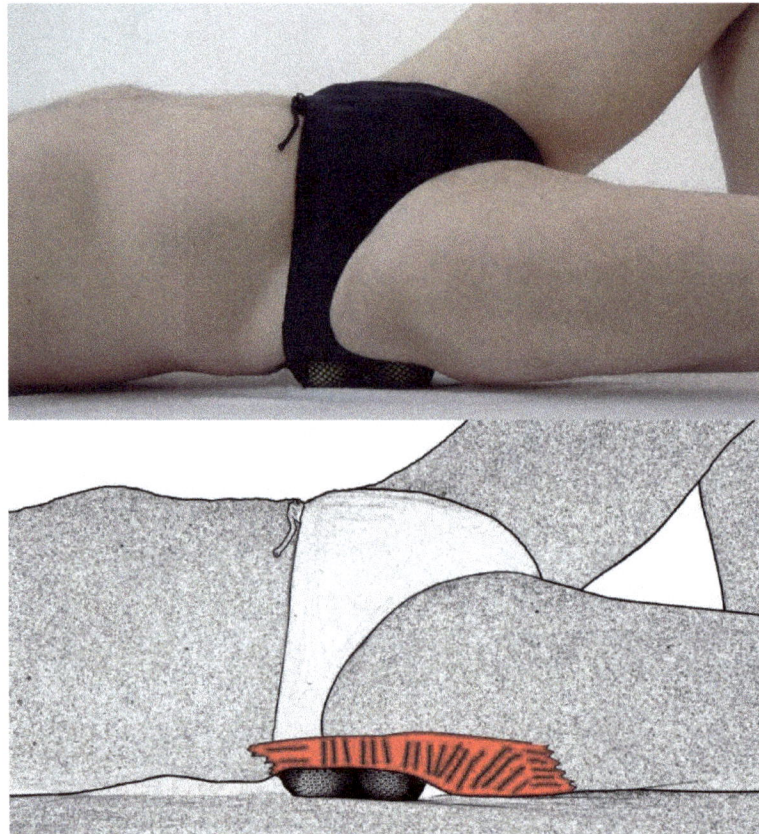

- Focus on letting go of the muscle if it tenses up with the initial pressure.
- Straighten your right leg but do not lock it - keep it slightly flexed for controlling your balance and stability.
- Lift the left side of your pelvis so your pelvis is tilted a few degrees right.
- Move your left knee to the right until your pelvis and the muscles are balanced directly over the balls.
- Move your pelvis from side to side and allow the balls to roll a few centimetres along the floor and over a small area of muscle.
- After completing this rolling action two or three times, lift your pelvis off the floor and reposition the balls on a muscle further down your pelvis.
- Repeat the rolling and movement of the balls down the pelvis, down a line parallel with the sacroiliac joint and sacrum and until you reach the bottom of the sacrum and beginning of your coccyx.

- Lift your pelvis off the floor and reposition the balls at the top of your pelvis a few centimetres in front of the original position.
- Return your pelvis and the balls to the floor but tilt your pelvis more to the right and move your left knee more to the right to take your weight directly over the balls.

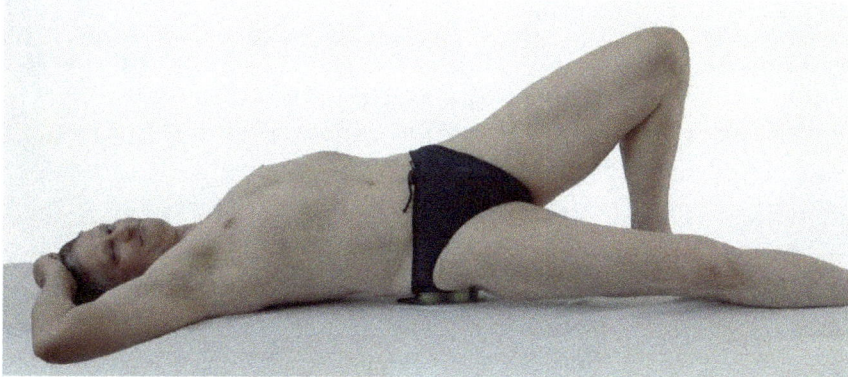

- Follow a second parallel line down the side of the pelvis to just above the right sit bone.
- Gluteus medius is at the top of the pelvis and gluteus maximus and the deeper hip external rotator muscles are further down the pelvis.
- As you move down a third or fourth line tilt your pelvis and move your left leg further to the right to keep the weight of your pelvis directly over the balls and muscle.

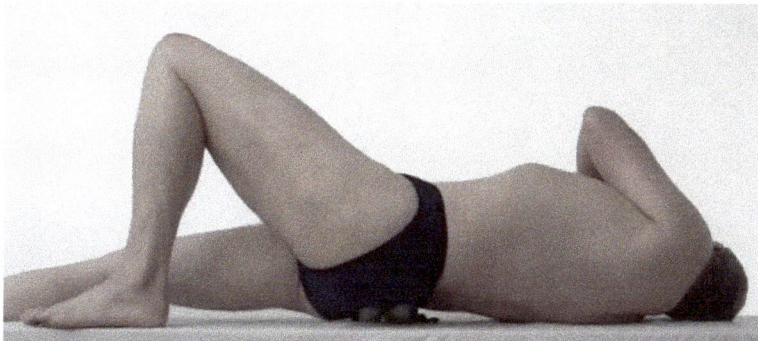

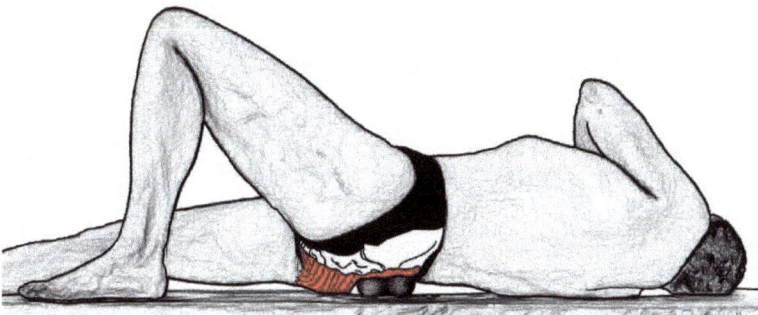

- Gluteus minimus lines up with the shaft of the femur so you will need to tilt your pelvis to about 45 degrees and further for tensor fasciae to keep your weight over the muscle for greater pressure on the muscle.
- Your head, right shoulder, the outside of your right thigh, leg and foot and the sole of your left foot remain in contact with the floor.

3.0c Kneading tensor fasciae latae using the tip or pad of your thumb

- Lie on your left side on a mat or carpeted floor with your head on a pillow or supported in your left hand.
- Flex your hips about 60 degrees and your knees about 90 degrees.
- Move your right knee backwards and allow it to drop to the floor behind your left thigh.
- Lift your left foot off the floor, then flex your left knee and place your left ankle on the outside of your right knee to hold it to the floor.
- Flex your right elbow, lift your arm about 45 degrees out to the side, then internally rotate it and place the tip of your thumb on the top of the tensor fasciae latae muscle - this is located at the top, front and outside of the pelvis, under the iliac crest, a ridge at the top and outside of the pelvis.

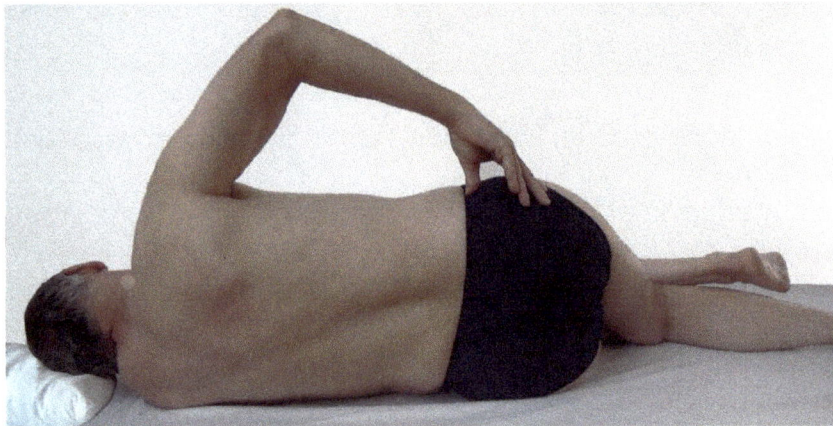

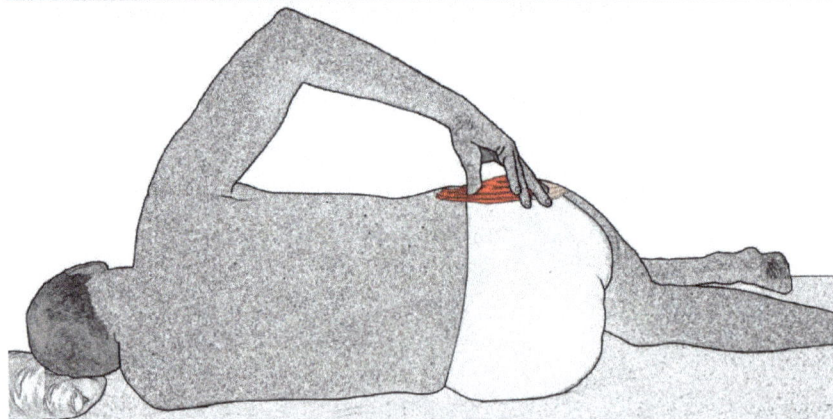

- Push your thumb into the muscle while simultaneously moving the right side of your pelvis backwards to stretch the muscle and act as a counterforce against your thumb.
- Reposition your thumb about one centimetre lower down the muscle and repeat the action, working down the muscle until you reach its attachment on the iliotibial band.
- Return to the top of the muscle and work down to the iliotibial band again along a line just behind and parallel with the first and treat the entire muscle.

3.0d Inhibition or kneading tensor fasciae latae using two balls in a net

- Lie on your back, on a carpet or mat on the floor.
- Flex your left hip and knee and place the sole of your foot on the floor.
- Rotate your body to the right so it is tilted about 45 degrees.
- Grasp the two balls in your left hand and place them, in a head-to-toe direction, against the right side of your pelvis, at the top and in front of your hip joint.
- The ball closest to your head, is in the small depression at the top and front of your pelvis.

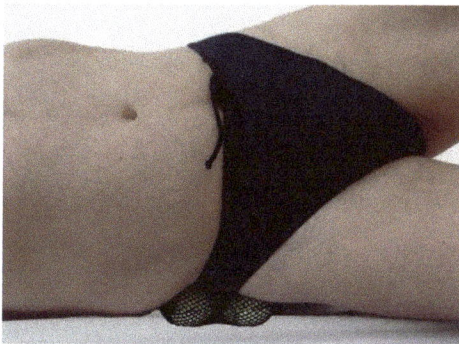

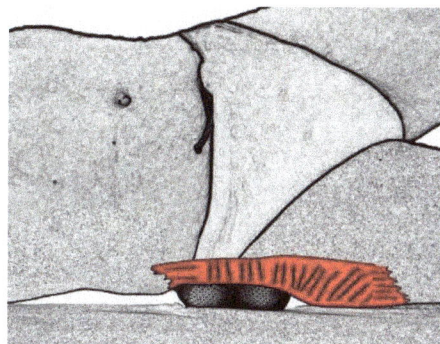

- The ball that is closest to your feet, is in front of the prominent bone (greater trochanter) of the hip joint.
- Hold the balls in place.
- Lift your pelvis off the floor and rotate your body further to the right until the right side of your pelvis is directly over the balls.
- Lower your pelvis and the balls to the floor.

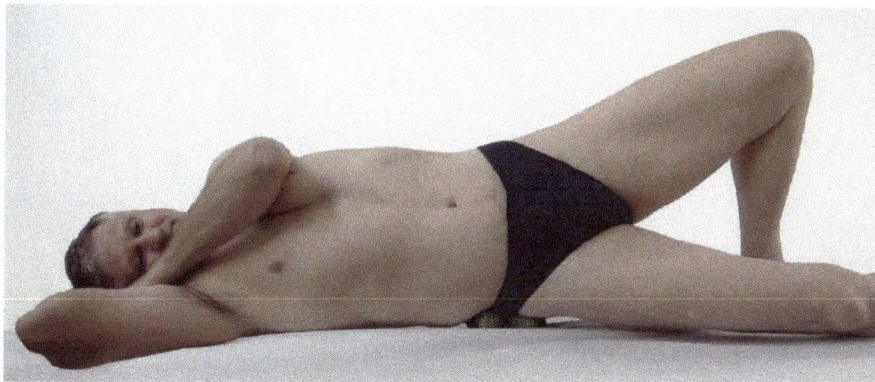

- Let go of the balls with you left hand.
- Adjust the angle of your pelvis so it is directly over the balls - when it is in position it is about 70 degrees with the floor.
- Rotate your left hip outwards so it is vertical.
- The sole of your left foot and most of the right side of your body are in contact with the floor.
- Keep your right leg straight or flex it a bit if it helps with balance.
- Support your head in the palm of your right hand or use a pillow.
- Take a deep breath in, then exhale and relax the muscle.
- As you sink into the balls allow the balls to push into the muscle.

- Repeat the breathing and letting go two or three times.
- Lift your pelvis off the floor again and reposition the balls about two centimetres further down the front and side of your pelvis and repeat the breathing and letting go action.
- Continue down the length of the muscle until you reach the iliotibial band.
- An alternative to the inhibition technique is to move your pelvis forwards and backwards so the balls roll over the muscle.
- Use deep breathing and exhale as you move across the entire width of the tensor fasciae latae muscle two or three times.
- Relaxing this muscle may be difficult while there is movement and strong pressure, and the rolling technique may not suit some people.

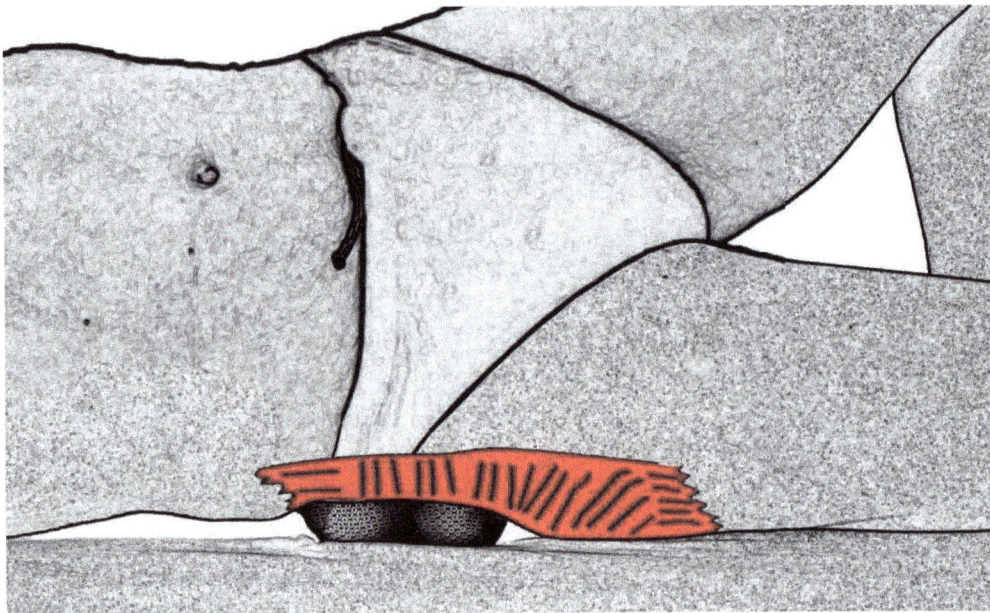

The hip adductors

Massaging the hip adductor muscles can be useful for thigh, hip, groin and lower back pain caused by ligament sprains and muscle and tendon strains. Adductor longus strains are the most common but strains can occur in adductor magnus and gracilis. The strain is usually in the upper part of the adductor longus muscle, in the tendon or at the junction between the tendon and the pubic bone of the pelvis. There may be groin pain and swelling and tenderness at the site of injury and there may be a limp when walking.

The hip adductors are arranged in three layers, with pectineus and adductor longus at the front of the thigh, adductor brevis and gracilis in the middle and adductor magnus at the back. The adductor longus and its tendon are easy to find on the inner thigh as you bring your leg outwards.

Hip adductor muscles - anterior view showing muscle layers

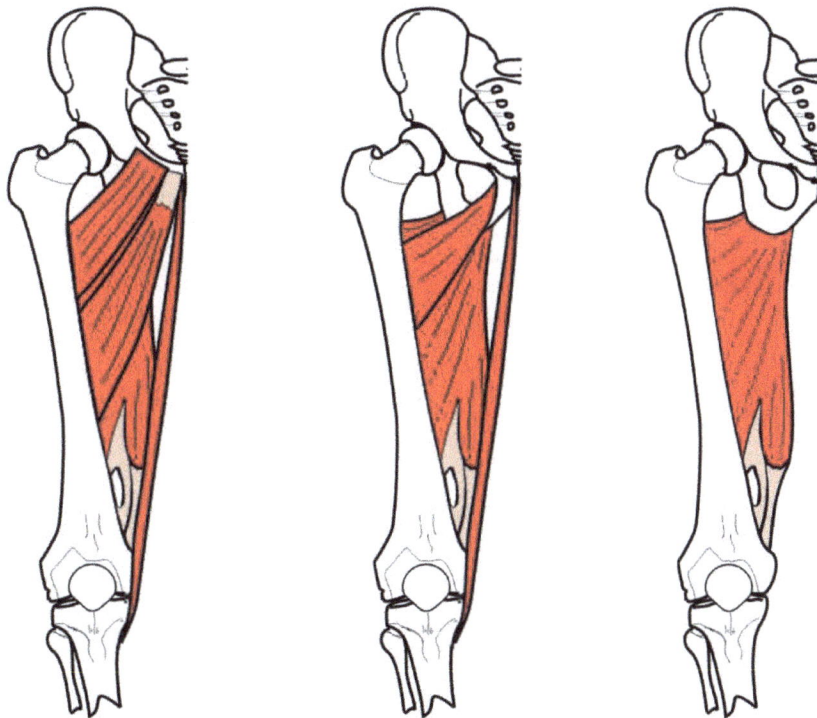

Pectineus and adductor longus - layer one

Adductor brevis and gracilis - layer two

Adductor magnus - posterior layer three

143

Pectineus is a flat four-sided muscle arising on the crest of the pubis. Its fibres run downwards and outward to attach along the linea aspera, at the top of the femur.

The muscle flexes the thigh and assists with adduction, especially when the hip is flexed. During standing it has minimal activity. Its main role is in controlling posture during walking.

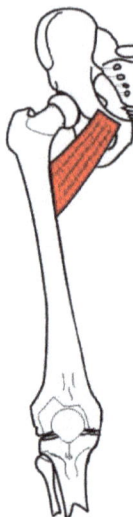

Adductor longus arises as a flat narrow tendon on the front of the pubis and runs downwards and backwards to attach on the middle third of a ridge running down the back of the femur, the linea aspera.

The muscle produces adduction, flexion and rotation of the thigh, depending on the position of the limb.

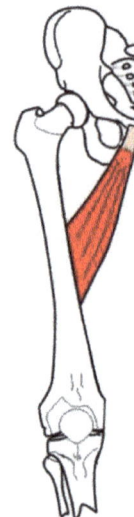

Adductor brevis arises on the outside and lower part of the pubis and runs downwards to attach on the upper part of the ridge running down the back of the femur, the linea aspera. It is deep and is not directly palpable.

The muscle produces hip adduction, and it is a weak hip flexor.

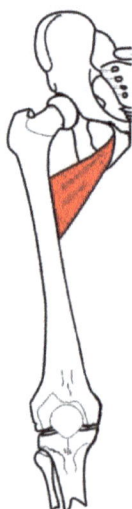

Gracilis arises along the bottom of the pubis and passes down the inside of the thigh to attach on the inside of the condyle of the tibia. It can be felt as a thin muscle running down the inside of the thigh.

The muscle flexes and internally rotates the leg. It is a weak adductor of the thigh.

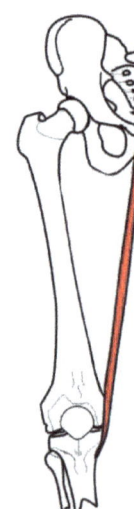

Adductor magnus arises on the lower part of the pubis and on the sit bone or ischial tuberosity. Its fibres fan out to attach along the entire length of the linea aspera, a ridge running down the back of the femur.

The longest fibres run almost vertically from the ischial tuberosity to a round tendon attaching onto the adductor tubercle on the medial condyle at the bottom of the femur.

The muscle adducts, flexes and extends the thigh, depending on the position of the limb. Because of its attachment on the ischial tuberosity the muscle acts like a hamstring.

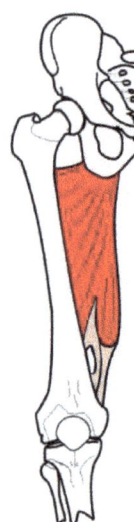

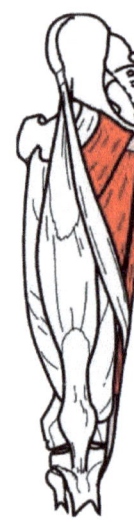

144

Pectineus

Adductor
longus

Adductor
brevis

Gracilis

Adductor magnus

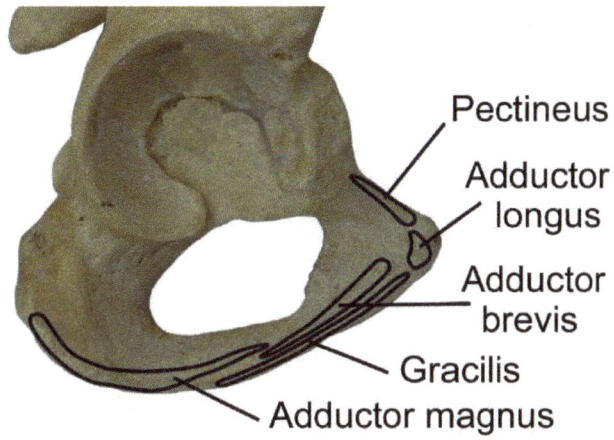

Lower ilium - lateral view

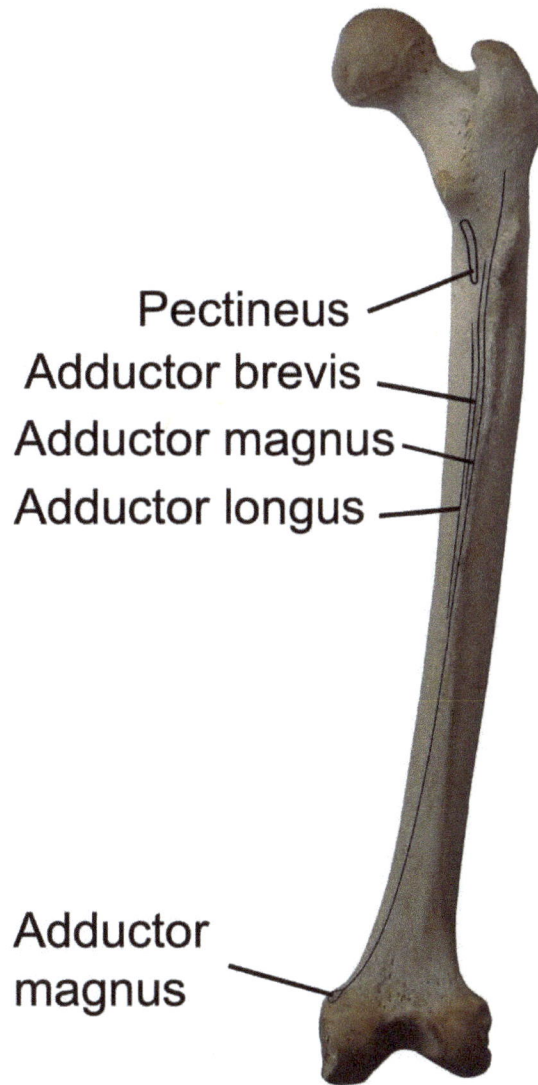

Pectineus

Adductor brevis

Adductor magnus

Adductor longus

Gracilis

Semi-
tendinosus

Sartorius

Adductor
magnus

Femur - posterior view

Tibia - anterior and medial view

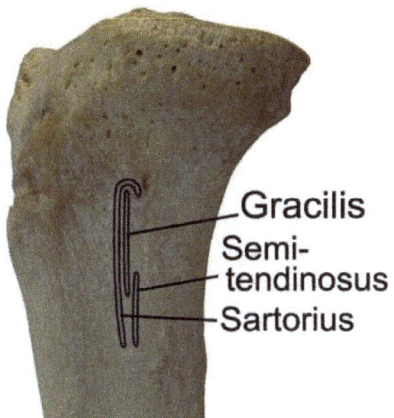

3.1a Kneading the hip adductor muscles using your thumb, fingers or the heel of your hand

- Stand straight and hold a wall or post with your left hand for balance.
- Lift your right leg and place the heel of your right foot on a table with your foot pointing upwards.
- Keep both legs straight.
- Rotate your left hip so that your foot points forwards.

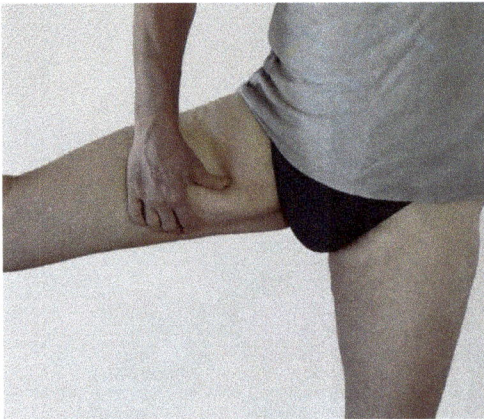

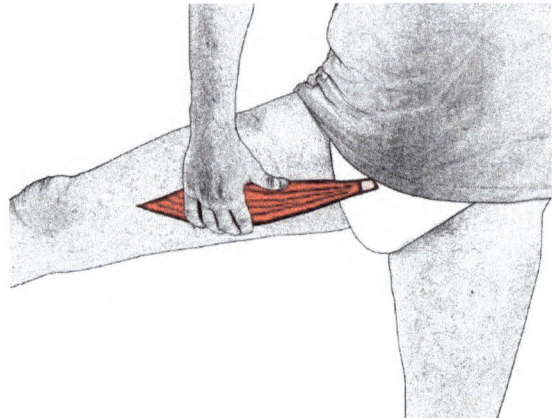

- Rotate your trunk and pelvis to the left to give your right hip adductor muscles a mild stretch.
- Place the side and pad of your right thumb against the outer border of your adductor muscles.
- Hook the fingers of your right hand under the inner border of your hip adductor muscles.

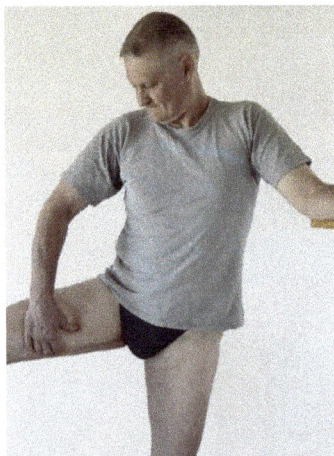

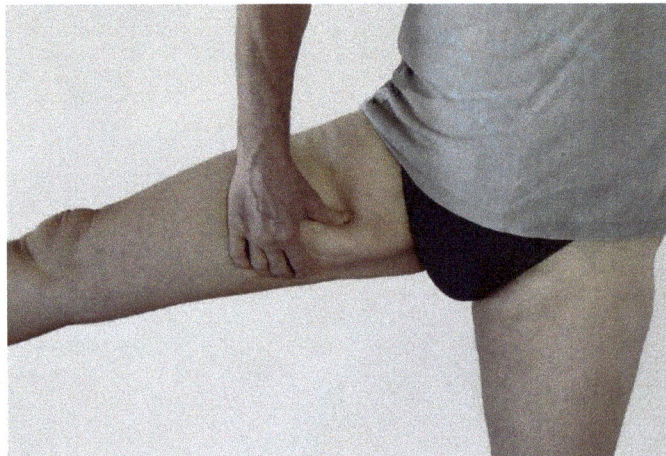

- Push the pad of your thumb down and into the muscle or pull the pads of your hooked fingers up and into the muscle or combine fingers and thumb with a twisting action of your wrist.
- Start at your groin and work down the inside of your thigh to where gracilis attaches just below the knee.
- Strong thumb pressure may be required in the lower half of the thigh because adductor longus and magnus pass under other muscles.

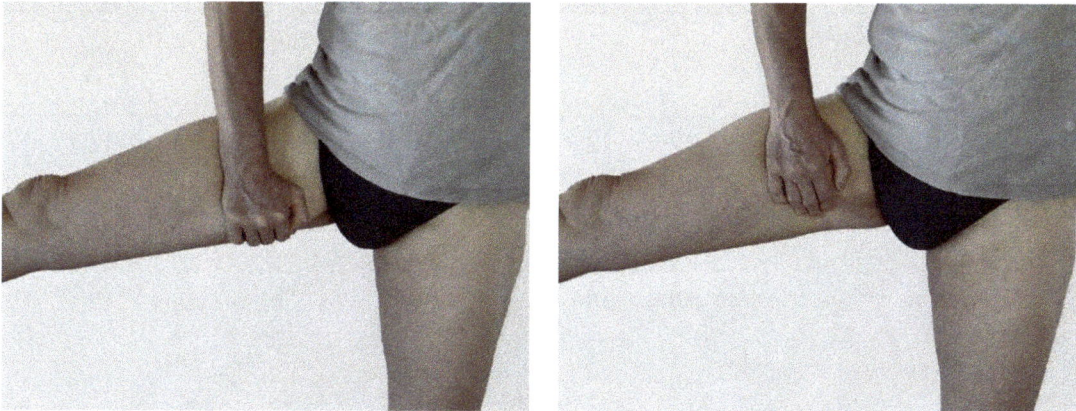

- This can be done sitting on a chair or the floor with your legs wide apart.
- An alternative to pushing with the thumb is to push the heel of your hand down and against the outer border of the adductor muscles.

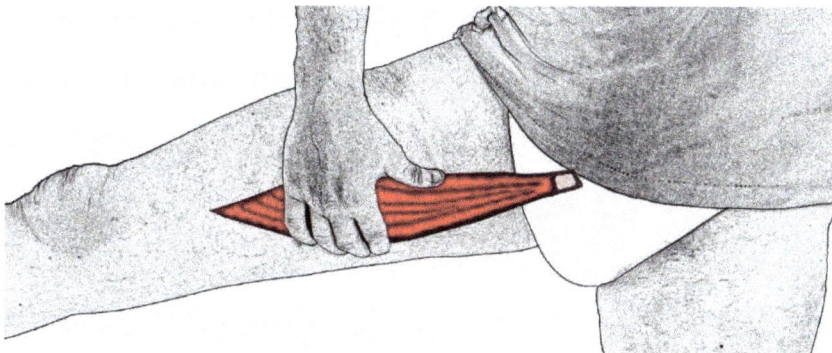

3.1b Transverse friction over the tendon of the adductor longus muscle using the tip of your thumb

- Sit on a chair with your legs wide to access the adductor longus tendon.
- The tendon can easily be found crossing the middle of the groin and attaching on the pubic bone.
- Place the tip of your right thumb or middle finger on the tendon.
- The tendon is about 11 mm long and 4 mm thick, blending with muscle.
- Feel for areas of tenderness.
- Apply transverse friction across the tendon for about 30 seconds.

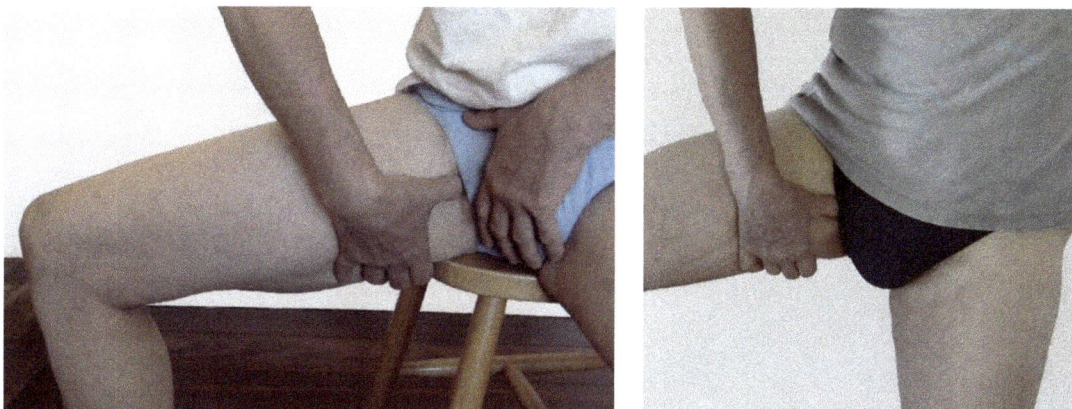

3.1c Kneading the hip adductor muscles using your fingers, thumb or the heel of your hand

- Stand straight and hold a wall or post with your left hand for balance.
- Lift your right leg, place the sole of your foot on a chair or low table and keep your right knee flexed.
- Allow your knee and thigh to drop towards the table.
- When the hip rolls outwards there is hip external rotation and abduction, and your hip adductors are put on stretch.
- Place the side and pad of your right thumb against the outer border of your hip adductor muscles.

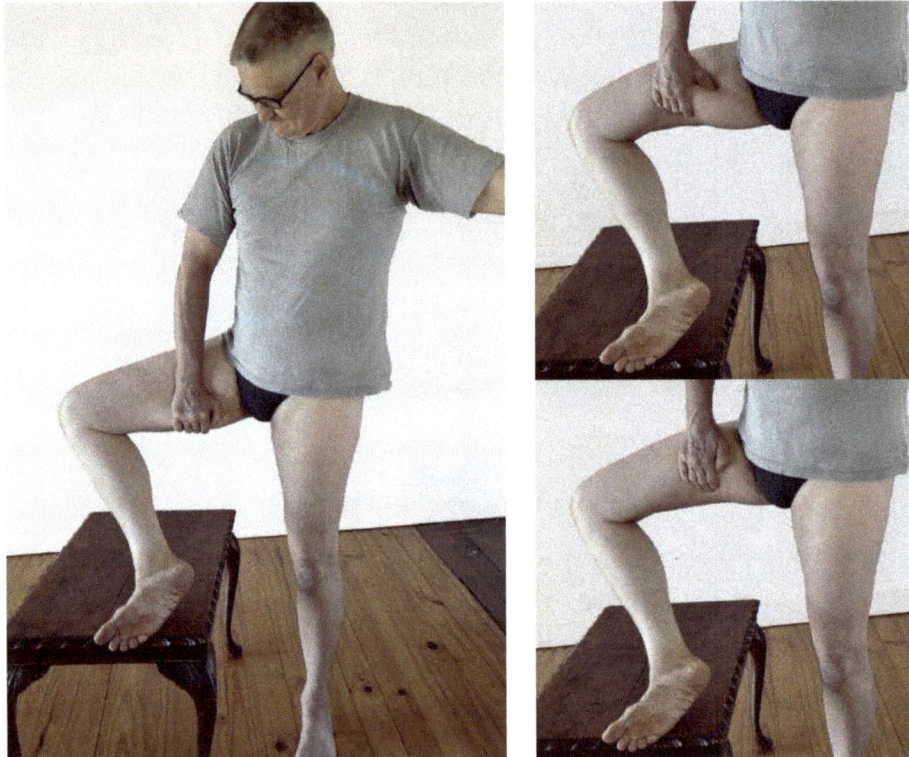

- Place the finger pads of your right hand against the inner border of your hip adductor muscles and hook your fingers under them.
- Push the pad of your thumb into the muscle and pull the pads of your fingers into the muscle with a push-pull twisting action of your wrist.
- Start at your groin and work down the inside of your thigh to your knee.
- About halfway down the thigh the adductors pass under other muscles and firmer thumb pressure is needed.
- Another option is to push down against the outer border of the adductors with the heel of your hand or pull up with fixed flexed fingers.
- This technique can also be done seated on a chair or sitting on the floor with your hip dropped out to the side or it can be used to treat the hamstrings and quadriceps muscles on the inside of the thigh.

THE HIP, THIGH AND KNEE

The hamstrings

Massaging the hamstrings can be useful when there is pain from a muscle strain, cramp, spasm, tendon strain or bursitis.

A mild strain may be asymptomatic or result in tenderness and pain with activity whereas a severe strain may result in extreme pain and the inability to weight bear or walk. There may be swelling, bruising and weakness. The strain may occur in the muscle or tendon, or where the tendon attaches on the sit bone.

A cramp is a sudden involuntary muscle contraction. Commonly known as a charley horse, a cramp can last from a few seconds to several minutes. They often occur at night when the muscle is relaxed and short and the pain can be extreme.

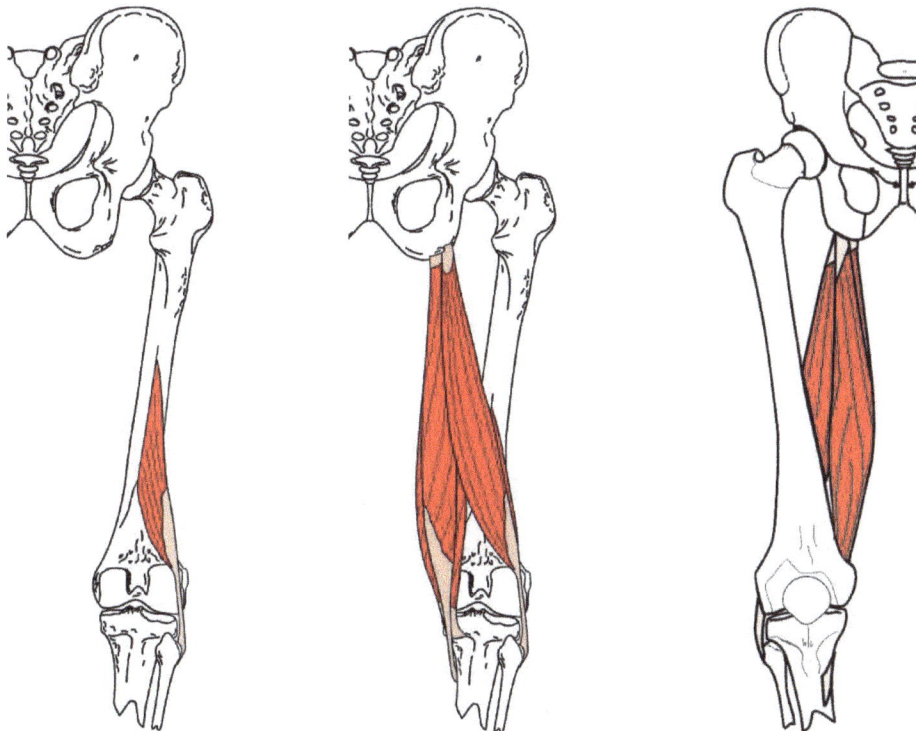

Bicep femoris short head - posterior view   Hamstrings - posterior view   Hamstrings - anterior view

The hamstrings consist of three muscles: semimembranosus, semitendinosus and biceps femoris.

Semimembranosus arises on the ischial tuberosity and remains a muscle to its insertion at the back of the medial tibial condyle.

Semitendinosus arises on the ischial tuberosity by a short tendon, which it shares with the long head of biceps femoris. The muscle ends about halfway down the posteromedial thigh as a long round tendon. The tendon curves around the medial tibial condyle and attaches onto the anteromedial tibia, posterior and inferior to the tendons of gracilis and sartorius.

Biceps femoris has two heads. The long head arises on the ischial tuberosity by a short tendon, which it shares with semitendinosus, and from the sacrotuberous ligament. The short head arises on a ridge running down the back of the femur and from fascia attaching to other muscles. Most of the tendon attaches onto the head of the fibula and the rest attaches on the lateral condyle of the tibia and the lateral collateral ligament.

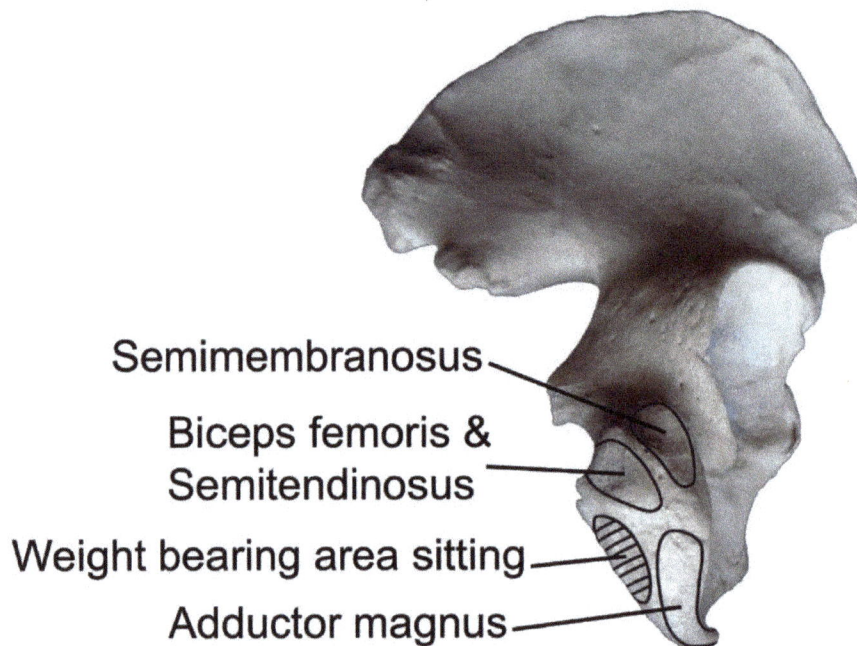

Ilium - inferior lateral view

The hamstrings flex the leg at the knee and in the semiflexed position they internally or externally rotate the leg. Semimembranosus, semitendinosus and the long head of biceps femoris extend the thigh and assist in stabilisation of the hip joint. The hamstrings also give support to the knee joint.

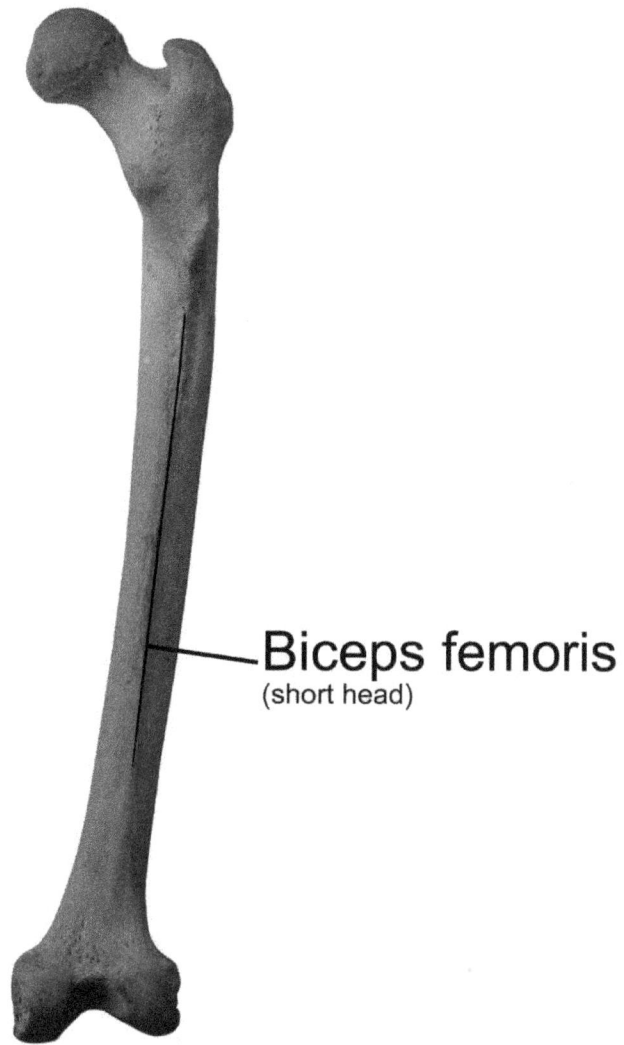

Biceps femoris
(short head)

Femur - posterior view

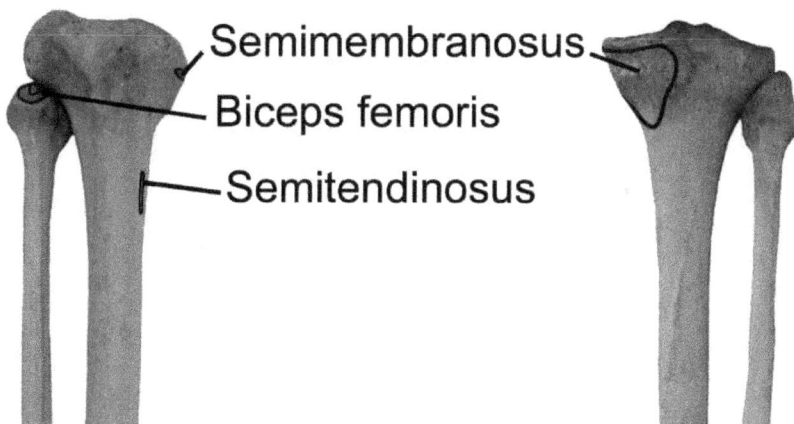

Semimembranosus

Biceps femoris

Semitendinosus

Tibia and fibula - anterior view (left) posterior view (right)

3.2a Kneading the hamstrings using your fingers and thumb sitting on the floor

- Sit on the floor with your right leg flexed at the knee.
- Reach around the outside and under your right thigh with your right hand and grasp the back of your thigh between your fingers and thumb.
- Hook your fingers around the hamstrings on the inside of your thigh.

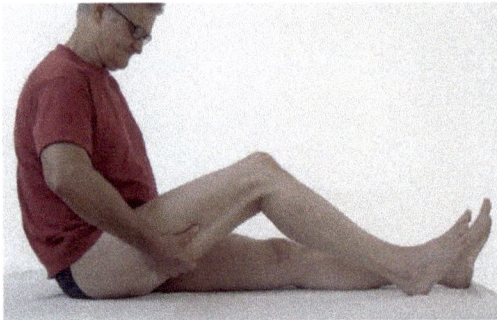

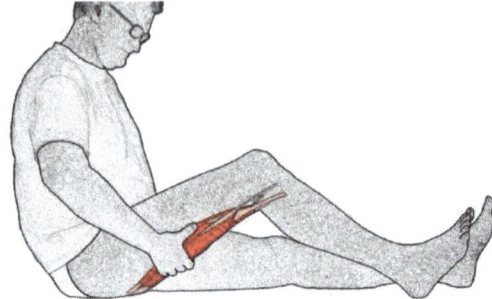

- Place the pad or tip of your thumb on the hamstrings on the outside of your thigh. Pull the muscles with your fingers and simultaneously push with your thumb using a squeezing action.
- To produce greater leverage and pressure on the hamstring muscles, lift your right elbow and tilt your wrist to the side.
- Keep your right leg in a fixed flexed position.

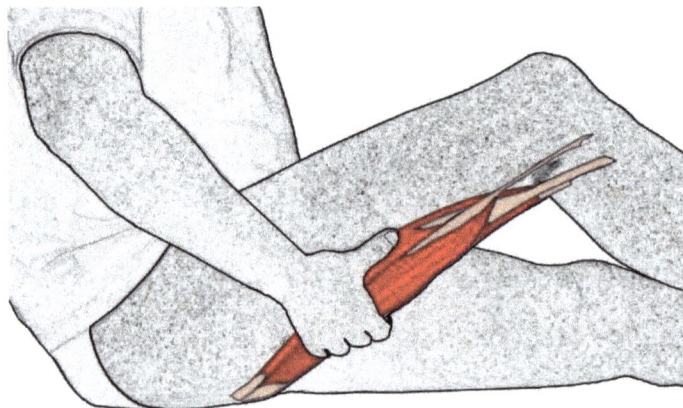

- Start where the hamstrings attach on the sit bone and work down the length of the muscles to the knee.
- As you move towards your knee the hamstring muscles spread out, and so your thumb and fingers will need to be wider.

3.2b Kneading the hamstrings using your hooked fingers sitting on the floor

- Sit on the floor with your right leg flexed at the hip and knee.
- Reach around the outside and under your right thigh with your right hand and hook your fingers around the hamstrings on the inside of your thigh.
- Pull the muscle with your fixed flexed fingers while simultaneously straightening your right leg by sliding the heel of your right foot away.

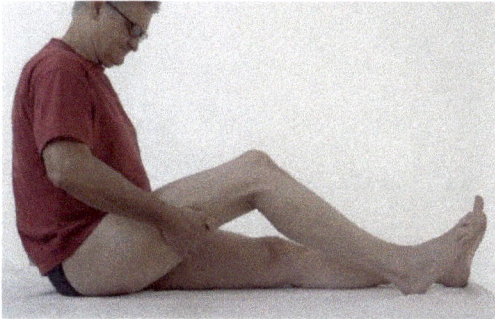

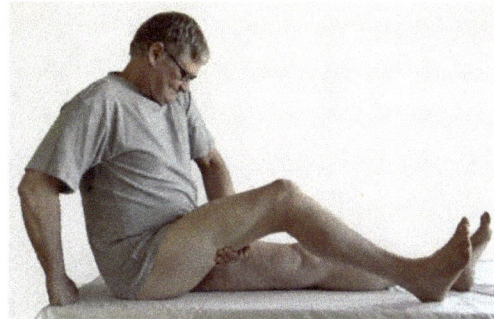

- Lift your right elbow and tilt your wrist to increase leverage.
- Straightening your right leg stretches the hamstrings and adds a counterforce to the pulling action of your fingers.
- Start where the hamstrings attach on the sit bone and work down the entire length of the muscles to the knee.

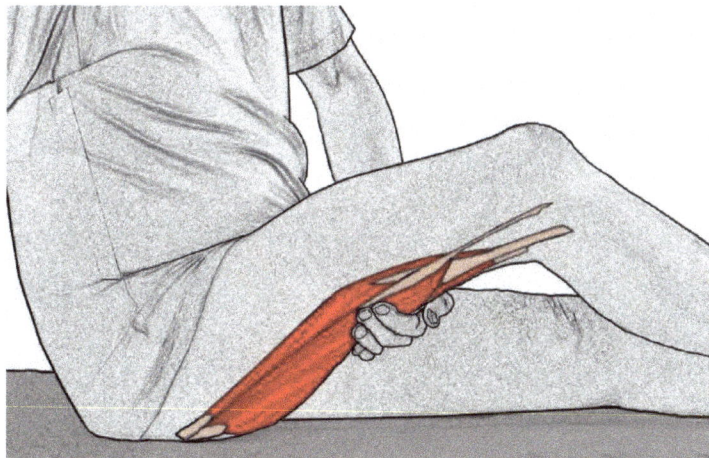

- Reach around the inside and under your right thigh with your left hand and hook your fingers around the hamstrings on the outside of your thigh.
- Pull the muscle with your fixed flexed fingers while simultaneously straightening your right leg by sliding the heel of your right foot away.
- Coming from the inside of the thigh treats the biceps femoris but more of the hamstring muscles are treated when coming from the outside.

3.2c Kneading the hamstrings using your hooked fingers lying on the floor

- Lie on your back with your head on a pillow and your hips and knees flexed.
- Flex your right hip more so your thigh is about vertical.
- Reach around the outside and back of your right thigh with your right hand and hook your fingers around the inner hamstring muscles.

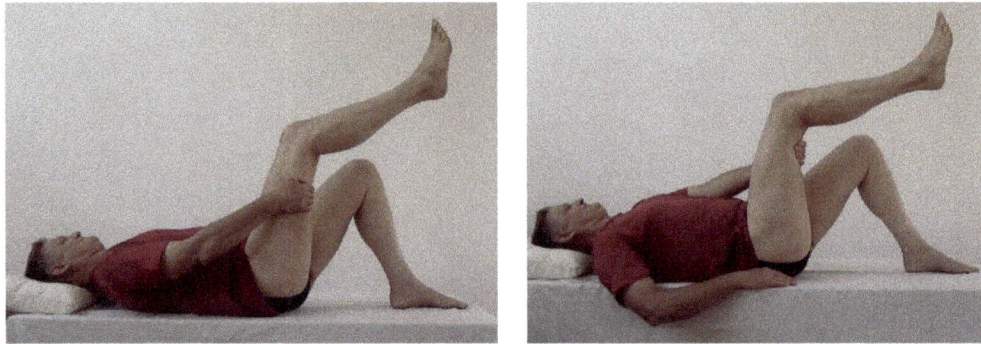

- Pull on the inner hamstrings with the fingertips of your fixed flexed fingers while simultaneously straightening your right knee and hip.
- Straightening your knee stretches the hamstrings.
- Straightening your hip produces a counterforce against the pull of your fingers and increases your fingertip pressure on the muscle.
- Start where the hamstrings attach on the sit bone and work down the entire length of the inner muscles to the knee.

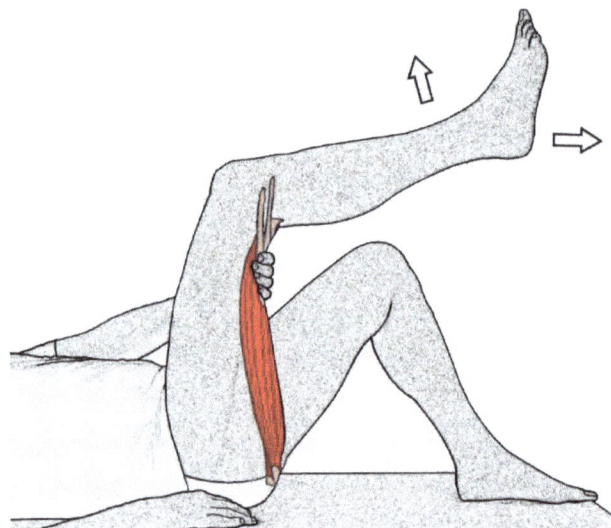

- Reach around the inside and back of your right thigh with your left hand and hook your fingers around your outer hamstring muscles.
- Pull on the outer hamstrings with your fingertips while simultaneously straightening your hip and knee.
- Work along the entire length of the outer hamstring, the biceps femoris.
- More hamstrings are available by coming from the outside of your thigh.

3.2d Kneading the hamstrings using your fingers and thumb lying on the floor

- Lie on your back with your head on a pillow and hips and knees flexed.
- Flex your right hip so your thigh is about vertical.
- Reach around the outside and back of your right thigh with your right hand and hook your fingers around your inner hamstring muscles and place the pad of your thumb against your outer hamstring muscles.
- Pull on the inner muscles with your fingertips and push on the outer muscles with your thumb while straightening your right knee.

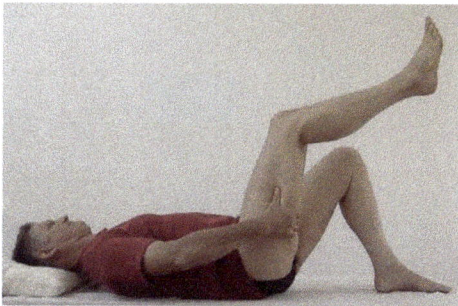

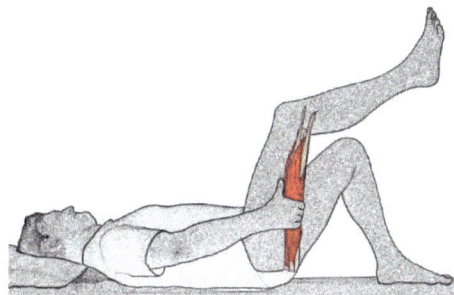

- Straightening your leg stretches the hamstrings and adds a counterforce to the pull of your fingers.
- To produce greater leverage and pressure on the muscles lift your right elbow and tilt your wrist to the side.
- Work along the entire length of the muscle.
- Reach around the inside and underside of your right thigh with your left hand and hook your fingers around your outer hamstrings and place the tip of your thumb against your inner hamstrings.
- Pull on the outer hamstrings with your fingertips and push on the inner hamstrings with your thumb while straightening your right knee.
- Work along the entire length of the muscle.

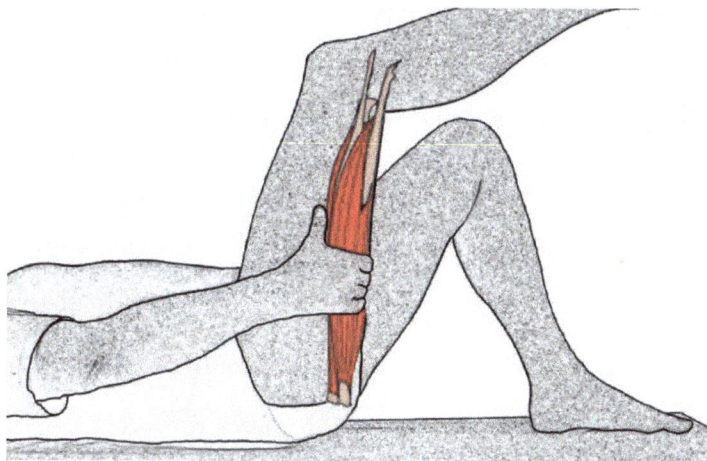

- An option is to use both hands, one on either side of the thigh, and to press your fingertips into the middle of the thigh while simultaneously straightening your right knee - this is particularly effective for treating the short head of biceps femoris.

3.2e Pin and stretch technique for the hamstrings using two balls in a net

- This is similar to the pin and stretch technique for the calf muscles 3.4b
- Sit on the floor with your legs straight out in front.
- Flex your right hip and knee and place the two balls under your thigh, with one ball against or near the inner hamstrings and the other against or near the outer hamstring.
- Place the balls near where the hamstrings originate on the sit bones.
- Return your leg and the two balls to the floor.

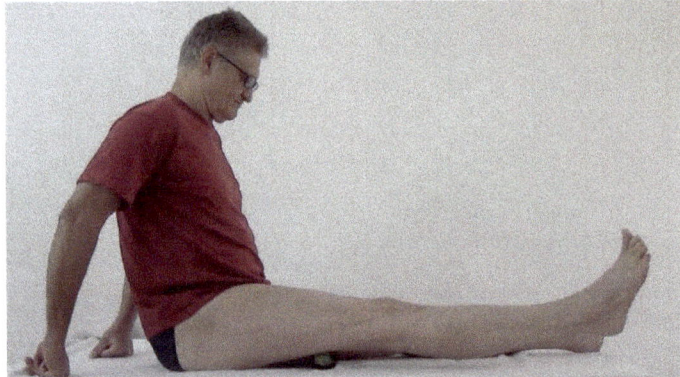

- Press the back of your thigh against the balls and pin the muscle, and while maintaining the downward pressure on the balls contract your quadriceps and straighten your knee.
- Pull up your kneecap and hold the contraction for a couple of seconds.
- Relax your quadriceps and allow your foot to return to the floor.

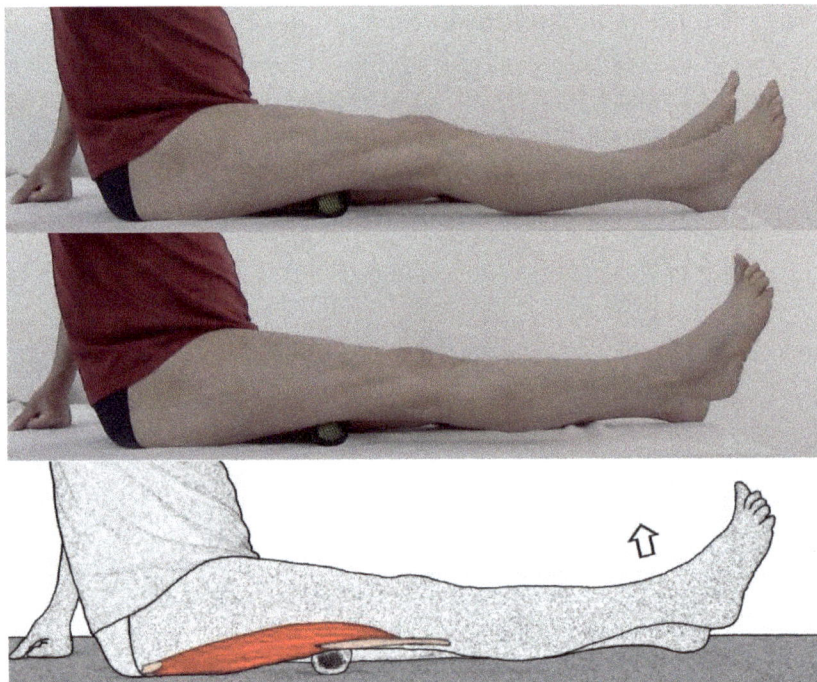

- Reposition the balls further down your thigh and repeat the action.
- Continue down the back of the thigh, along the entire length of the muscle from the sit bone to just above the knee.

3.2f Kneading the hamstrings using a rolling action of two balls in a net

- This is similar to the rolling technique for the calf muscles 3.4a.
- Sit on the floor with your legs straight out in front.
- Flex your right hip and knee and place the balls under your thigh, with one ball under the inner hamstrings and the other under the outer hamstrings.

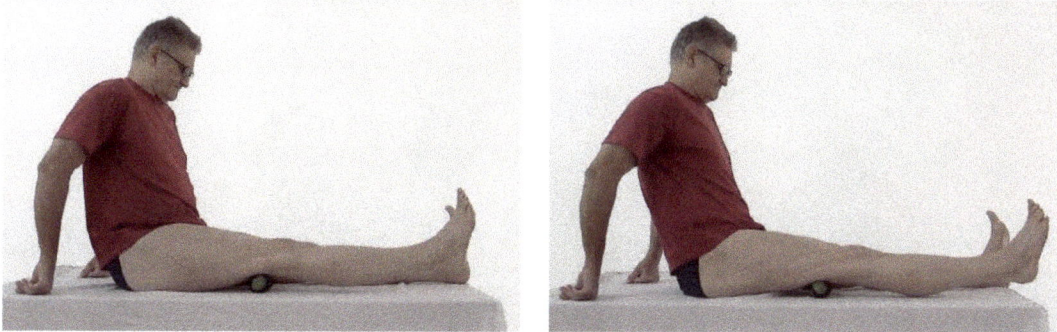

- Place the balls near where the hamstrings originate on the sit bones.
- Contract your quadriceps so your leg is straight, and heel lifts off the floor.
- Move the right side of your pelvis and leg forwards and then backwards and allow a small section of your hamstrings to roll over the balls.

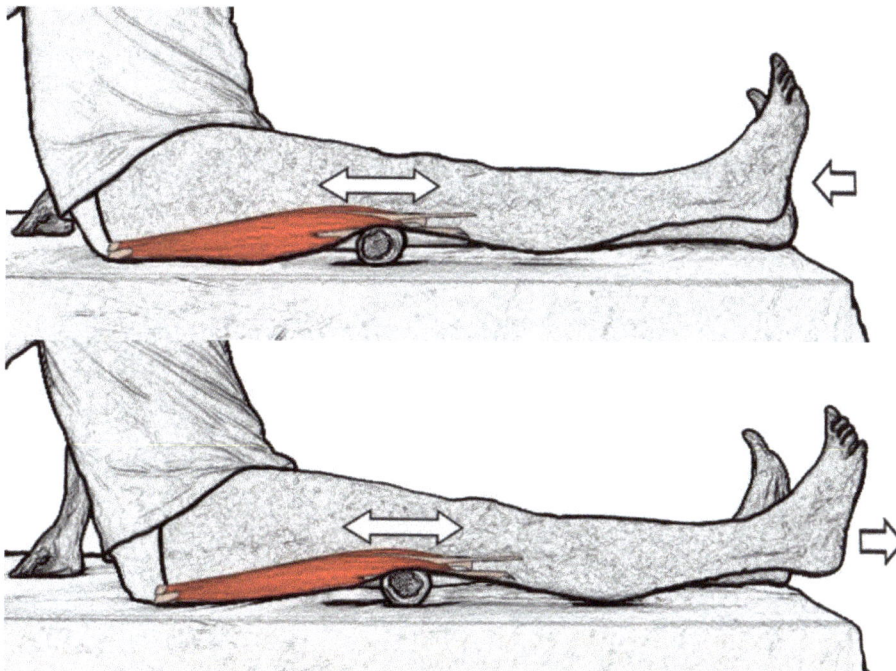

- Roll up and down the thigh several times and then relax your quadriceps and allow your heel to return to the floor.
- Reposition the balls further down your thigh and repeat the rolling action until you reach the end of the hamstrings at the knee.

3.2g Transverse friction on the hamstring attachment on the sit bone using two balls in a net

- Sit on a chair with your feet planted on the floor.
- Grasp the two balls in your right hand.
- Lift the right side of your pelvis so your sit bone raises off the chair.
- Place one of the balls at the points the hamstrings originate on the right sit bones and return your right sit bone to the chair so that it rests on the ball.

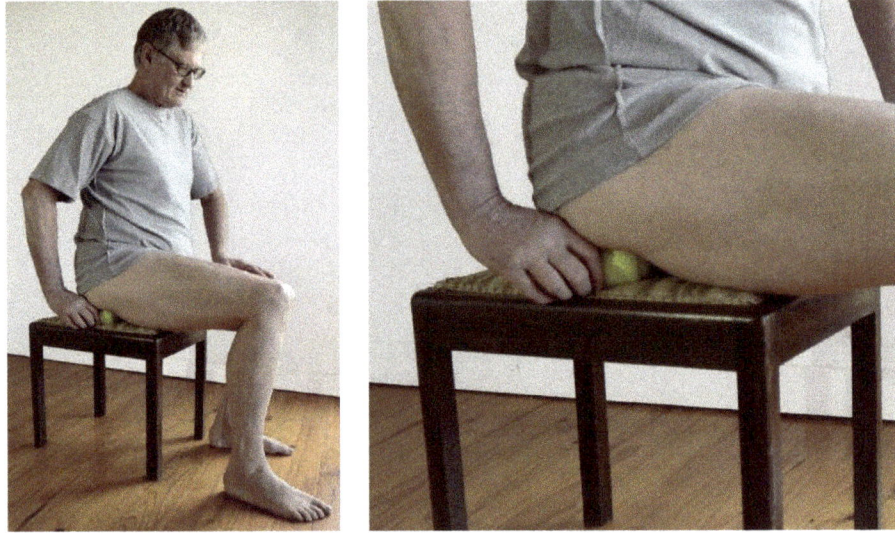

- With the full weight of your body over one of the balls move your pelvis forwards and backwards and side to side over the balls.
- Apply transverse friction over the hamstring origin on the sit bone and cover the entire area for about thirty seconds

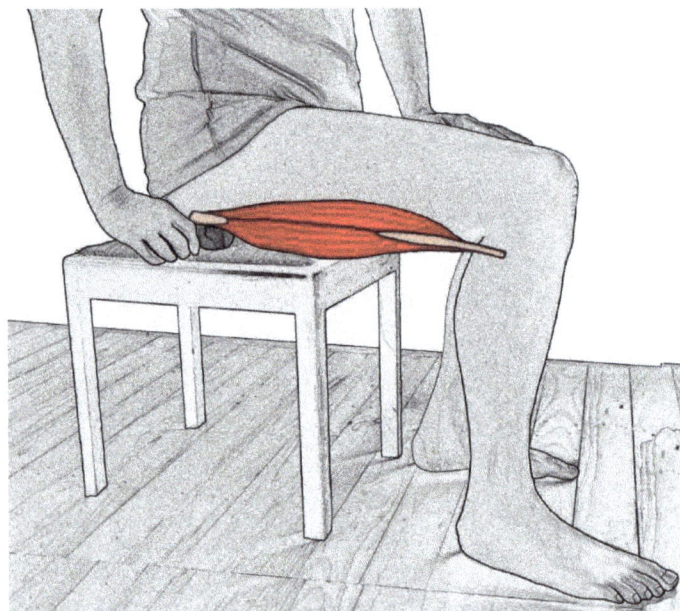

The quadriceps

Massaging the quadriceps can be useful for knee pain and pain from bruises, spasms, muscle and tendon strains, ligament sprains and bursitis.

A bruise or contusion is the most common quadriceps injury and usually occurs from a direct blow to rectus femoris because it is closest to the surface. A severe bruise should not be massaged aggressively because this may result in bleeding and bone formation in the muscle, a condition called myositis ossificans.

A quadriceps strain can occur in the muscle, tendon above the kneecap or patella ligament below the kneecap. The fibres can be stretched but not torn, partially torn or completely torn. Symptoms include pain, especially with knee movement, swelling, tenderness, weakness and stiffness in the knee joint. Medial or lateral collateral ligament sprains of the knee are usually the result of a direct blow to the outside or inside of the knee or sustained stretching. Symptoms include pain, swelling and tenderness on one side of the knee.

Quadriceps femoris

The four muscles that make up quadriceps femoris are rectus femoris, vastus lateralis, vastus medialis and vastus intermedius.

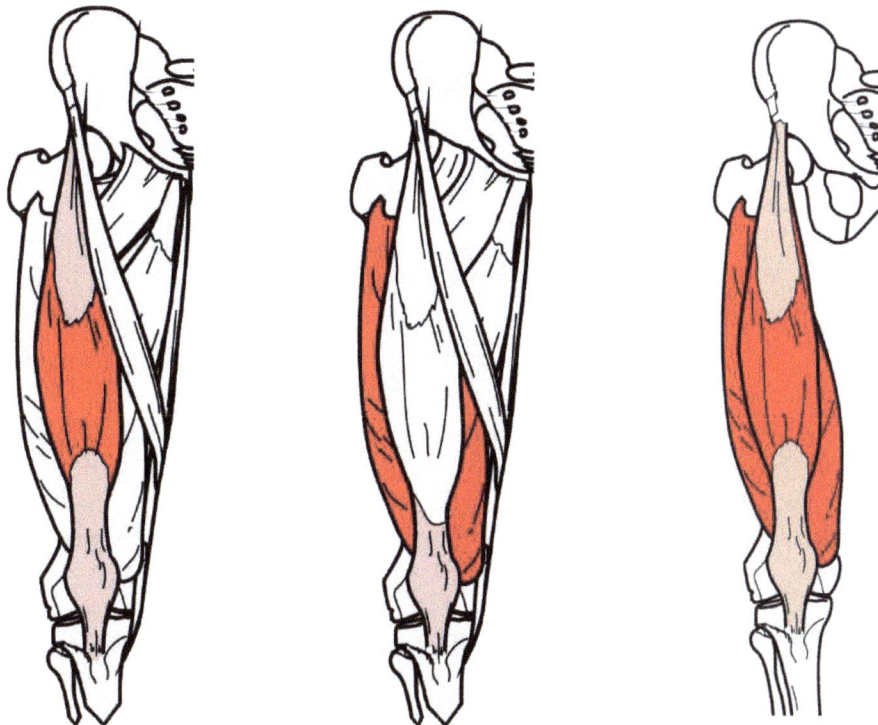

Rectus femoris   **Vastus lateralis & medialis**   **Quadriceps**

Vastus lateralis arises on a broad aponeurosis attached to the intertrochanteric line, greater trochanter, lateral lip of the gluteal tuberosity and the upper linea aspera. The aponeurosis covers a large part of the muscle. The muscle also arises on the tendon of gluteus maximus and on the lateral intermuscular septum. Inferiorly a thick aponeurosis emerges from the deep part of the muscle which becomes a flat tendon attaching onto the lateral patella. Some fibres of the tendon also blend with the capsule of the knee joint and the iliotibial band.

Vastus medialis arises on a lower area of the intertrochanteric line, the medial lip of the linea aspera and the medial supracondylar line. The muscle also arises on the tendons of adductor longus and magnus and the medial intermuscular septum. The muscle attaches onto an aponeurosis emerging from a deep part of the muscle which attaches on the medial border of the patella and the quadriceps tendon. Some fibres of this aponeurosis blend with the capsule of the knee joint and the medial tibial condyle. The muscle is prominent above the medial aspect of knee and is important for knee stability.

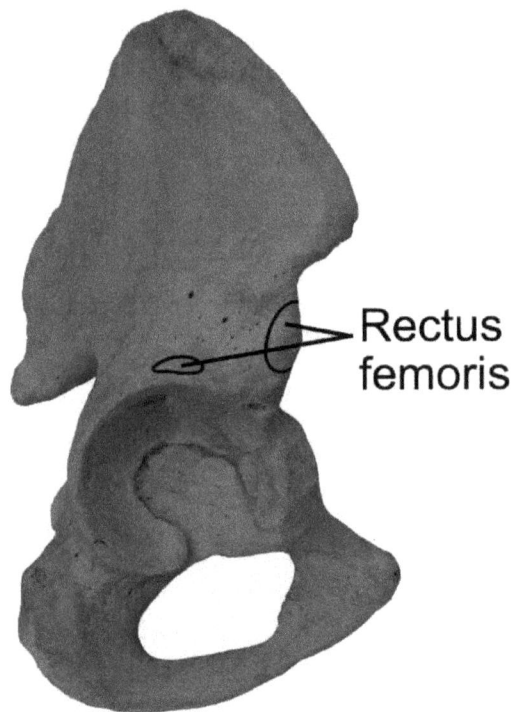

Ilium - lateral view

Vastus intermedius arises on the upper anterior and lateral shaft of the femur and a lower part of the lateral intermuscular septum. The muscle attaches on an aponeurosis which forms the deep layer of the quadriceps tendon, and on the lateral border of the patella and the lateral condyle of the tibia. The muscle is deep to rectus femoris.

Rectus femoris arises by two tendinous heads. The straight head arises from the anterior inferior iliac spine of the ilium and the reflected head arises from an area just above the acetabulum and from the hip joint capsule. The two heads form an aponeurosis, and the muscle arises from this. Inferiorly another thick aponeurosis emerges from the posterior part of the muscle which becomes a flat tendon attaching onto the base of the patella. Rectus femoris is the most superficial quadriceps muscle running down the anterior thigh and is easily palpable.

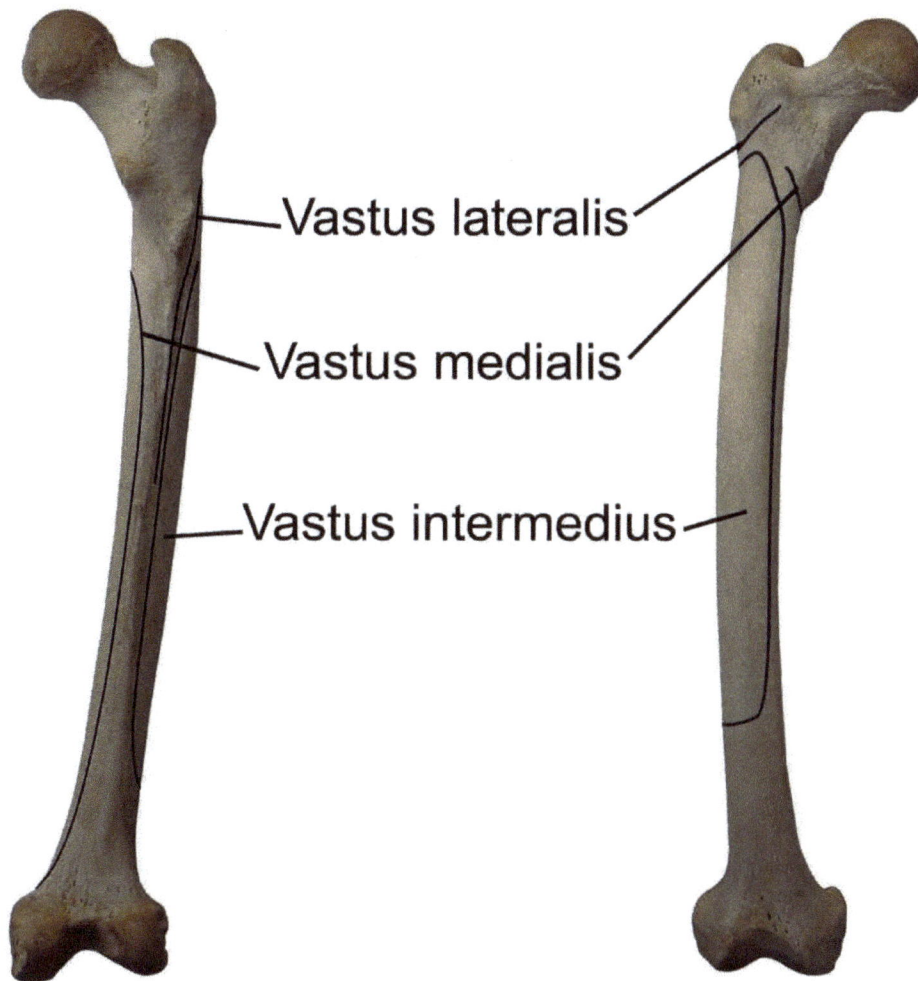

Femur - posterior view (left) and anterior view (right)

Vastus lateralis

Vastus medialis

Vastus intermedius

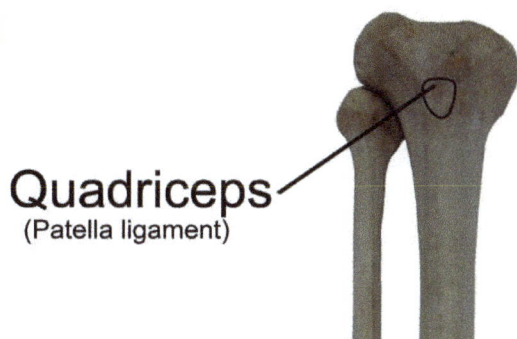

Quadriceps
(Patella ligament)

Fibula and tibia - anterior view

Quadriceps femoris extends the leg on the thigh. Rectus femoris is also a weak hip flexor, flexing the thigh on the pelvis or, if the thigh is fixed, flexing the pelvis on the thigh. The lowest fibres of vastus medialis are important in maintaining the patella in its groove during the final phase of knee extension. Ligaments stabilize the knee and vastus medialis and lateralis may also help with knee stability. The medial and lateral collateral ligaments prevent lateral and medial knee movements, and the anterior and posterior cruciate ligaments prevent the tibia from sliding too far forward or backward.

3.3a Kneading the quadriceps between your fingers and heel of hand or between your fingers and thumb or just using the tip of your thumb

- Stand straight, flex your right hip and knee, and place the sole of your foot on a stool or chair in front of you.
- Place the tip of the thumb of your right hand against the outer quadriceps muscle, vastus lateralis, situated just below and in front of the bony mass (greater trochanter) projecting from the side of your hip.
- Push the tip of your thumb from right to left into the muscle while simultaneously flexing your right knee by lunging forwards.
- Keep your body straight as you pivot around your ankle.

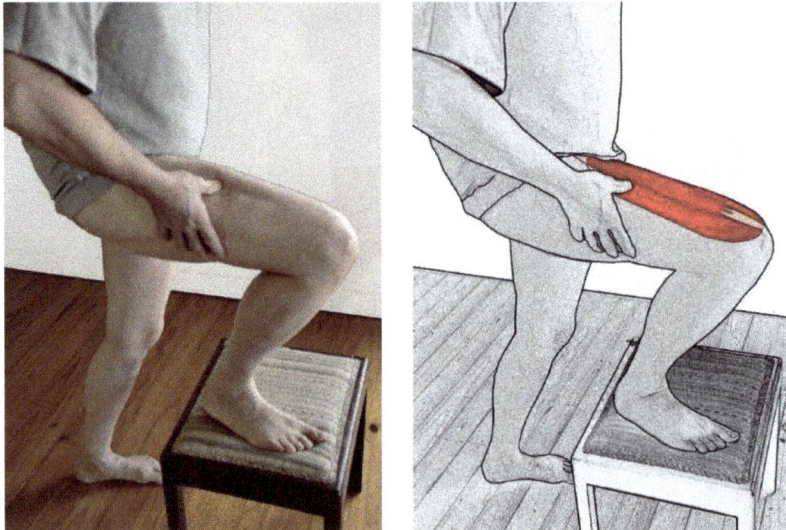

- Start at the top and right of your thigh and work down the outside thigh to the muscle attachment on the top and outside of your kneecap.
- Stay in front of the iliotibial band, the thick tendon passing down the outside of your thigh.
- Cover a series of consecutive parallel strips down vastus lateralis on the outside of your thigh, then work down rectus femoris in front of your thigh and then down vastus medialis on the inside and lower half of your thigh.
- The sartorius muscle passes diagonally down and across the front of the thigh and only the lower half of vastus medialis is available for kneading.

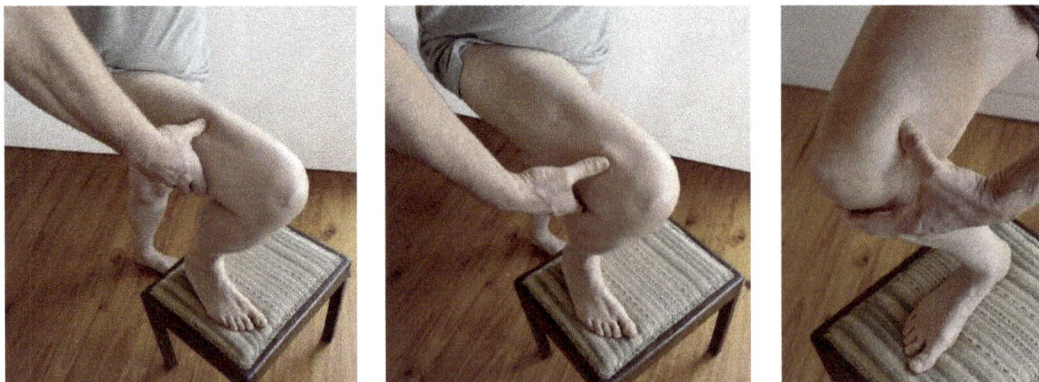

- After kneading the quadriceps muscles in a right to left direction place the tip of the thumb of your right hand on vastus lateralis again and repeat the technique pushing your thumb in a left to right direction.
- As you knead the muscle flex your right knee by lunging forwards.
- Work down all three quadriceps muscles like before.
- The muscle fibres are nearly parallel with the thigh for most of its length but curve inwards near the kneecap so to keep perpendicular with the muscle fibres your kneading should follow an arc around your kneecap.

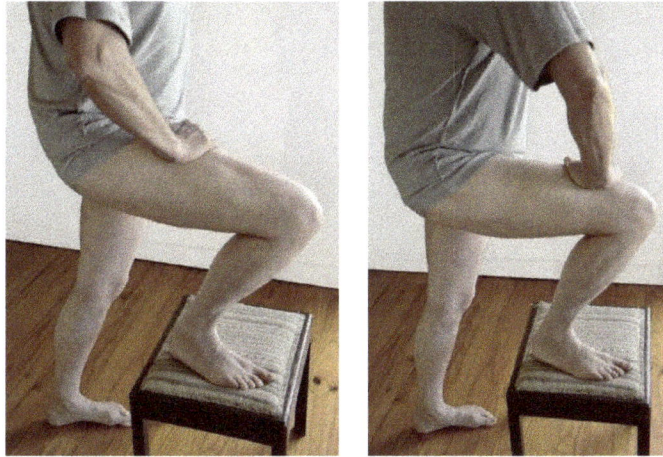

- An alternative to using the tip of your thumb is to place the heel of your hand on the outside of your thigh and your fingertips on the inside and squeeze the muscle, adding a twist of your wrist as you lunge forwards.
- The fingers of your hand point inwards when kneading vastus medialis and rectus femoris but outwards when kneading vastus lateralis.
- Another option is to place your fingertips on one side of your thigh and the tip of your thumb on the other side.
- Squeeze the muscle between your fingertips and thumbs, adding a twist of your wrist as you flex your right knee by lunging forwards.
- The fingers of your hand point inwards when kneading vastus medialis and rectus femoris and outwards when kneading vastus lateralis.

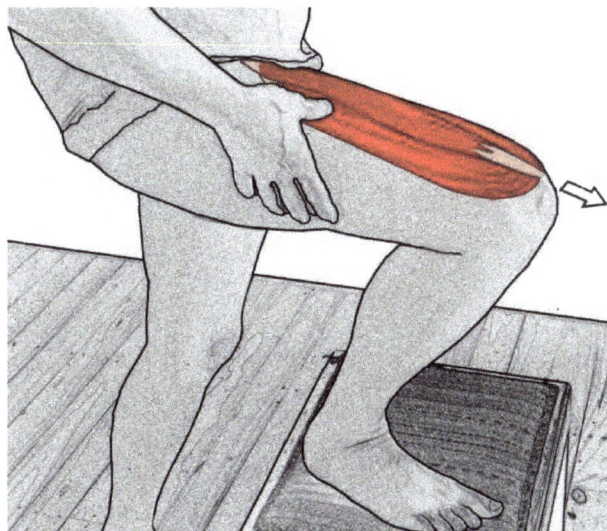

3.3b Transverse friction on the quadriceps tendon attachments on your kneecap using the tip of your thumb

- Stand straight, flex your right hip and knee and place the sole of your foot on a stool or chair in front of you.
- Place the tip of the thumb of your right hand, part of the way down the outside of your right kneecap.

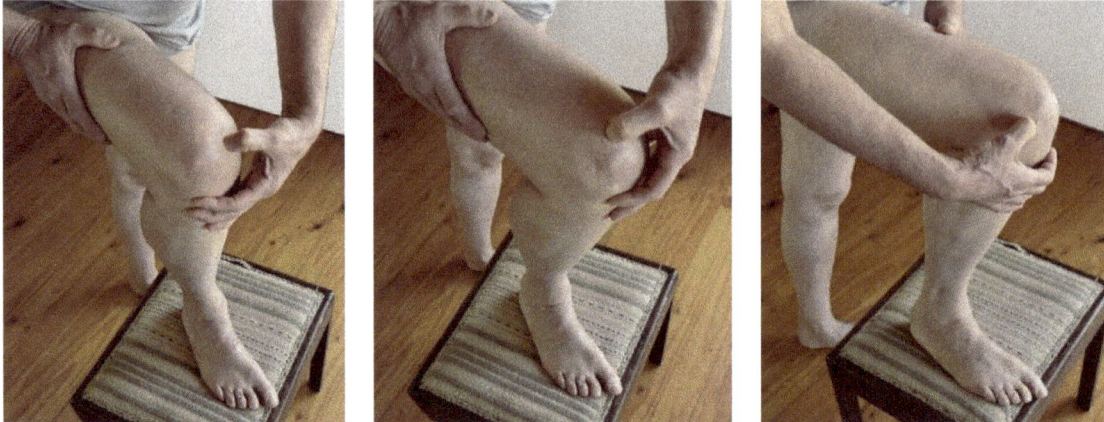

- Move your thumb up and down the edge of the kneecap and apply transverse friction on the quadriceps tendon.
- Reposition the tip of your thumb a few millimetres further up the side of the kneecap and apply transverse friction again.
- Work over the top of the kneecap and then down the inside and cover the whole tendon with transverse friction.
- The thickest part of the tendon is at the top of the kneecap.

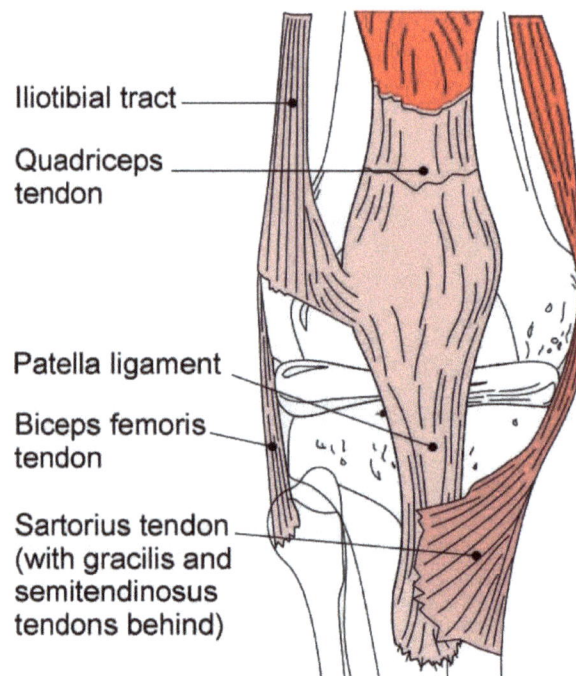

Iliotibial tract

Quadriceps tendon

Patella ligament

Biceps femoris tendon

Sartorius tendon (with gracilis and semitendinosus tendons behind)

Knee - anterior view
Femur, fibula, tibia and tendons

3.3c Transverse friction on the patella ligament attachment on the tibial tuberosity with the tip of your thumb or index finger

- Stand straight, flex your right hip and knee and place the sole of your foot on a stool or chair in front of you.
- Lean forwards and place the tip of the thumb or the tip of the index finger of your right hand on the tibial tuberosity, the large bump a few centimetres below the front of your knee.

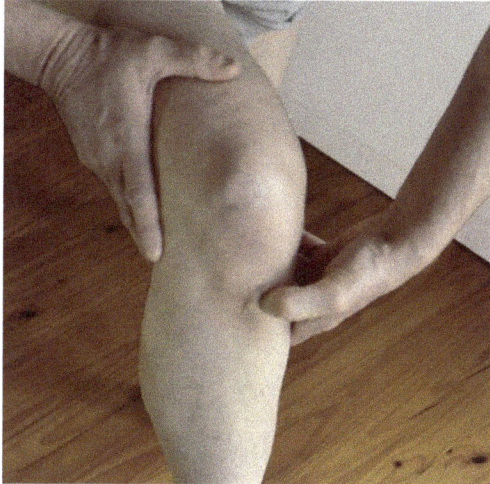

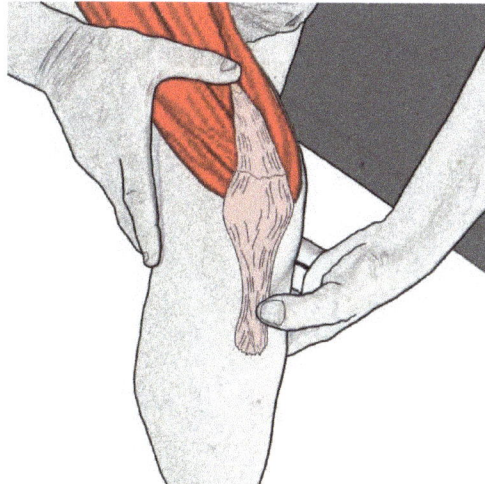

- Apply transverse friction across a small area of the quadriceps tendon which attaches on the tibial tuberosity.
- Cover the entire area of the quadriceps tendon attachment by repositioning the tip of your thumb or finger on different locations and apply transverse friction.

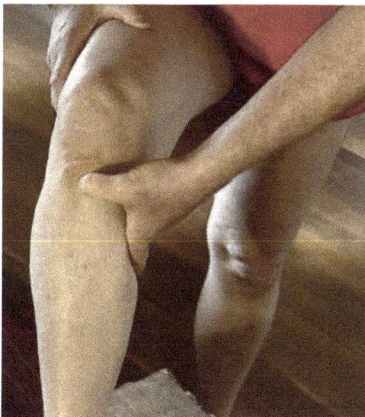

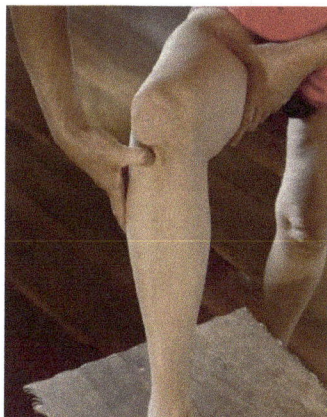

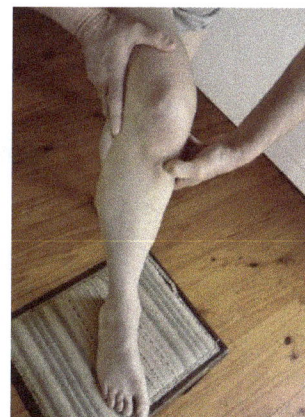

3.3d Transverse friction over the medial collateral ligament of the knee using the tip of your thumb

- Sit on a chair with your feet planted on the floor.
- Raise your right foot off the floor, externally rotate your right hip and place the outside of your leg or ankle on your left knee or lower thigh.

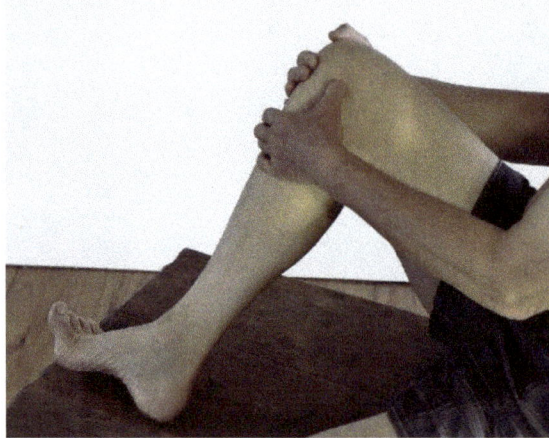

- Allow your right hip to relax so your knee drops toward the floor. Grasp your thigh just above the knee with your right hand and grasp your leg just below the knee with your left hand.
- Place the tip of your left thumb against your medial collateral ligament, which is on the inside of your knee joint.

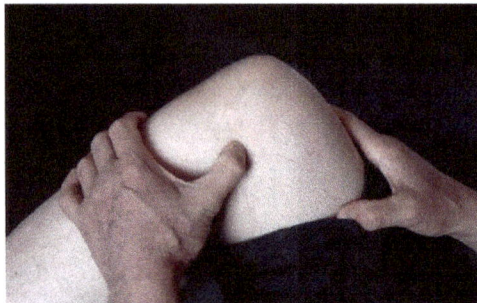

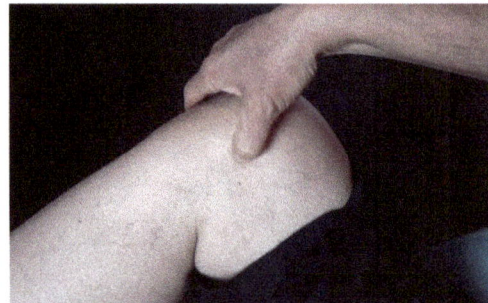

- Work across the ligament with a firm pressure with the tip of your thumb.
- Move along the joint line and then along strips parallel to the joint line.
- Points of tenderness may indicate the location of a ligament sprain.
- An alternative to crossing your legs is to place your foot on a stool or sit on the edge of a table with your foot in front of you.

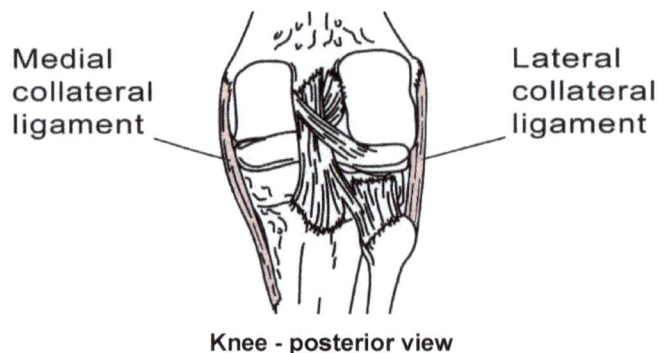

Medial collateral ligament

Lateral collateral ligament

Knee - posterior view

3.3e Transverse friction over the lateral collateral ligament of the knee using the tip of your thumb

- Sit on a chair or stand straight, flex your right hip and knee and place the sole of your foot on a stool in front of you.
- Move you right knee to the left so your thigh rotates inwards and the outside of your knee and thigh turns more upwards and there is better access to the lateral collateral ligament on the outside of your knee joint.

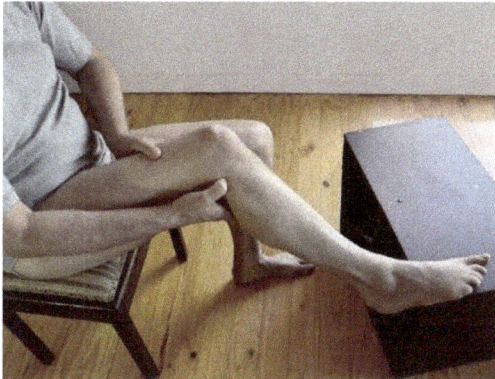

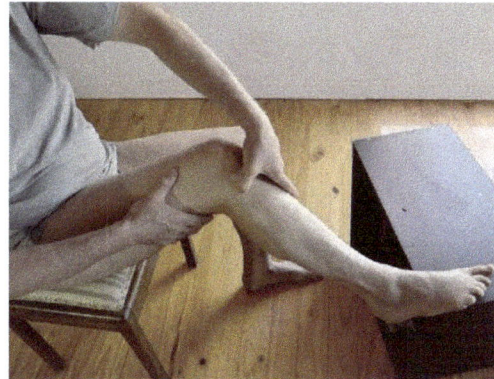

- Place the palm of your left hand on top of your knee to steady it.
- Place the thumb of your right hand on the large bump on the lower part of the outside of the knee - this is the head of the fibula.
- The lateral collateral ligament attaches here and passes over the outside of the knee joint to attach on the lateral epicondyle of the femur.
- Place the tip of the thumb of your right hand on the point the ligament attaches on the fibula head.
- Apply transverse friction with the tip of your thumb across the ligament.
- Reposition your thumb further up the ligament and apply transverse friction along the joint line.
- Repeat the transverse friction along parallel strips above the joint line and ensure you cover the whole ligament.
- Points of tenderness may indicate the location of a ligament sprain.

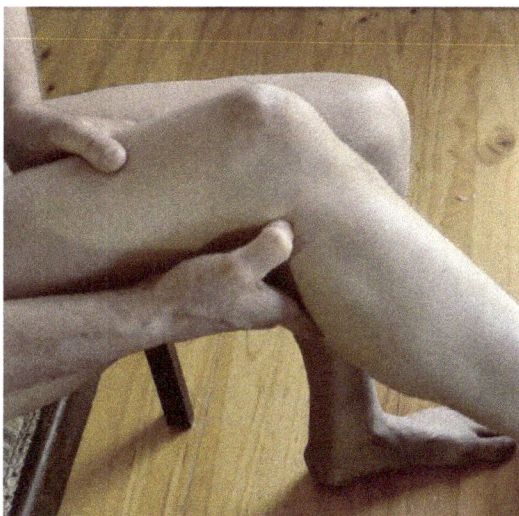

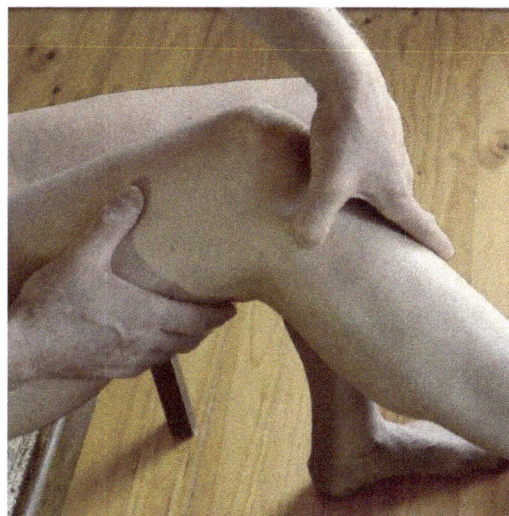

THE KNEE, LEG AND ANKLE

The calf and the posterior compartment muscles

Massaging the calf muscles can be useful for pain caused by calf muscle cramps, spasm or bruising, muscle and tendon strains, including Achilles tendon strains, knee and ankle ligament sprains and pain referred from the knee, foot or lower back, for example in sciatica. Massaging the much deeper posterior compartment muscles can be useful for pain caused by posterior shin splints.

Calf pain and lumps in the back of leg can be the result of serious problems like a blood clot (deep vein thrombosis). This can develop at any age, but your risk is greater after age 40 and in people who are physically unfit or sedentary. If you have doubts about massaging a painful calf, get a diagnosis from your doctor.

A cramp is an involuntary muscle contraction that usually starts as extreme pain for a few minutes then milder pain and stiffness. Repeated cramping may leave fibrous masses within the muscle. A calf strain is a tear in the muscle. It may be acute from overstretching or over-contraction or chronic from repetitive injuries. A mild acute strain can produce pain, swelling, bruising or stiffness whereas a chronic strain can also affect your ability to walk.

A calf muscle bruise may occur after a direct blow to the lower leg. A severe bruise should not be treated aggressively with massage because of the danger of causing further bleeding and unwanted bone formation within the muscle.

Achilles tendon strains can occur when the tendon is over-stretched. Repeated strains and overuse can lead to Achilles tendinitis with symptoms of pain and inflammation at the site of injury. Tendinitis and tenosynovitis can also develop as the tibialis posterior tendon passes behind the medial malleolus.

Posterior shin splints, also known as medial tibial stress syndrome, is a strain at the muscle-tendon-bone junction of tibialis posterior at the back and inside of the leg brought on by exercises such as running and jumping. Symptoms include dull pain, swelling and tenderness down the lower half of the back of the leg.

The calf muscles

Gastrocnemius is the most superficial muscle running down the back and outside of the leg and **soleus** is deeper. Both attach on the Achilles tendon.

The Achilles tendon extends about half the length of the leg. It is broad and flat superiorly and becomes thicker and rounded as it descends. Its fibres spiral and give the tendon elastic properties which facilitate gait. The tendon is strong but may be ruptured.

168

Gastrocnemius forms the bulk of the calf and arises by two heads attached to the medial and lateral femoral condyles by strong flat tendons and from the knee joint capsule. Fibrous expansions from the tendons of both heads extend inferiorly over the posterior surface of the muscles. The heads are separated by an aponeurosis which attaches to its posterior surface, and this tendinous expansion forms the Achilles tendon.

The muscle produces foot and ankle plantar flexion and knee flexion and assists with balance and knee stability. It exhibits only intermittent contraction during standing.

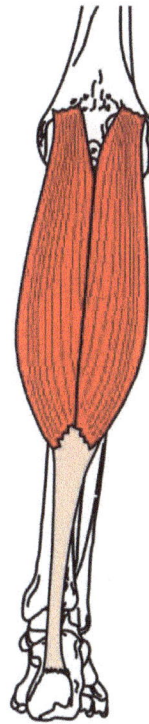

Soleus arises from a posterior area of the upper fibula, the head of the fibula, the soleal line at the back of the tibia and the upper medial tibia, and from the posterior surface of an aponeurosis which spans between the tibia and fibula. The muscle fibres insert on the anterior surface of the Achilles tendon, which then inserts onto the middle of the posterior calcaneus. Soleus is deep to gastrocnemius and only directly palpable at the bottom and sides of the leg.

The muscle produces plantar flexion and assists with balance. Soleus is continuously active during standing.

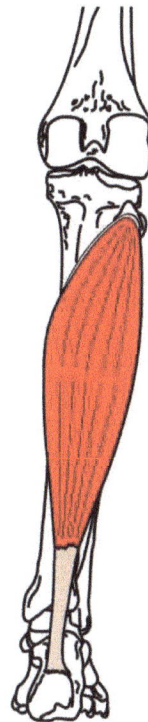

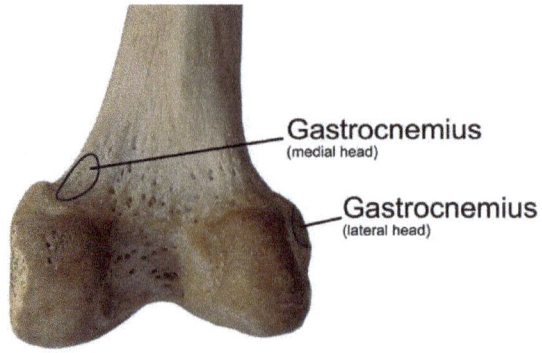

Gastrocnemius
(medial head)

Gastrocnemius
(lateral head)

Femur - posterior view

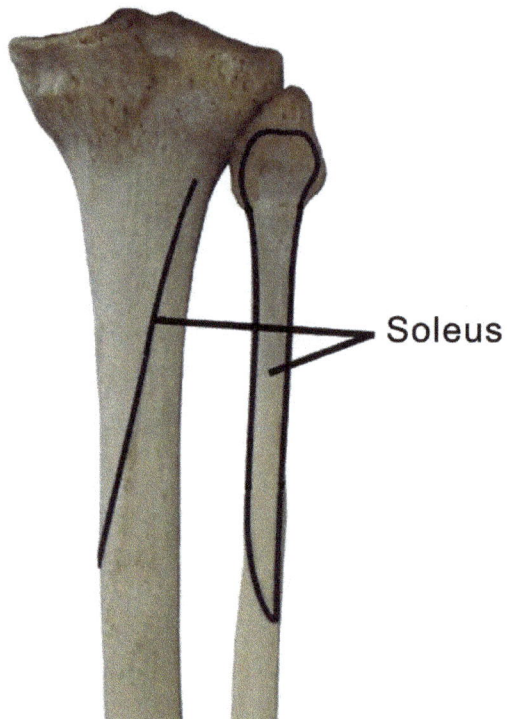

Soleus

Tibia and fibula - posterior view

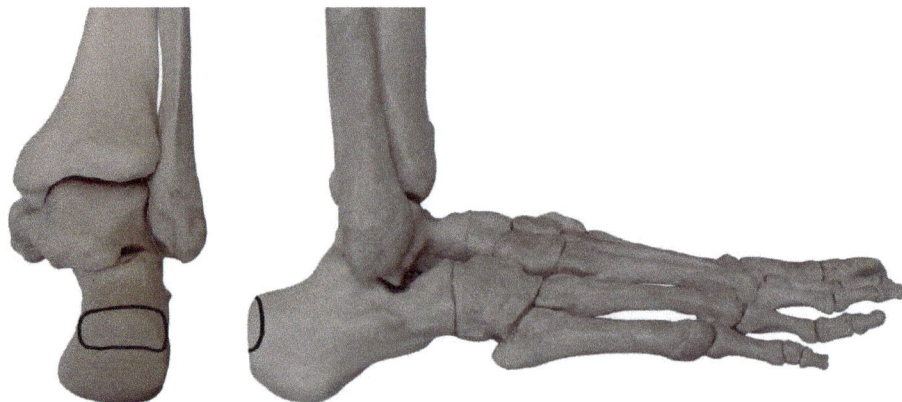

Lower leg, ankle and foot showing attachment of Achilles tendon

3.4a Kneading gastrocnemius and soleus using a rolling action of two balls in a net

- This is similar to the rolling technique for the hamstrings 3.2f.
- Sit on the floor with your legs straight out in front.
- Flex your right hip and knee and place the two balls or a rolled-up towel across the top of the gastrocnemius muscles behind the knee.
- Place one ball under one gastrocnemius head and one under the other.
- Return your leg and the balls to the floor so the back of your calf rests on the balls and the balls rest on the floor and relax your hip and knee.
- Contract your quadriceps, straighten your knee and allow your heel to come off the floor.
- Do not push your leg into the balls - solely use the weight of your leg to apply sufficient pressure on the muscles.
- Point your heel and bring your toes towards you to stretch the muscle.
- Roll your leg a few centimetres up and down over the balls by moving your pelvis forwards and backwards.

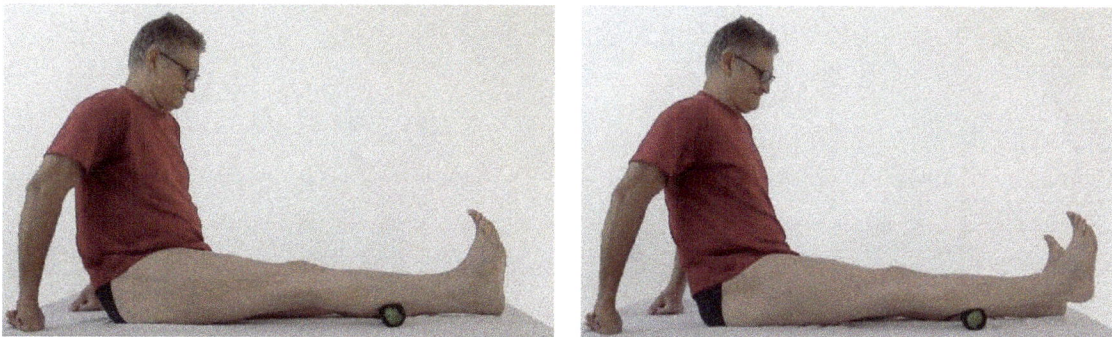

- Relax your calf muscles as you move your leg over the balls.
- After rolling a few times over the muscles return your heel to the floor and reposition the balls on a new part of the muscle further down your leg.
- Contract your quadriceps and point your heel away again and repeat the rolling action.
- Repeat the rolling action on different areas of the calf until you are at the end of the muscle and the beginning of the Achilles tendon.
- To knead the soleus muscle, reposition the balls or rolled-up towel across the muscle, starting a couple of centimetres below the back of the knee.
- Keep your right knee bent, quadriceps relaxed and your heel on the floor.
- Point your heel and bring your toes towards you to put the calf on stretch.
- Roll your leg up and down over the balls by moving your pelvis forwards and backwards but keep your heel on the floor and pointed away.
- Relax your calf muscles as you move over the balls.
- After rolling a few times over the muscles reposition the balls on a new part of the muscle further down the leg and repeat the rolling action.
- Repeat the rolling action over different areas of the soleus until you are at the end of the muscle and the beginning of the Achilles tendon.

3.4b Pin and stretch gastrocnemius and soleus using a tightly rolled-up towel or two balls in a net

- This is similar to the pin and stretch technique for the hamstrings 3.2e.
- Sit on the floor with your legs straight out in front.
- Flex your right hip and knee and place the two balls or a rolled-up towel across the calf muscles, a couple of centimetres below the knee.
- Position the two balls so that one ball rests on one gastrocnemius head and the other ball rests on the other.
- Return your leg and the balls to the floor and relax your hip and knee.
- Contract your quadriceps, straighten your knee and allow your heel to come off the floor.
- Point your toes away so your foot is in full plantar flexion.
- Press your leg down towards the floor and onto the balls to pin the muscle against the balls.
- Maintain the downward pressure against the balls and slowly point your heel away until your foot is in full dorsiflexion and hold it there.
- After about three seconds relax your quadriceps, return your heel to the floor and reposition the balls further down your leg.

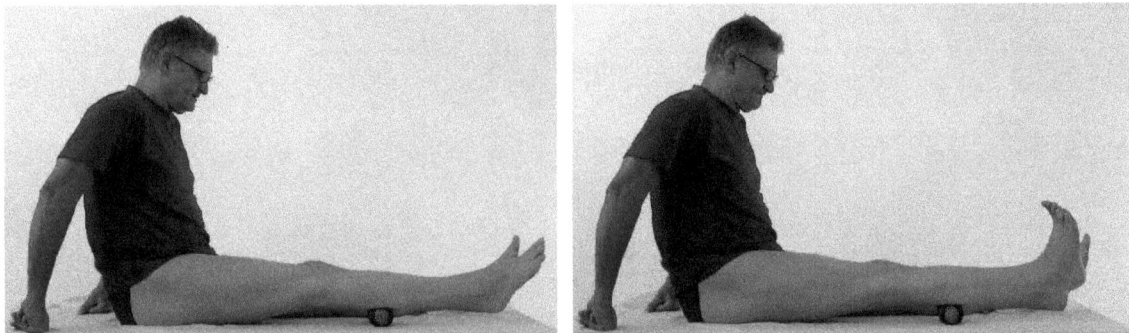

- Repeat the pin and stretch action and then work down the muscle using pin and stretch until you are at the start of the Achilles tendon.
- Pin and stretch on the soleus muscle is best done with the rolled-up towel placed across the muscle, a couple of centimetres below the knee.
- Keep your right knee bent, quadriceps relaxed and your heel on the floor.
- Point your toes away so your foot is in full plantar flexion.
- Press your leg down towards the floor and onto the rolled-up towel to pin the muscle against the rolled-up towel but do not straighten your knee.
- Maintain the bent knee and downward pressure on the rolled-up towel and slowly point your heel away until your foot is in full dorsiflexion and hold it.
- After about three seconds relax your muscles, flex your knee, reposition the rolled-up towel further down your leg and repeat the pin and stretch.
- Repeat the pin and stretch action on different parts of the muscle until you are at the end of the muscle and the beginning of the Achilles tendon.
- Towards the lower half of soleus you may need to flex your knee to prevent your heel lifting off the floor - but keep your leg pressed down against the rolled-up towel.

3.4c Kneading gastrocnemius using your fingertips and the tip of your thumb

- Sit on the floor with your legs out in front.
- Flex your right hip and knee.
- Reach towards your right leg with both hands.
- Place the tip of the thumb of your right hand against the back of your knee, near the outside and behind the lateral head of gastrocnemius.
- Place the tip of the thumb of your left hand against the back of your knee, near the inside and behind the medial head of gastrocnemius.

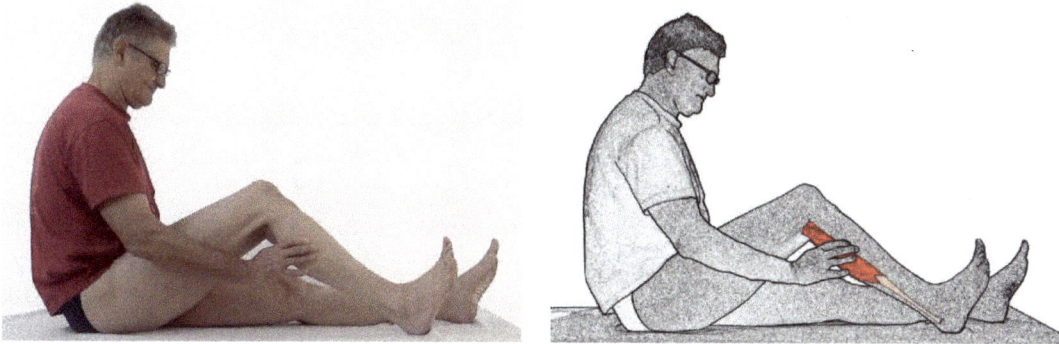

- Place the fingertips of your right hand in front of the muscle, which is just around the outside of the knee.
- Place the fingertips of your left hand in front of the muscle, which is just around the inside of the knee.
- Hook your fingers and thumbs around both heads of gastrocnemius, close to where they attach behind the knee.
- Push into the muscles with your thumbs and pull back on them with your fingertips while simultaneously pointing your heel away and bringing your toes towards you to puts the muscle on stretch.

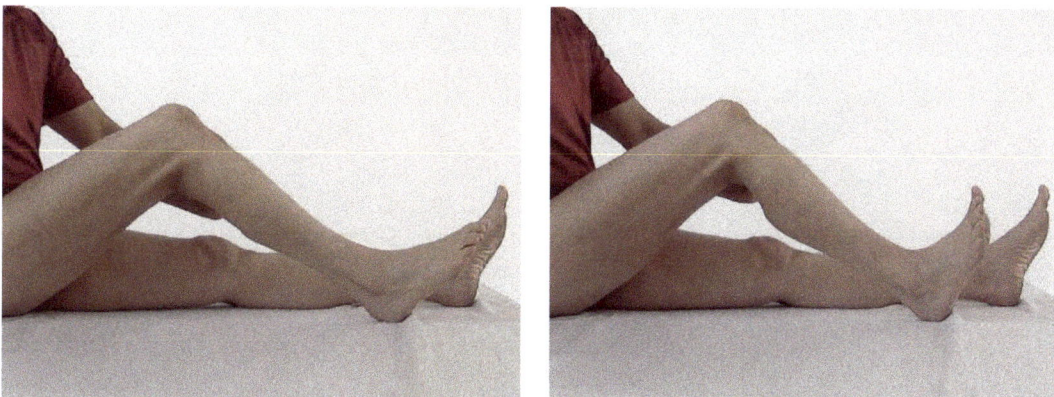

- Add a little rotation with a push-pull twisting action of the wrists.
- Work down the muscle from the knee to the start of the Achilles tendon.
- This technique can be done using just the thumb and fingers of one hand to knead one of the heads of gastrocnemius.

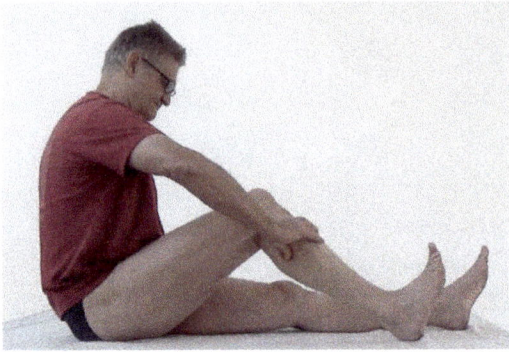

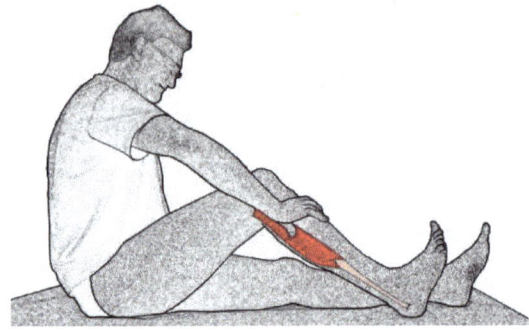

Other options for kneading gastrocnemius include:

- Rest your fingers in front of your leg and push the tip of the thumb of your right hand in a medial direction against the outside of the lateral head of gastrocnemius while pointing your heel away
- Push the tip of your left thumb in a lateral direction against the inside of the medial head of gastrocnemius while pointing your heel away
- Reach under your right knee with your left hand and pull against the outside of the lateral head of gastrocnemius with your fingertips
- Similarly pull against the inside of the medial head of gastrocnemius with the fingers of your right hand

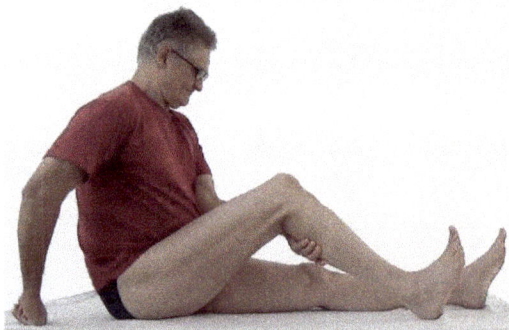

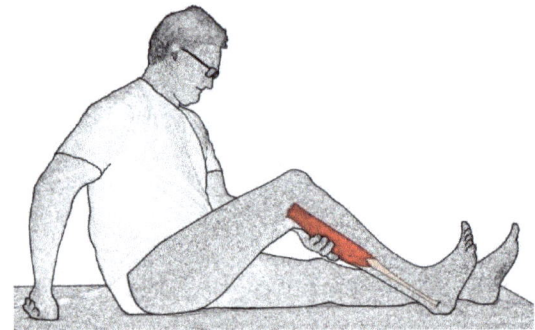

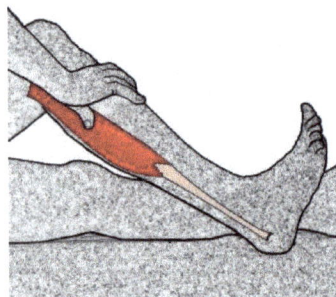

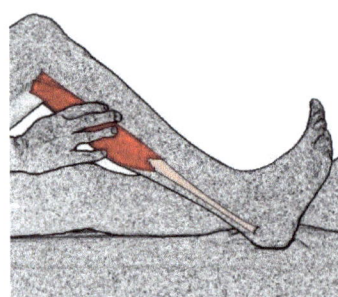

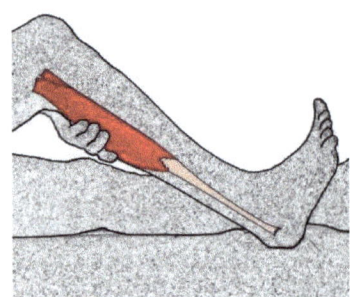

The posterior compartment muscles

The posterior compartment consists of **tibialis posterior,** the deepest muscle, **flexor digitorum longus** and **flexor hallucis longus.** The tendons of the deep posterior muscles pass behind the medial malleolus and into the foot. From medial to lateral they are the tibialis posterior tendon, flexor digitorum longus tendon and the flexor hallucis longus tendon. The calf muscles and deeper posterior compartment muscles are separated by a thick layer of deep transverse fascia in the back of the leg.

Tibialis posterior arises on the lateral side of the proximal half of the posterior shaft of the tibia, along the medial side of the proximal two thirds of the posterior shaft of the fibula and the posterior interosseous membrane, deep transverse fascia and intermuscular septa. It is the deepest of the flexor muscles.

The tendon passes over a groove behind the medial malleolus and then goes under the foot. It splits and attaches on the navicular bone, first and second cuneiforms, calcaneus and metatarsals 2, 3, and 4. The tendon is prominent below the malleolus with resisted inversion and plantar flexion of the foot.

The muscle produces inversion of the foot and assists with plantar flexion and adduction. It supports the arch during gait.

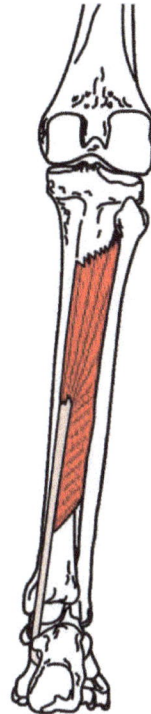

Flexor Digitorum longus arises along the medial side of the posterior shaft of the tibia, just below the soleal line, and on the fascia covering tibialis posterior. The tendon passes over a groove behind the medial malleolus. It attaches onto the bases of the distal phalanges of the lateral four toes. The tendon is palpable behind and below the medial malleolus and is prominent with resisted toe flexion. The muscle flexes toes and assists in inversion, adduction and plantar flexion of the foot.

Flexor Hallucis longus arises along two thirds of the medial side of the posterior shaft of the fibula, the interosseous membrane and the fascia covering tibialis posterior. The tendon attaches on the plantar surface of the base of the distal phalanx of the big toe. The muscle flexes the big toe and assists in inversion, adduction and plantar flexion of the foot. It is most active in the push off phase of gait.

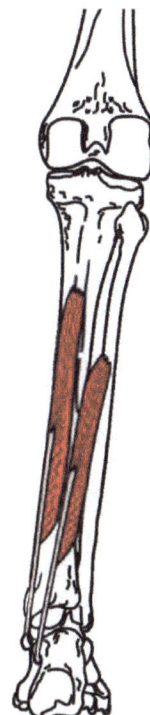

175

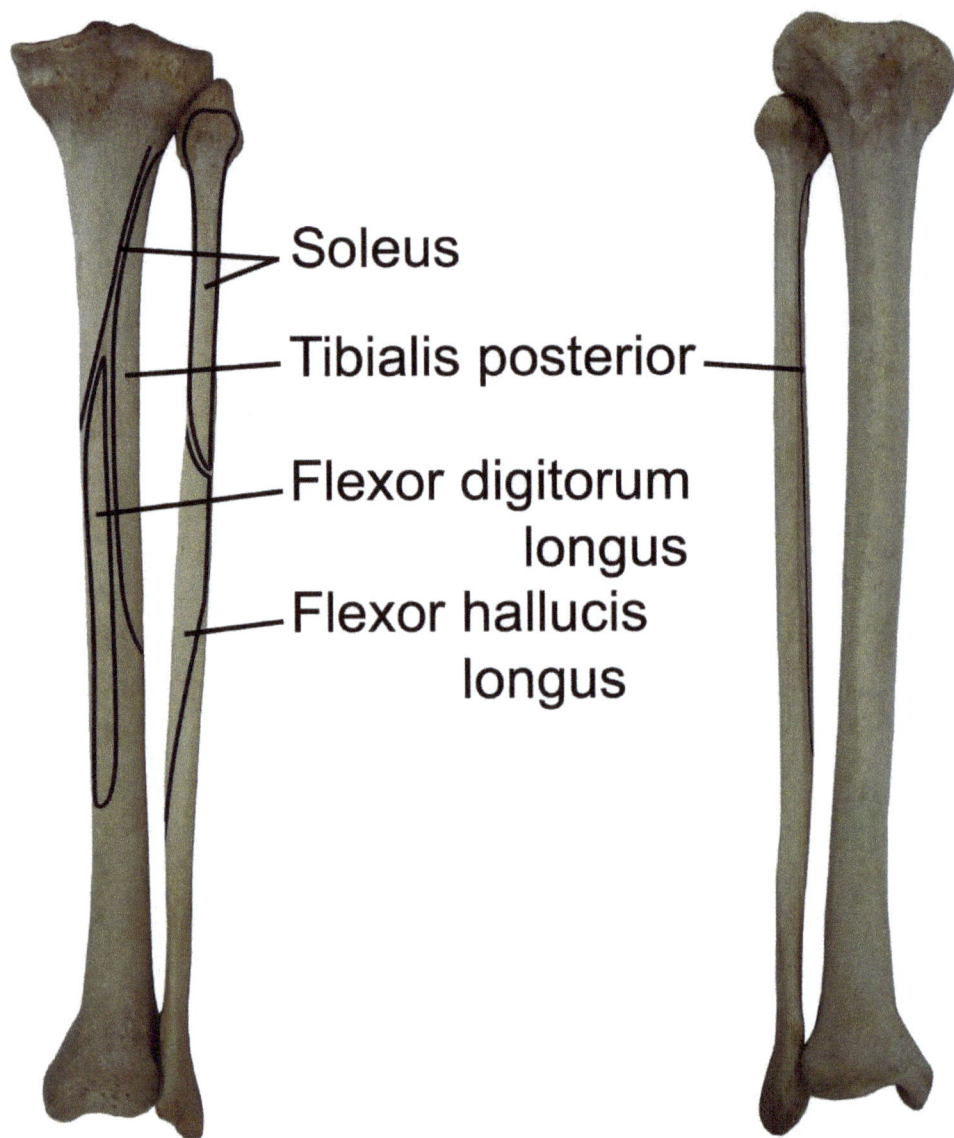

Soleus

Tibialis posterior

Flexor digitorum longus

Flexor hallucis longus

Tibia and fibula - posterior view (left) anterior view (right)

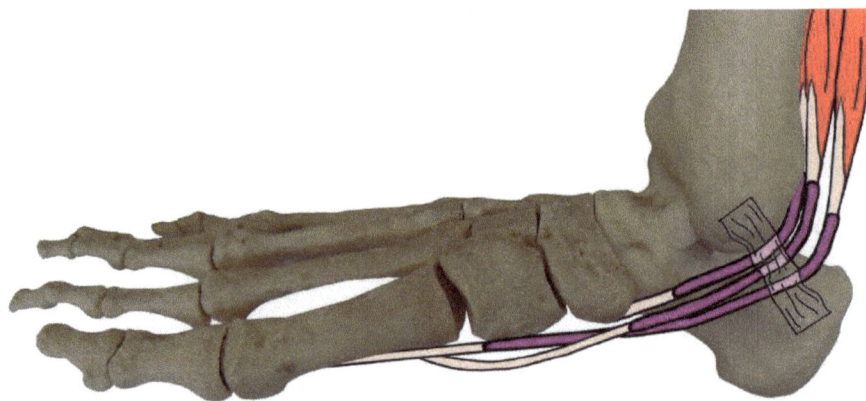

Right foot - medial view - tendons and synovial sheaths of tibialis posterior, flexor digitorum longus and flexor hallucis longus

3.4d Kneading soleus and the posterior compartment muscles using the tips of your thumbs

- Sit on the floor with your legs out in front of you.
- Flex your right hip and knee.
- Reach towards your right leg with both hands.
- Bring your thumbs together and place the tips of both thumbs against the back of your leg, near the top and towards the outside.

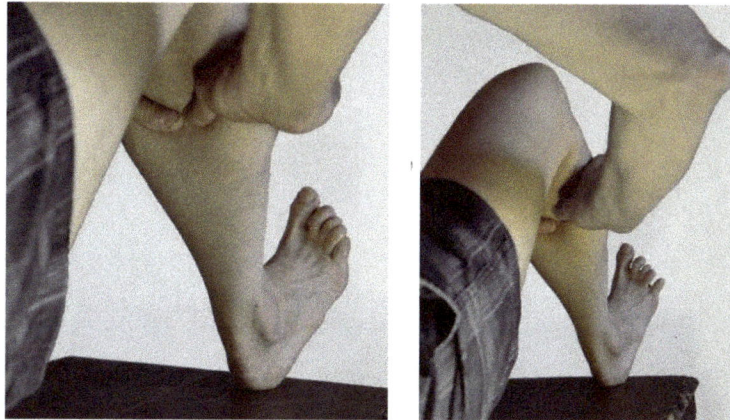

- Place the pads of the fingers of your right hand against the outside of your leg and the pads of the fingers of your left hand against the inside.
- Push into the muscles with both thumbs while simultaneously pointing your heel away to put the muscle on a mild stretch.
- Work from the knee, down the lateral part of soleus and deeper posterior compartment muscles on the outside and back of your leg, to the start of the Achilles tendon.

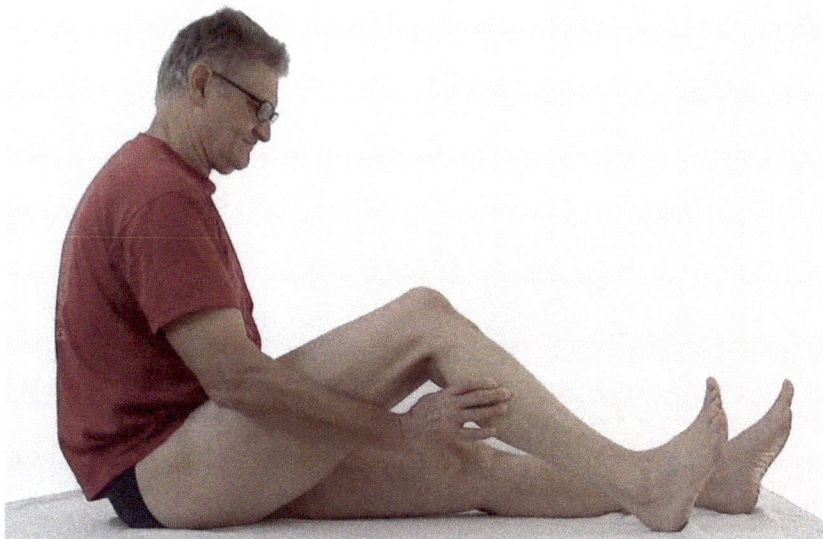

- Place the tips of both thumbs against the back of your leg, near the top and towards the inside.
- Place the pads of your fingers towards the front of your leg.
- Push into the muscles with both thumbs while simultaneously pointing your heel away to put the muscle on a mild stretch.

- Work from the knee, down the medial part of soleus and deeper posterior compartment muscles on the inside and back of your leg, to the start of the Achilles tendon.
- Repeat the technique down the middle of the back of your leg.
- To reach the soleus and the posterior compartment muscles you must push through gastrocnemius and overlying fascia.
- Do not dorsiflex your foot so hard that it makes gastrocnemius too tight to work through.
- Keep the knee flexed to relax gastrocnemius.
- Use a firm but broad pressure.

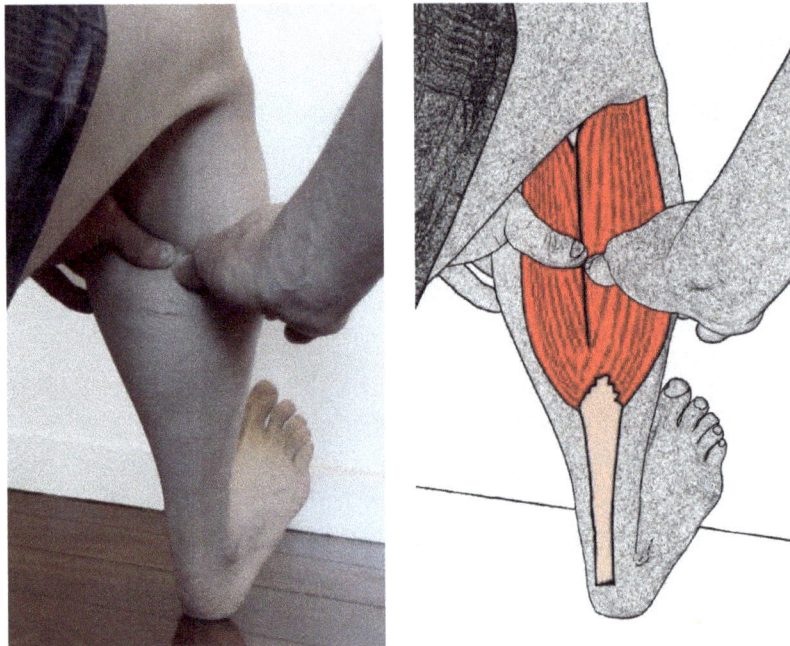

View of gastrocnemius muscle and posterior leg

In the lower half of the leg lateral fibres of soleus arise from the lateral side of the Achilles tendon and from under the lateral head of gastrocnemius. Similarly, medial fibres of soleus arise from the medial side of the Achilles tendon and from under the medial head of gastrocnemius. These two parts of soleus can be kneaded on either side of your leg using the tip of your thumb.

- o Place the fingertips of your right hand against the front of your right leg and the tip of your right thumb against the outside of the lower part of soleus and push your thumb in a medial direction while simultaneously pointing your heel away
- o Place the fingertips of your left hand against the front of your right leg and the tip of your left thumb against the inside of the lower part of soleus and push your thumb in a lateral direction while simultaneously pointing your heel away.

The Achilles tendon

The Achilles tendon arises from the calf muscles as a broad flat structure and becomes thicker and rounded as it descends the back of the lower half of the leg. Its fibres spiral which gives the tendon elastic properties which facilitate gait.

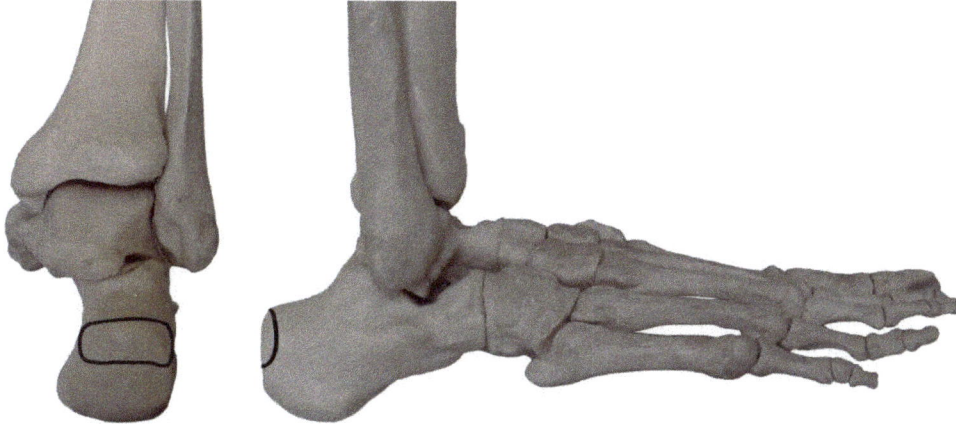

Lower leg, ankle and foot showing attachment of Achilles tendon

3.4e Transverse friction on the Achilles tendon

- Sit on a chair or stool.
- Lift your right foot off the floor, rotate your hip and place the outside of your ankle on the top of your left thigh, just above your knee.
- Allow your right knee to drop down towards the floor.
- Reach forward and grasp your right ankle with your right hand.
- Reach forward and grasp the heel of your right foot with your left hand.

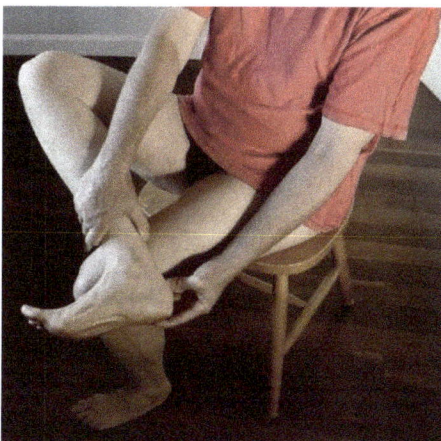

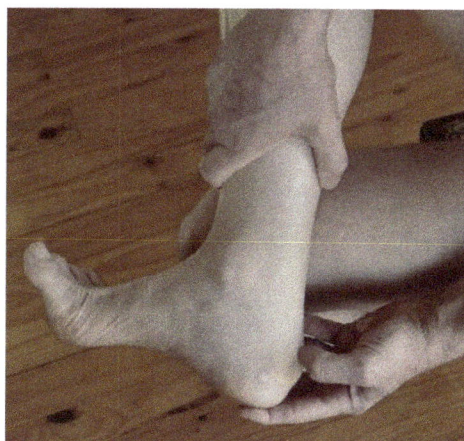

- Place the tip of the thumb of your left hand on the top and inside of the back of your heel - the Achilles tendon attachment on the calcaneus.
- Use a firm pressure and move the tip of your thumb a few millimetres across this part of the tendon attachment for three to five seconds.
- Apply transverse friction across the top of the tendon attachment and then along parallel lines below this until the entire Achilles tendon attachment on the calcaneus is covered.

Popliteus

Massaging popliteus can be useful when there is pain at the back of the knee caused by a popliteus muscle strain or a strain of another lower limb muscle or one of the knee ligaments or tendons.

Popliteus can be strained when the partially flexed knee is subject to forced hyperextension, rotation or sidebending during walking, running or skiing downhill or navigating a sloping terrain. The strain may be accompanied by an injury to another structure such as a knee ligament. Symptoms may also include joint stiffness, swelling and a feeling of fullness in the back of the knee.

Popliteus is a small, thin, flat, triangular shaped muscle situated deeply at the back of the knee. It arises on the lateral femoral condyle and runs diagonally across the back of the knee joint to attach on a broad area at the top and back of the tibia, above soleus.

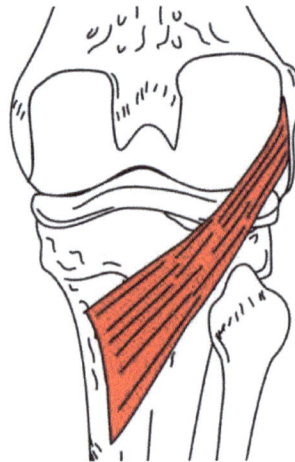

Popliteus - posterior view of knee

Popliteus is a flexor and internal rotator of the knee, and it prevents the femur from slipping forwards on the tibia during squatting. It initiates knee flexion from the fully extended position and unlocks the knee by laterally rotating the femur on the tibia at the start of flexion. It is important for knee stability and function.

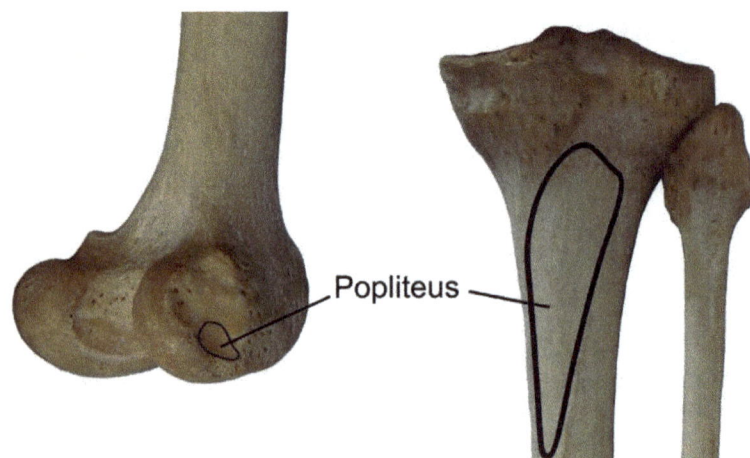

Femur - posterior lateral view (left) Tibia and fibula - posterior view (right)

3.5a Kneading popliteus using your fingertips, while sitting on the floor

- Sit on the floor with your legs out in front of you.
- Flex your right hip and knee.
- Reach towards your right leg with both hands and grasp your knee.
- Place the palm of your right hand against the outside of your knee and your fingertips behind the back of your knee, towards the outside.
- Place the palm of your left hand against the inside of your knee and your fingertips behind the back of your knee, towards the inside.

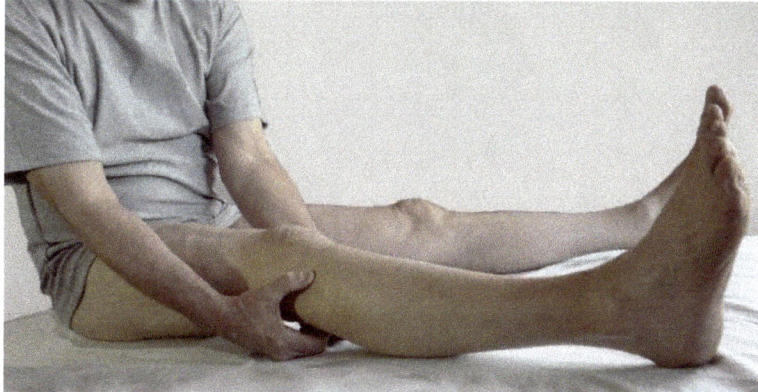

- Place your thumbs in front of your knee, one on either side.
- Return your knee and both hands to the floor so the back of your fingers rest on the floor and the back of your knee rests on your fingertips.
- Keep your fingers flexed.
- Attempt to straighten your leg by pushing the back of your knee into your fingertips and towards the floor.

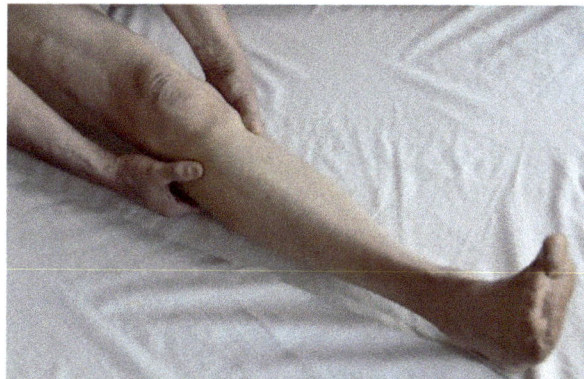

- Do not straighten your knee completely or bring your heel off the floor.
- As you push harder with your knee this increases the fingertip pressure on the popliteus muscle.
- Relax your calf muscles by keeping your ankle in a neutral position.
- Slowly push down and then hold your fingertip pressure on the popliteus muscle for three to five seconds.
- Relax your leg, flex your hip and knee and reposition your fingertips on another part of the popliteus muscle.
- Follow a diagonal line across the back of the knee from the top and outside to the bottom and inside until the entire muscle is covered.

3.5b Kneading popliteus using your fingertips, while laying on your back

- Lie on your back with your hips and knees flexed.
- Flex your right hip so your thigh is about vertical.
- Reach around the outside of your right knee with your right hand and reach around the inside of your right knee with your left hand and place the tips of your hooked fingers against the back of your knee.
- Place the pads of your thumbs against the front and sides of your knee.

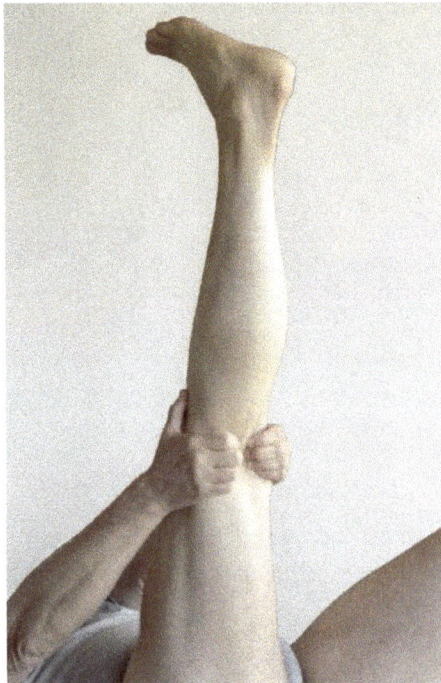

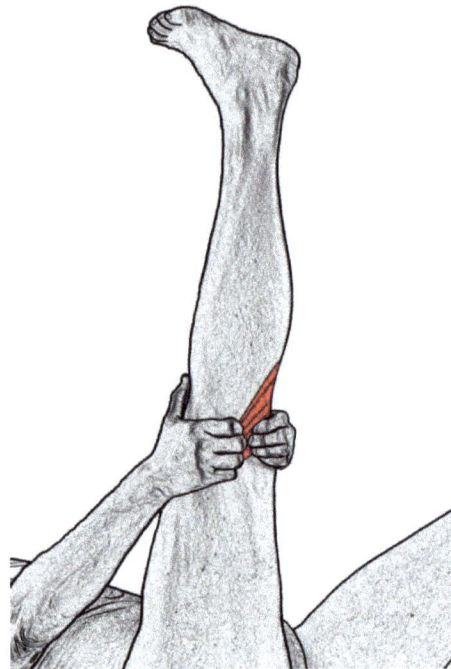

- Push your fingertips into the popliteus muscle situated at the back of your knee while simultaneously straightening your right knee.
- Straightening your leg stretches the popliteus muscle and adds a counterforce against the pressure of your fingertips.
- Keep your arms in a fixed position, with your elbows straight or slightly bent.
- Work over the entire popliteus muscle behind and just below your knee.

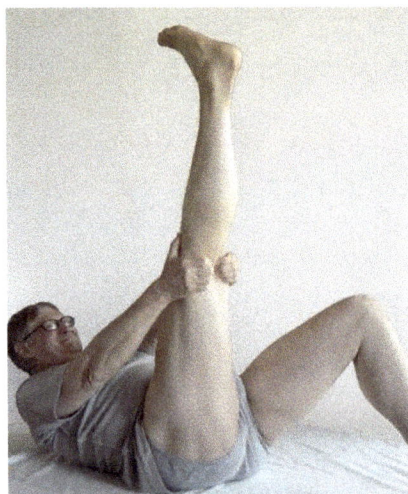

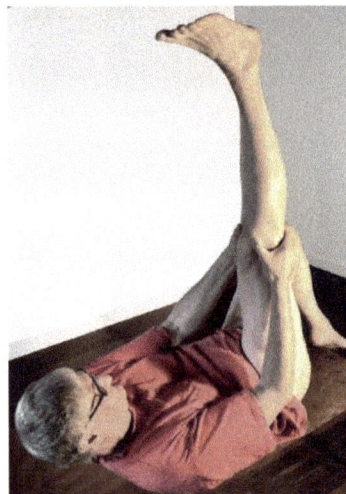

The anterior compartment muscles

Massaging tibialis anterior and other anterior compartment muscles can be useful when there is pain in front of the leg as a result of a tibialis anterior muscle or tendon strain, stress fracture, chronic exertional compartment syndrome or anterior shin splints. These conditions have similar characteristics, and it is important to get an accurate diagnosis before using massage.

Tibialis anterior tendinitis may be caused by repetitive kicking or running or running on uneven surfaces or from wearing badly designed shoes. Symptoms include ankle stiffness, swelling, weakness and pain at the top of the foot.

Chronic exertional compartment syndrome is a painful condition resulting from the build-up of pressure in a muscle compartment during exercise. It usually occurs in the anterior compartment of the lower leg in young adult runners. The pain is described as burning, aching, tight, cramping or squeezing pain. There may be tenderness in the muscle or tendon and swelling in front of the leg.

Anterior shin splints are a strain at the muscle-tendon-bone junction of tibialis anterior, brought on by exercises. Cumulative stress from overuse or repetitive use causes pain and swelling. The pain is usually dull but may be sharp. There may be tenderness along the sharp edge of the bone at the front of the leg. Small stress fractures can develop leading to muscle weakness, foot drop and problems with gait. It may occur in someone who is unfit and just starting exercise, or during stop-start activities, running on uneven or hard surfaces or over long distances. Stress fractures of the tibia can occur with overuse or repetitive use and they can develop with relatively mild force if there is an underlying pathology, such as osteoporosis.

Tibialis anterior arises on the lateral tibial condyle and proximal two thirds of the anterolateral surface of the tibia, the interosseous membrane, the intermuscular septum between it and extensor digitorum longus, and on the deep surface of the deep fascia of the leg. The tendon attaches on the medial and inferior side of the first cuneiform and the base of the first metatarsal.

Tibialis anterior is the most superficial muscle in the anterior compartment and lies lateral to the sharp subcutaneous border of the tibia. Its tendon is prominent with resisted dorsi flexion of the foot.

The muscle dorsiflexes and inverts the foot and helps supports the arch. It is active during gait by slowing plantar flexion after heel strike, so the foot does not slap down onto the ground, and by maintaining dorsiflexion and holding the foot upwards so it does not drag along the ground during the swing phase.

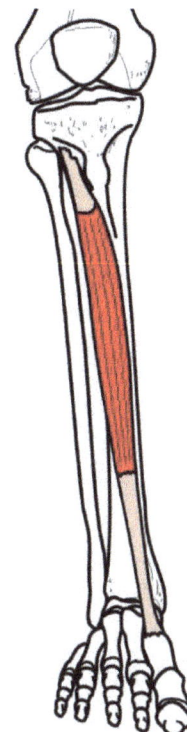

Extensor hallucis longus (left) arises on the middle of the fibula shaft and interosseous membrane and attaches onto the base of the distal phalanx of the big toe. The muscle lies deep in the anterior compartment. The tendon is prominent with resisted extension of the big toe.

The muscle extends the big toe and dorsiflexes the foot.

Extensor digitorum longus (right) arises on the lateral tibial condyle, upper two-thirds of the anterior fibula, interosseous membrane, and on deep fascia of the leg. The tendon splits into four tendons which attach onto the bases of the middle and distal phalanges of the lateral four toes.

The muscle extends the toes and dorsiflexes the foot.

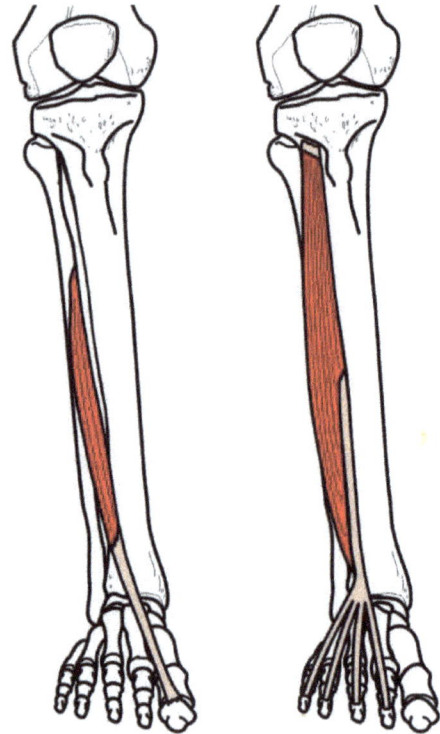

Extensor digitorum longus

Extensor hallucis longus

Tibialis anterior

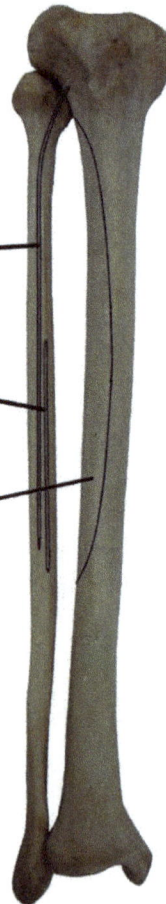

Tibia and fibula - anterior view

184

3.6a Kneading tibialis anterior and other anterior compartment muscle using two balls in a net or a tightly rolled-up towel

- Kneel on a carpet or mat on the floor.
- Grasp two balls in a net with your right hand.
- Raise your right knee off the floor, reach under your leg with your right hand and place one of the two balls under the muscles at the top and front of your leg and near your knee.

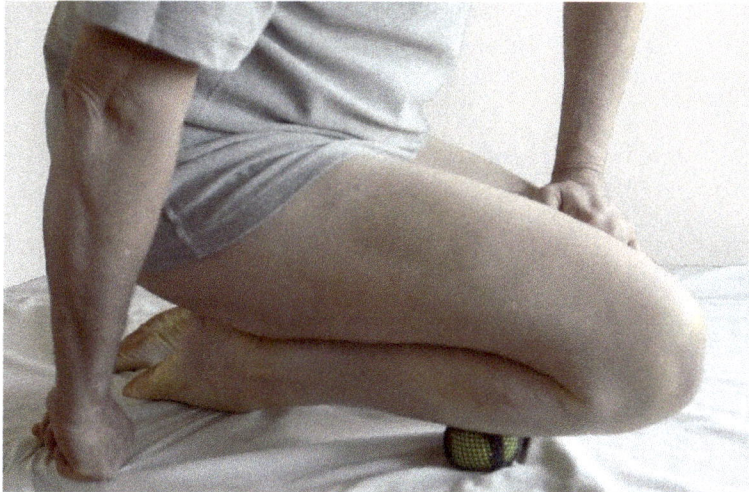

- Return your knee and the balls to the floor so the muscles at the front of your leg rest on one of the balls.
- Attempt to dorsiflex your foot by pushing the top of your foot and toes into the floor and lean your body backwards.
- Allow the ball to push into the muscles in front of your leg.

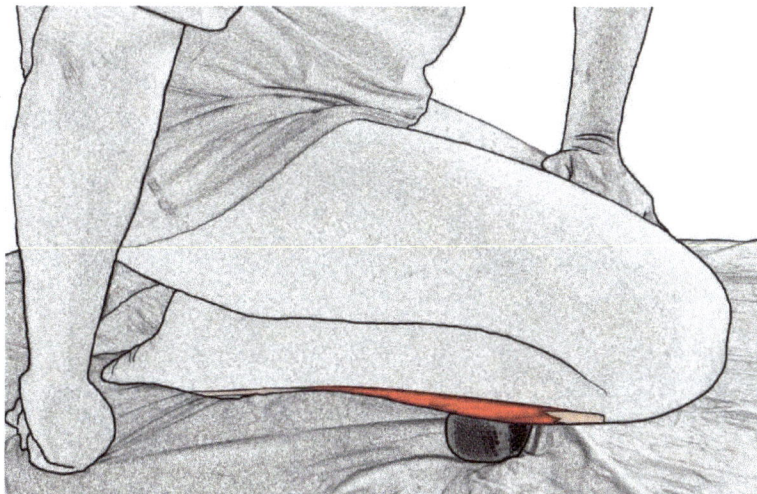

- After a few seconds cease the contraction, relax, lean forwards and allow the weight of your body to increase the downward pressure into the ball.
- After a few seconds of passive pressure on the ball lift your knee off the ball on the floor and reposition it further down the front of your leg.
- Work from just below your knee, down the front of your leg, almost to your ankle until the entire anterior compartment is covered.

3.6b Kneading tibialis anterior and other anterior compartment muscle using the tips and pads of your fingers while seated in a chair

- Sit on a chair or stool with your feet planted on the floor.
- Flex your right knee and place the top of your toes on the floor.

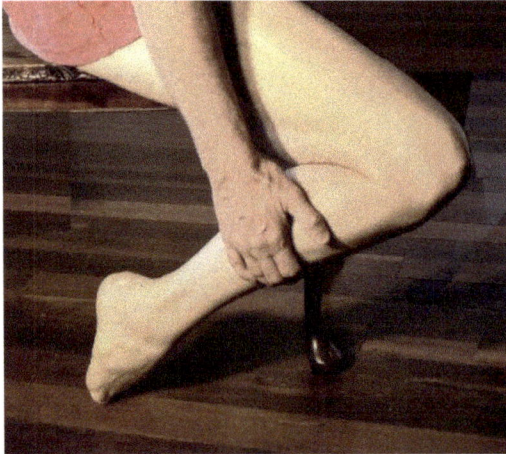

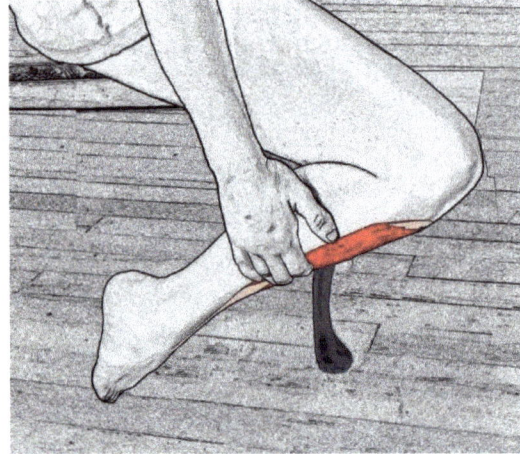

- Lean forwards and place the pads of the fingers of your right hand on the muscles in the front of your leg and the tips of your fingers against the sharp border of your tibia - start at the top of your leg near your knee.
- Curl your fingers until they are in a fixed hooked position.
- Lean backwards, allow your arm to straighten a bit and feel the pads of your finger press into the muscles running down the front of your leg.

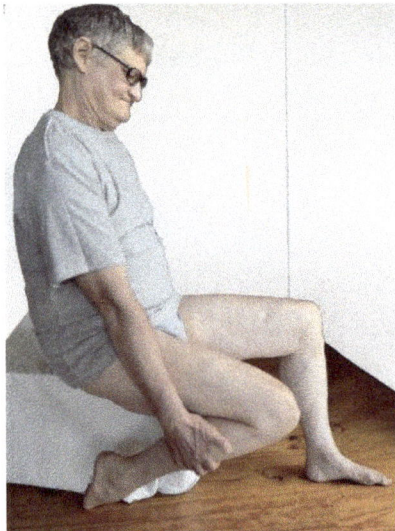

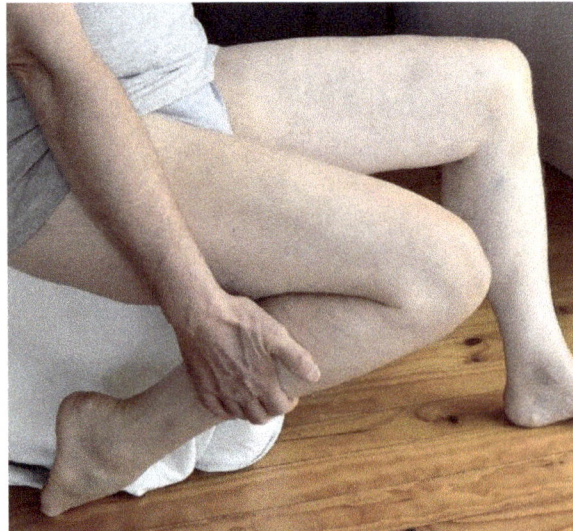

- Attempt to dorsiflex your foot by pushing the top of your toes into the floor for a few seconds then cease the contraction, relax your foot, lean backwards and allow your fingertips to slide across the front of your leg.
- Reposition your fingers further down the front of your leg and repeat the kneading action.
- Work down the front of your leg almost to your ankle until the entire anterior compartment is covered.

The lateral compartment muscles

Massaging the lateral compartment muscles, fibularis longus and fibularis brevis, can be useful when there is pain down the outside of the leg from fibularis tendinitis, lateral compartment syndrome and muscle overuse and tightness.

Fibularis tendinitis can occur in the fibularis longus or brevis tendons as they pass around the back of the lateral malleolus and over the side of the foot. The tendinitis usually occurs when overuse combines with an underlying foot or ankle problem and causes irritation of the tendon. There may be pain, swelling and tenderness over the tendon. The pain may be worse when walking or running.

Lateral compartment syndrome is rare but can occur when intense or repetitive activities such as running and jumping cause the fibularis muscles to swell. If the compartment walls are tight then pressure can build up within the compartment causing nerve and muscle damage, foot numbness, burning and tingling. There may be pain down the outside of the leg and ankle stiffness. A foot or ankle problem such as a lateral ankle ligament strain can cause fibularis muscle overuse because the muscle tries to compensate for the problem, resulting in pain, tightness and fibrous changes within the muscles.

Fibularis longus arises on the head and upper two-thirds of the lateral shaft of the fibula and from the deep fascia. The tendon is long and passes over a groove behind the lateral malleolus, which it shares with the fibularis brevis tendon. It runs over the side of the calcaneus and then goes deep under the foot. It attaches on the first metatarsal and first cuneiform.

Fibularis brevis arises on the middle third of the lateral shaft of the fibula and intermuscular fascia of the leg. The tendon attaches on the tuberosity or styloid process of the fifth metatarsal.

Fibularis longus and brevis produce eversion and plantar flexion of the foot, support the lateral ligaments and stabilise the leg on the foot during side swaying. Fibularis longus also supports the arch, especially during the toe off phase of gait.

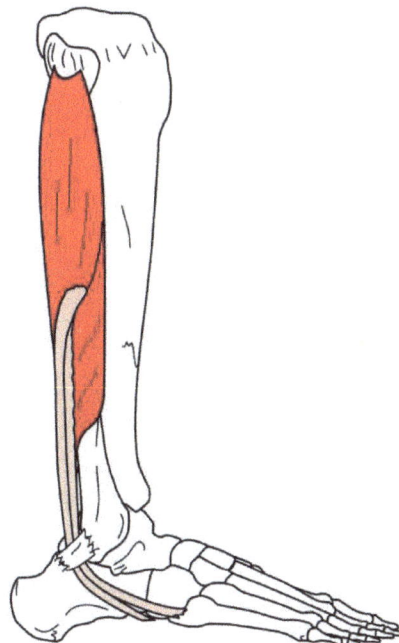

3.7a Kneading fibularis longus and brevis using the tip of your thumb while seated in chair

- Sit on a chair or stool with your feet planted on the floor.
- Flex your right hip and place the middle of the sole of your foot on a brick or block of wood and let your heel drop over the edge and onto the floor.

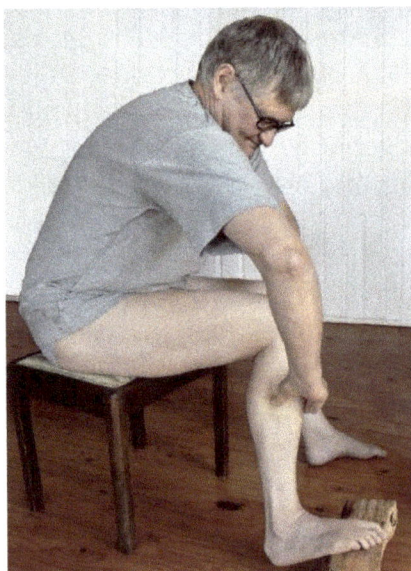

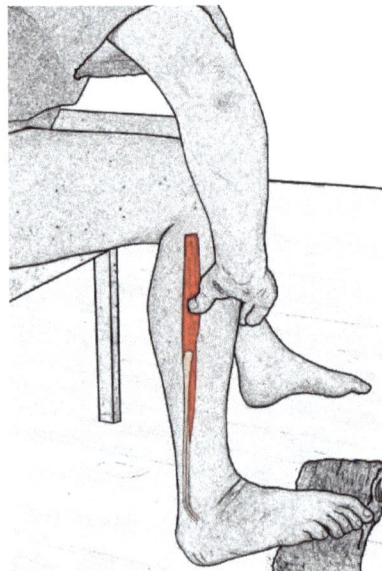

- Lean far forwards, lift your right arm, flex your elbow and then internally rotate your arm and extend your hand at the wrist so that your thumb points backwards and towards your body.
- Place the pad of your thumb on the outside of your knee and then slide it down the outside of your leg towards the foot until you feel the round bony bump just below the knee - this is the head of the fibular.
- Go over the bump until your thumb is on the outside of the shaft of the fibular - there is a nerve just after the bump, so do not press hard here.

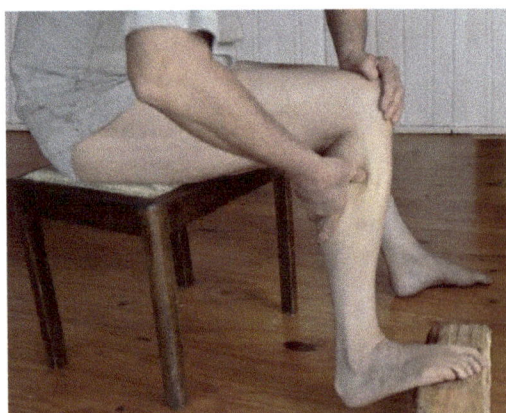

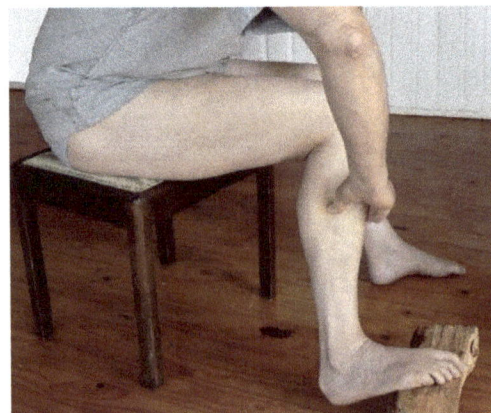

- Just below the nerve feel the fibres of the fibularis longus muscle.
- Place the tip of your thumb against the front of the muscle.
- Adjust the position of your right shoulder, elbow and wrist so your thumb points backwards towards you.
- Push into the muscle with the tip of your thumb while simultaneously dropping your heel further towards the floor and dorsiflexing your foot.

- Reposition your thumb about one centimetre further down the outside of your leg and repeat the kneading action.
- Work down the side of your leg across fibularis longus and then brevis.
- Pull across the muscles with the tips of your hooked fingers if you are unable to reach your lower leg with your thumb.

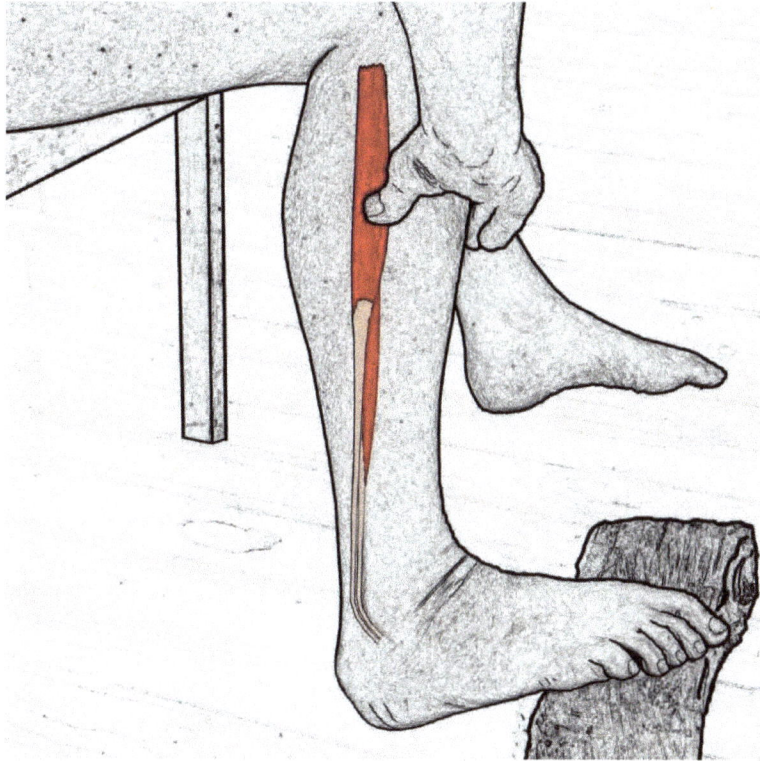

- Return to your knee and place the tip of your thumb behind the muscle.
- Drop your right elbow so your arm rotates outwards, and your thumb points forwards and away from you.
- Push into the muscle with the tip of your thumb while simultaneously dropping your heel further towards the floor and dorsiflexing your foot.
- Repeat the kneading action with your thumb until you have covered both fibularis longus and fibularis brevis along the whole outside of your leg.

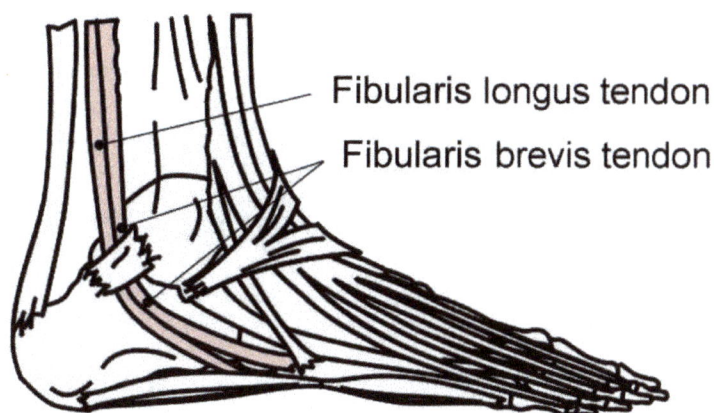

Fibularis longus tendon

Fibularis brevis tendon

Foot lateral view - fibularis tendons

3.7b Transverse friction over the fibularis longus and brevis tendons using the tip of your thumb while sitting on the floor

- Sit on the floor with your hips and knees flexed, feet planted on the floor in front of you and the palms of both hands flat on the floor behind you.
- Twist your hips to the left and drop your knees to the floor.

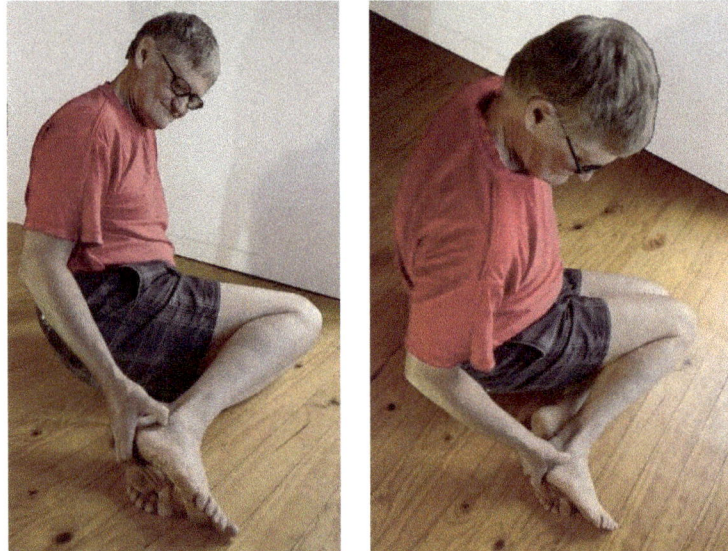

- Flex and sidebend your trunk to the right and lean towards your feet.
- Lift your right arm and flex your elbow to about 90 degrees, then internally rotate your arm and place the tip of your thumb on the outside of your right foot and the pads of your fingers underneath your heel.

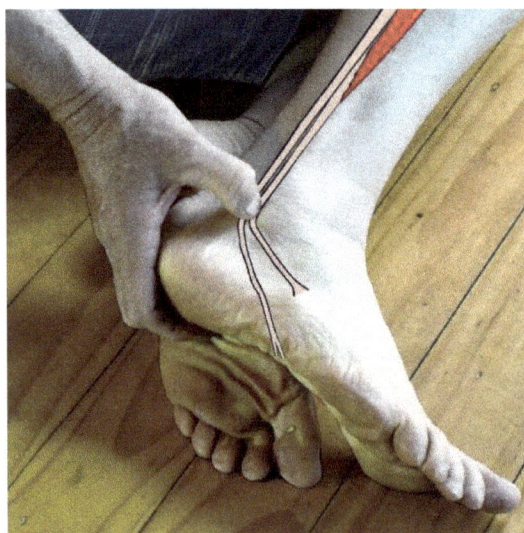

Lateral view of foot and the fibularis tendons passing around the lateral malleolus

- Find the large bump, the lateral malleolus, on the outside of the ankle and the fibularis tendons that pass under it.
- If this is the location of the pain and if the tendons are tender to touch here, then this may be the site of tendinitis.

- Find the small bump just below the lateral malleolus and about one centimetre towards the little toe - this is the peroneal tubercle of the calcaneus.
- If this is the location of the pain and if the tendons are tender to touch here, then this may be the site of tendinitis.

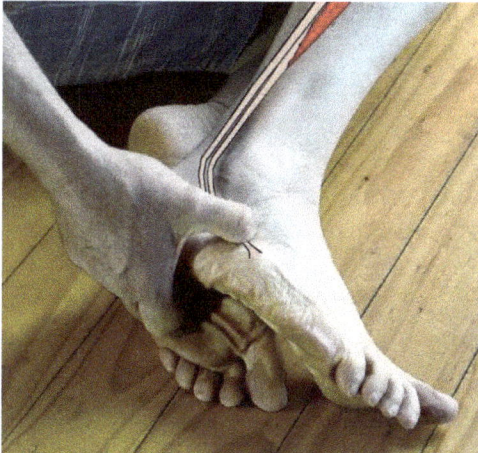

Fibularis tendons passing either side of the peroneal tubercle

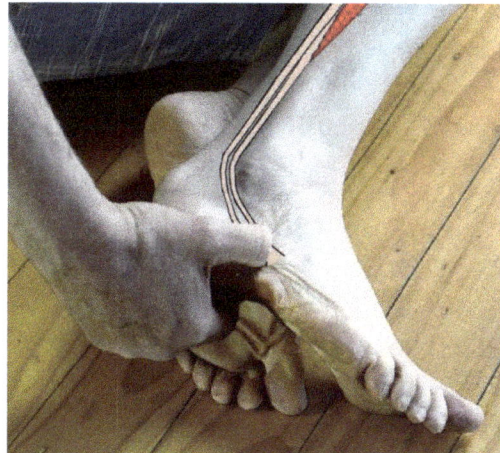

Fibularis brevis tendon attaching on the styloid process

- Find the medium size bump about halfway down the outside of the foot and in line with the little toe - this is the styloid process of the fifth metatarsal bone.
- Move your thumb back towards your heel and into the depression at the side of your foot - this is the cuboid bone where the fibularis longus tendon passes around the outside of the foot and under it.
- If this is the location of the pain and if the tendons are tender to touch here, then this may be the site of tendinitis.
- Apply transverse friction on any of these points if they are tender.

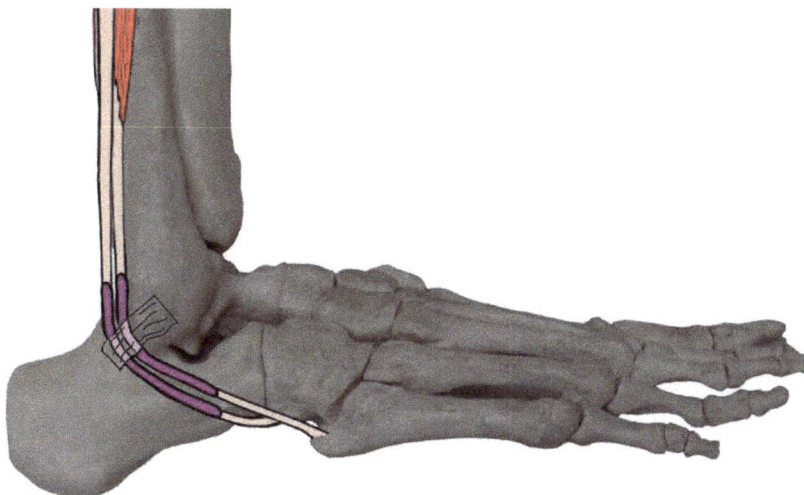

Lateral view of foot showing the fibularis tendons and the tendon sheath

The ankle and foot

Massaging the foot muscles can be useful for foot muscle cramps and strains, tendinitis, heel spurs, plantar fasciitis, ankle ligament sprains and problems resulting from fallen arches (pes planus) or abnormally high arches (pes cavus).

A muscle cramp is a sudden involuntary painful muscle contraction. In the foot they can occur from prolonged sitting or holding the foot in a fixed position, extreme cold, over-working the muscles or wearing badly fitting shoes. Muscle and tendon strains in the foot can occur from overstretching or a direct blow to the foot, stepping on a hard object or repetitive forces such as running and kicking. Symptoms include pain, swelling and stiffness and difficulty walking.

Tenosynovitis is the inflammation of the synovial sheaths that surrounds tendons. Ankle overuse, repetitive use, injury or infection can cause the problem. The tendon of tibialis anterior or posterior or fibularis longus or brevis becomes irritated, inflamed and painful and there may be ankle stiffness.

A heel spur or calcaneal spur is an outgrowth of bone from the heel, projecting down and along the sole of the foot. Plantar fasciitis is inflammation of the band of fascia running down the sole of foot. In both cases there is heel pain with weight bearing and they are caused by tight calf muscles, wearing old, ill-fitting shoes and unsupported shoes like sandals, repeatedly stressing the heel during running and jumping, overweight and osteoarthritis.

Ligament sprains can occur at any joint but one of the most common sprains is of the anterior talofibular ligament, the weakest of the lateral collateral ligaments supporting the outside of the ankle. The sprain usually occurs when walking or running on uneven ground and the foot lands awkwardly and rolls inwards resulting in pain and swelling over the outside of the foot, ankle and lower leg.

The foot has three aches the transverse arch, and the medial and lateral longitudinal arches which act like springs, storing and releasing energy during walking and supporting the weight of the body. The arches are maintained by ligaments, fascia, muscles and tendons and the failure of any of these tissues can change the arches and cause problems in the foot, knee, hip and spine. Changes can be acquired (short calf muscles) or congenital (ligament laxity).

Pes planus (flat feet) is the loss of the medial longitudinal arch. There may be pain in the midfoot, heel or ankle. Pes cavus is the elevation of the longitudinal arch of the foot or a fixed high arched foot. It usually begins in childhood and only becomes a rigid deformity later in life. It can be caused by neurological diseases, fractures, sprains, strains, tendinitis or burns. There may be pain under the heel or either side of the sole of the foot or in the knee and ankle. A failed transverse arch can lead to inflammation and pain in the forefoot and nerves between the toes can become irritated and inflamed.

The short muscles of the foot

Plantar aspect

Situated under the plantar fascia four layers of plantar muscles fan out, two from the heel to the toes and two deeper layers from below the middle of the foot to the toes.

Flexor digitorum brevis arises as a tendon on the medial process of the calcaneal tuberosity, plantar aponeurosis and fascia attached to adjacent muscles. It splits into four tendons which attach onto the middle phalanx of the lateral four toes. The tendon to the fifth toe is frequently absent. The muscle flexes the toes.

Flexor hallucis brevis arises on the plantar surface of the cuboid and third cuneiform bone and on the tibialis posterior tendon and plantar fascia. It attaches onto the base of the proximal phalanx and onto the abductor tendon. A small bone is found within the tendon. The muscle flexes the proximal phalanx of the big toe.

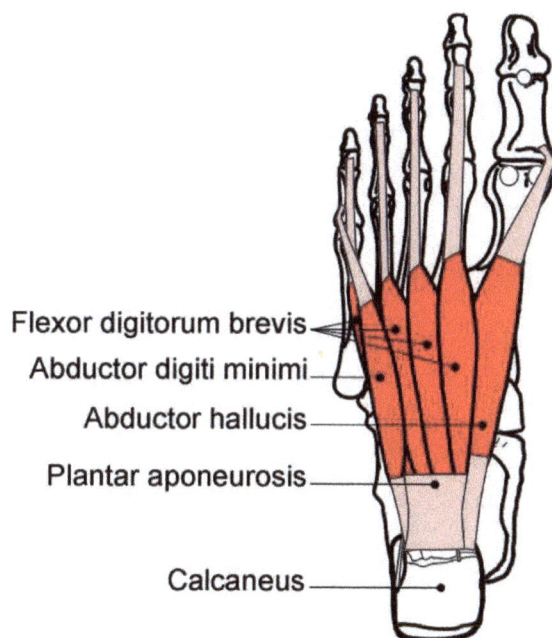

Flexor digitorum brevis

Abductor digiti minimi

Abductor hallucis

Plantar aponeurosis

Calcaneus

Short muscles of foot - inferior view

Abductor hallucis lies on the medial side of the foot and arises on the flexor retinaculum, medial process of the calcaneal tuberosity, plantar aponeurosis and fascia between it and flexor digitorum brevis. It attaches onto the medial side of the base of the proximal phalanx of the big toe. The muscle flexes and abducts the big toe.

Abductor digiti minimi arises on the lateral and medial processes of the calcaneal tuberosity and the area of bone between, plantar aponeurosis and fascia between it and flexor digitorum brevis. It attaches by a single tendon onto the lateral side of the base of the proximal phalanx of the fifth toe. The muscle is a flexor and abductor of the little toe.

Adductor hallucis arises by two heads. The oblique head arises from the base of the second, third and fourth metatarsal bones and the sheath of the peroneus longus tendon. The transverse head arises from capsules and overlying ligaments of the third, fourth and fifth metatarsophalangeal joints. It attaches onto the lateral side of the base of the proximal phalanx of the big toe. The muscle adducts and flexes the proximal phalanx of the big toe and is important for the internal strength of the foot.

Flexor digiti minimi brevis arises on the medial side of the plantar surface of the base of the fifth metatarsal bone and the sheath of the peroneus longus tendon. It attaches onto the lateral side of the base of the proximal phalanx of the fifth toe. The muscle flexes the proximal phalanx of the little toe.

The plantar interossei lie below the metatarsal bones. They arise on the base and proximal shaft on the medial sides of the third, fourth and fifth metatarsal bones and attach to the base on the medial sides of the proximal phalanx of the toes. The muscles abduct the toes and flex the proximal phalanx of the toes. They work together with the dorsal interossei to strengthen the metatarsal arch.

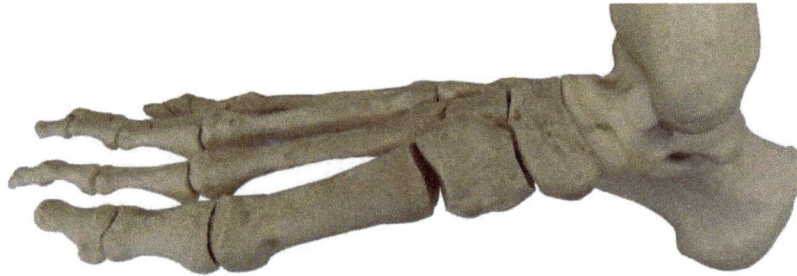

Foot, ankle and distal tibia - medial view

The plantar aponeurosis is a thick layer of fascia which helps support the longitudinal arch on the bottom of the foot by tightening as the foot bears weight. It lies superficially and fans out from the medial calcaneal tuberosity, the weight bearing part of the heel, to the heads of the metatarsal bones.

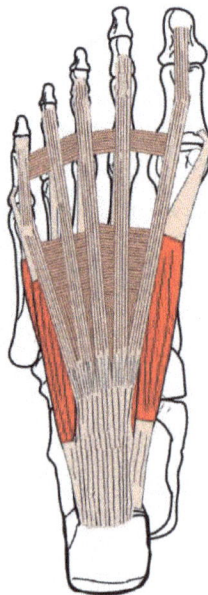

Plantar aponeurosis of foot - inferior view

194

3.8a Kneading the plantar fascia and short plantar muscles that flex the toes with the sole of your foot resting on a small ball on a mat on the floor

- Stand or sit on a chair or stool with your feet planted on the floor.
- Place a 4 cm diameter rubber ball on the mat on the floor in front of you.
- Lift your right foot and place the bottom of your heel on the ball.
- The pads of your toes and the ball of your foot remain on the floor.
- Lean forwards and bring your centre of gravity over the ball so that you can use your body weight to help push your foot against the ball.

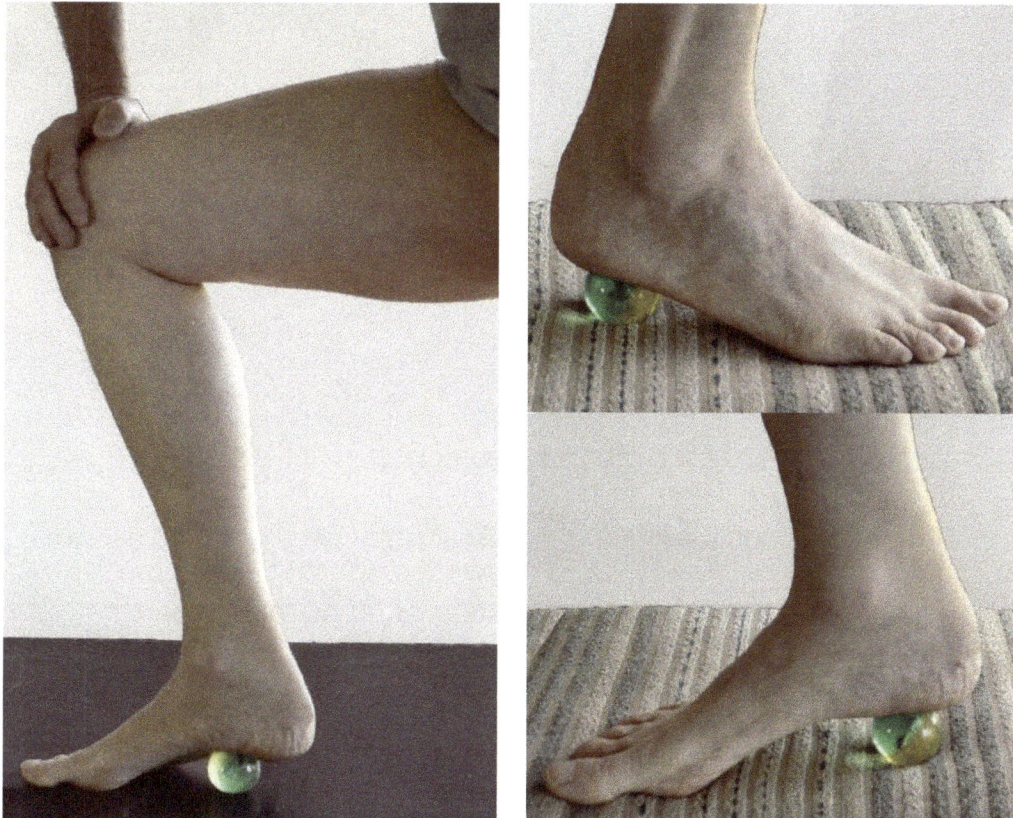

- Adjust your foot so the ball is directly under the point on the bottom of your heel where the plantar muscles and fascia emerge.
- Move your heel sideways left and right using a twisting action of your leg.
- Pivot around the end of your foot so the ball rolls across your foot.
- Push your heel down and let the ball press into the muscles and facia.
- Work down the foot along a consecutive series of parallel strips, starting at the heel and finishing at the base of the toes.
- The plantar muscles and fascia fan out as they pass down the sole of the foot and so the strips become wider.

3.8b Transverse friction over the plantar fascia using the tip of your thumb

- Sit on a chair with your feet planted on the floor.
- Raise your right foot off the floor, externally rotate your right hip and place the outside of your leg on your left knee.
- Allow your right hip to relax so your knee drops toward the floor.
- Grasp the toes of your right foot with your right hand and pull them back into extension.

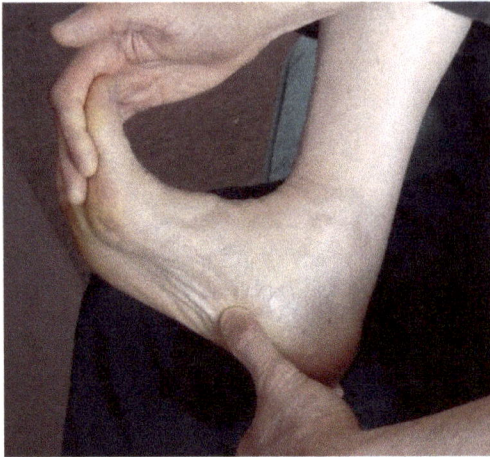

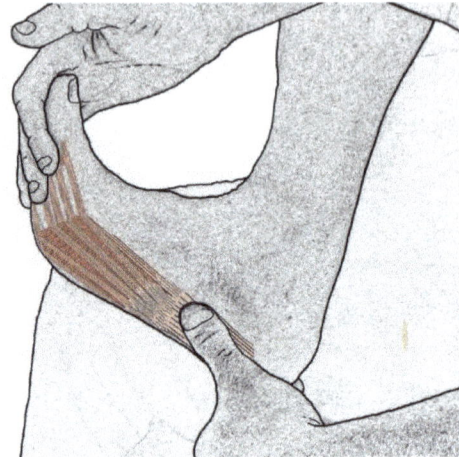

- Grasp the heel of your right foot between your fingertips and the tip of your thumb of your left hand.
- Place the tip of your left thumb on the plantar fascia, where it starts at the bottom of your heel and extends down the sole of the foot to your toes.
- Push into and across the plantar fascia using a firm pressure with the tip of your thumb.
- Keep your toes extended but relax them if the plantar fascia is very tight.
- Follow parallel strips across the sole of your foot.
- Points of tenderness may indicate plantar fasciitis

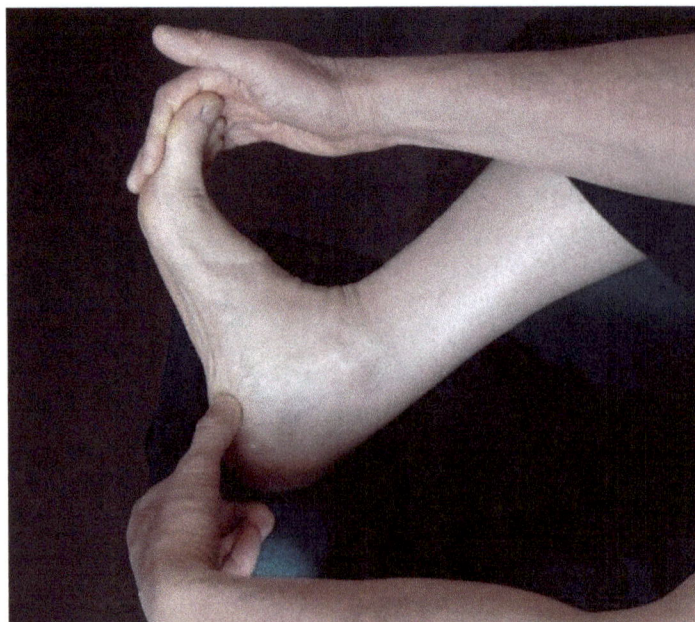

3.8c Transverse friction over the lateral collateral ligaments of the ankle using the tip of your thumb

- Sit on a chair or stool with your feet planted on the floor.
- Raise your right foot off the floor and place your heel on the edge of the chair.
- Reach forwards with your left hand and grasp your right leg and knee.
- Reach forwards with your right hand and place the tip of your thumb or index finger at the front of the ankle and just under the lateral malleolus, the large bony lump at the outside and end of your leg.

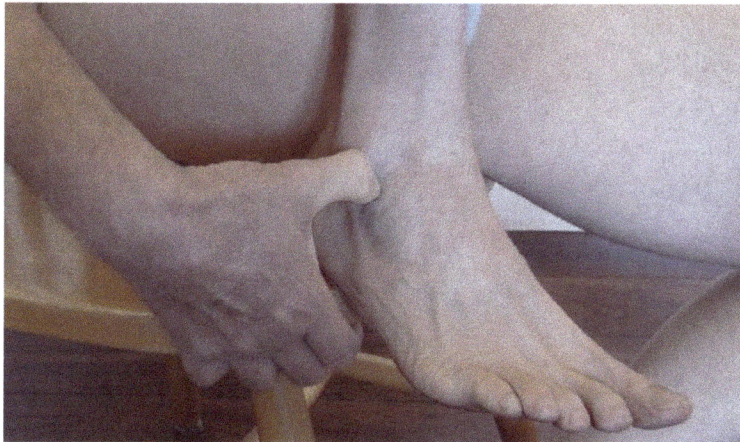

- Apply transverse friction on the anterior talofibular ligament which runs forwards from the front of the lateral malleolus to the talus.
- Move around the joint line from the front of the malleolus to just below it.
- Apply transverse friction on the calcaneofibular ligament which runs downwards from the bottom of the lateral malleolus to the calcaneus.
- Move around the joint line from the bottom of the malleolus to behind it.
- Apply transverse friction on the posterior talofibular ligament which runs backwards from the back of the malleolus to the talus.
- The ligaments will be tender if they have been sprained.

The **lateral collateral ligaments** of the ankle attach on the lateral malleolus of the fibular and go to the talus and calcaneal bones on the outside of the foot.

They limit plantar flexion and internal rotation at the ankle joint and are the primary support for the outside of the ankle.

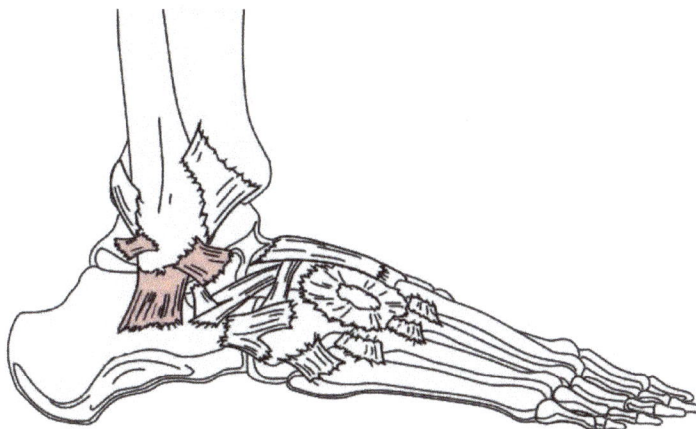

Anterior talofibular ligament, posterior talofibular ligament and calcaneofibular ligament

Dorsal aspect

Extensor digitorum brevis arises on the distal, lateral and superior surface of the calcaneus and the inferior extensor retinaculum. The medial part of the muscle, the **extensor hallucis brevis** attaches onto the dorsal aspect of the base of the proximal phalanx of the big toe. The other three tendons attach onto the lateral side of the long extensor tendons of the second, third and fourth toes. The muscles extend the toes.

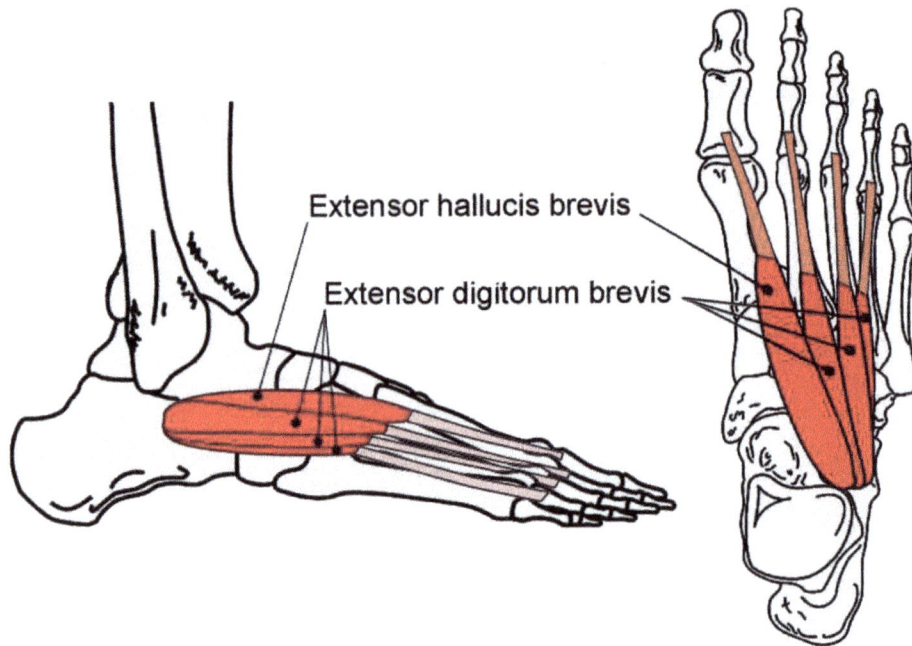

Foot - lateral view (left) superior view (right)

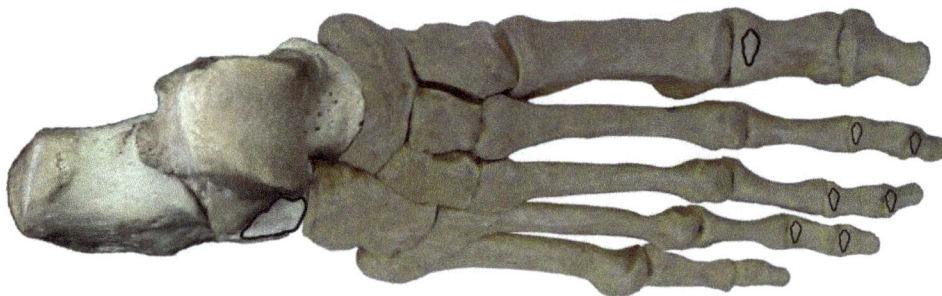

Dorsum of foot with short extensor muscle attachments marked

3.8d Kneading the short toe extensor muscles with the tip of your thumb

- Sit on a chair with your hips and knees flexed and your feet on the floor.
- Flex your right hip and knee and lift your foot off the floor and then place your heel on the edge of the chair with your foot and toes over the edge.
- Reach forwards with your left hand, grasp the front of your right leg and hold it firmly in your hand.

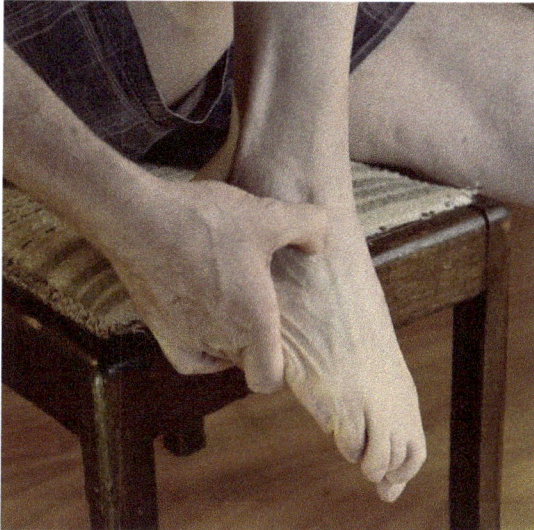

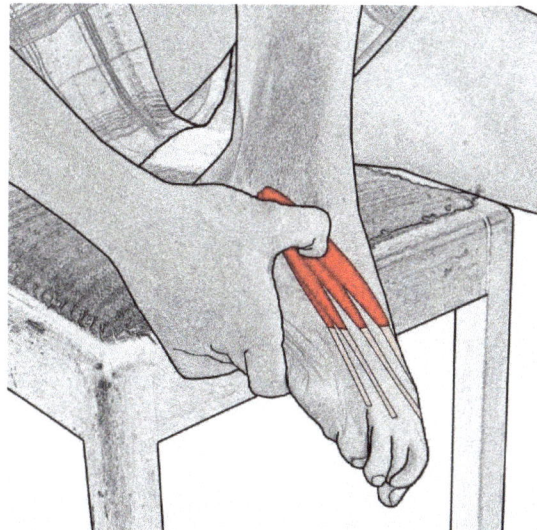

- Reach forwards with your right hand and grasp the outside of your foot.
- The pads of your fingers rest under the sole of your foot and the tip of your thumb rests on the top of your foot, near the front of your ankle.
- Feel the short dorsal toe extensor muscles which form a large mound over the top of the foot and find the most medial one going to the big toe.
- Push the tip of your thumb into this muscle - push in a medial to lateral direction while simultaneously flexing your toes.

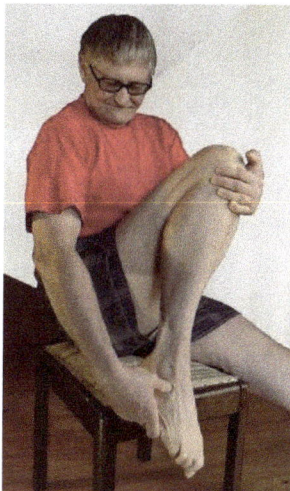

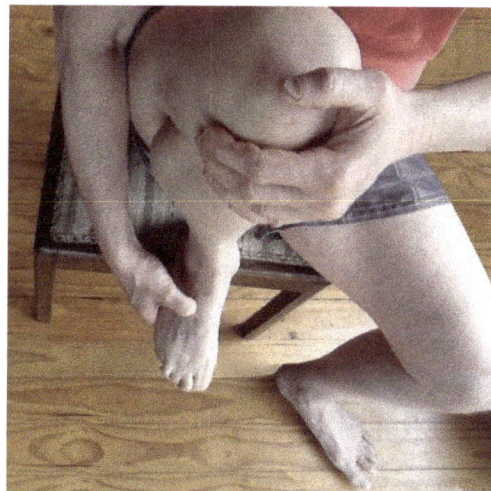

- After working down the big toe extensor muscle move the tip of your thumb to the muscle going to second toe.
- Start in front of your ankle and work down the muscle to its tendon.
- Work down the muscles going to the third and fourth toes.
- Repeat the technique pushing the tip of your thumb in a medial direction.

3.8e Kneading the dorsal interossei muscles that flex the toes using the tip of your thumb

- Sit on a chair with your hips and knees flexed and feet planted on the floor.
- Raise your right foot off the floor and place your heel on the edge of the chair with your foot and toes over the edge.
- Reach forwards with your left hand, grasp the front of your right leg and hold it firmly in your hand.
- Reach forwards and grasp the outside of your foot with your right hand.

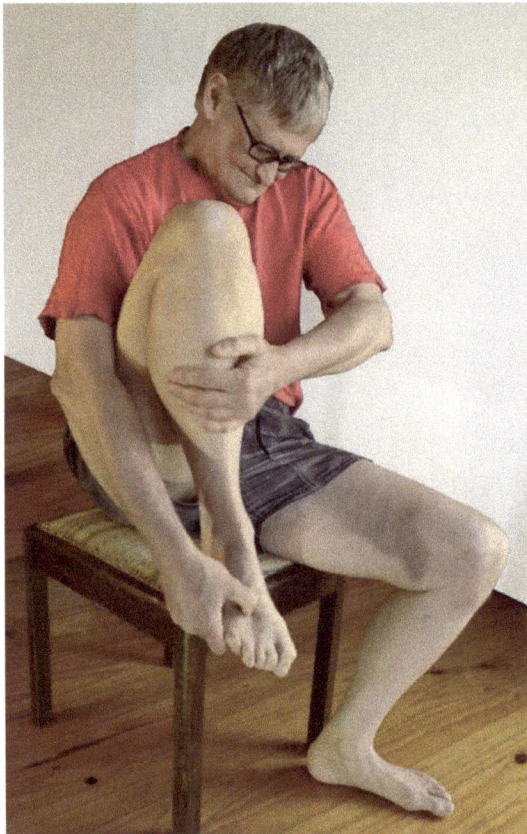

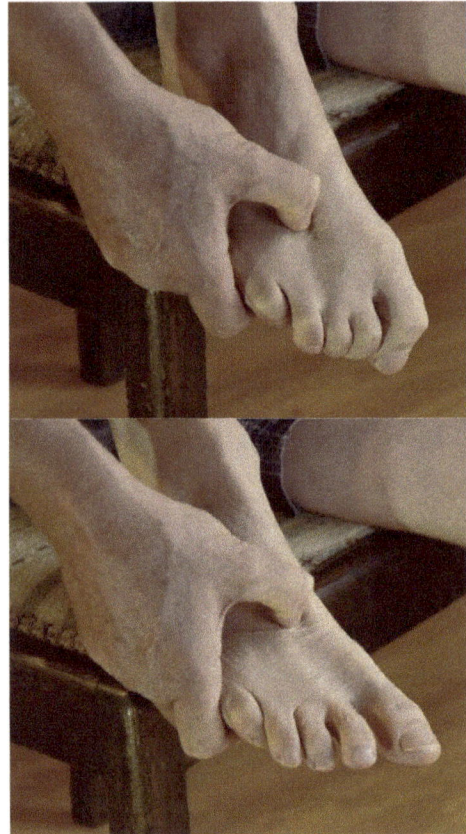

- The pads of your fingers rest under the sole of your foot and the tip of your thumb rests on the top of your foot in the depression between the first and second metatarsal bones - the long bones of the foot.
- Push the tip of your thumb firmly into the depression because the dorsal interossei muscle lies deep in the foot.
- Apply a strong counterforce with your fingers.
- As you increase the thumb pressure extend your toes.
- Work down the depression until you reach your toes and then reposition the tip of your thumb at the top of the depression between the second and third metatarsal bones and work down that dorsal interossei muscle.
- Repeat the action between all the metatarsal bones of the foot and cover all the dorsal interossei muscles.

The dorsal interossei lie deep between the metatarsal bones. They arise by two heads on adjacent sides of two metatarsal bones and attach onto the base of the proximal phalanx of the toes. These muscles abduct and flex the toes.

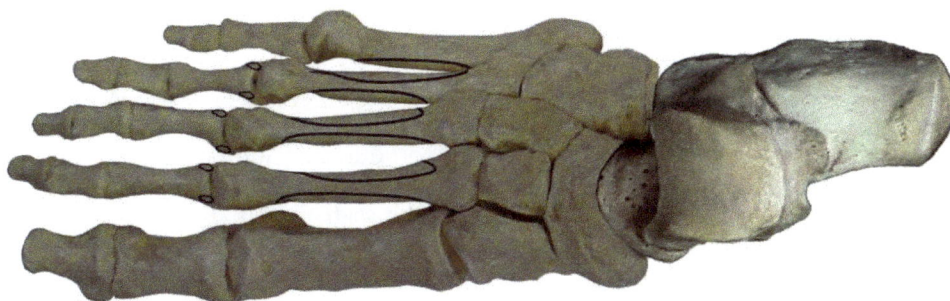

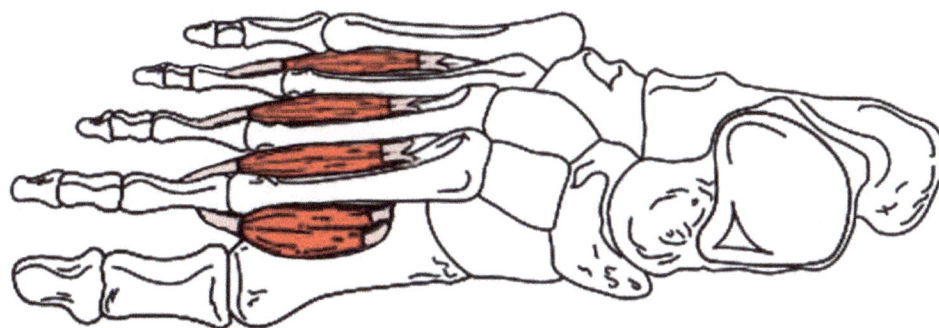

Foot dorsal interossei - superior view

Appendix 1

Glossary of terms used in this book

Abduction - taking the arm or leg sideways, up and away from the midline of the body or away from the midline of a limb. For the fingers and toes, it is moving the digits apart, away from the centreline of the hand or foot. Abduction of the wrist is also called radial deviation.

Acetabulum - a cup-shaped joint cavity on the lateral surface of the pelvis in which the head of the femur articulates.

Acromion process - a bony process on the upper and outer part of the scapula (shoulder blade).

Acute - a disease or illness with a rapid onset and short duration, for example a cold or sprain. Acute symptoms may range from mild to intense.

Adduction - taking the arm or leg down and towards the midline of body or towards the midline of a limb. For the fingers and toes, it is bringing the digits together, towards the centerline of the hand or foot. Adduction of the wrist is also called ulnar deviation..

Anatomy - a branch of biology dealing with the study of the structure of organisms, including human anatomy.

Anatomical position - erect with the arms at the side of the body and externally rotated, and the forearms fully supinated. For the superior aspect of the foot refer to dorsum or dorsal surface and for the sole of the foot refer to plantar surface.

Anterior - the front of the body or towards the front of the body or in front of something

Anterior occiput - where the head is positioned in front of the body's centre of gravity and the chin is protruding forwards. It can lead to neck pain, loss of head and neck movement, headaches, dizziness and pain in the shoulders and upper back. It is usually caused by slouching and poor sitting posture, especially while using a computer or mobile phone.

Anxiety - an unpleasant state of inner turmoil characterised by persistent feelings of nervousness, worry or dread of imminent death or future threats, real or perceived, plus physical symptoms including muscular tension, panic attacks, restlessness, fatigue, dizziness and poor concentration.

Anxiety disorders - a group of conditions including generalised anxiety disorder, social phobia, obsessive compulsive disorder, post-traumatic stress disorder, panic disorders and bruxism.

Applicator - a part of the hand or massage tool used to apply pressure on a part of the body, for example the wadi, two balls in a net, rolled-up towel, tip or pad of the thumb or finger.

Aponeurosis - a band of tough fibrous soft tissue that covers and invests muscles and other tissues and serves as support and attachment for muscles.

Asthma - an inflammatory disease, where the airways become narrow, swollen and produce extra mucus causing breathlessness, coughing, wheezing and tightness in the chest.

Atrophy - decrease in size or wasting of an organ or tissue, such as a muscle.

Bones - a dynamically active tissue that forms the skeleton. Bones have a complex structure, come in a range of shapes and sizes, and have many functions: they enable mobility, provide support, protect organs, produces blood cells and store minerals.

Breathing - the movement of the ribs and diaphragm produces inhalation and exhalation which moves air in and out of the lungs; part of the respiration process required to sustain life.

Bruxism - the habitual grinding of the teeth.

Bronchitis - inflammation of the larger airways in your lungs, from smoke, dust or a bacterial or viral infection, causing a cough, the production of mucus and shortness of breath.

Bruising - also known as a contusion, is a skin discoloration from an injury, where damaged blood vessels underneath the skin, causing them to leak into the soft tissue.

Bursitis - painful swelling of bursae that cushion the movement of tendons passing over joints. Bursae commonly become inflamed near joints that perform frequent repetitive movement such as the shoulder and hip or where there is a lot of pressure on a joint such as the elbow, knee, heel and the base of the big toe.

Buttock - rounded area at the back of the pelvis where the lower limb emerges, defined by gluteus maximus and gluteus medius, and containing the deeper hip external rotator muscles.

Capillary - the smallest of a body's blood vessels, capillaries are only one cell layer thick. They connect arterioles and venules, and enable the exchange of oxygen, carbon dioxide, water, nutrients and waste substances between the blood and the surrounding tissues.

Cartilage - a flexible connective tissue found in the joints, rib cage, nose, ear, bronchial tubes and the intervertebral discs. It is classified as fibrocartilage, elastic and hyaline cartilage.

Cervical spine - the upper seven vertebrae of the spine, usually forming a posteriorly concave lordotic curve and enabling the movement of the head.

Chin forward posture - see anterior occiput.

Chronic - a health condition or disease that persists for a long duration or at least three months, for example osteoarthritis, asthma, cancer and diabetes.

Clavicle - commonly known as the collar bone, this long, slightly S shaped bone sits over the top and front of the rib cage.

Collateral ligaments - ligaments running down the inside (medial collateral) or outside (lateral collateral) of the knee, elbow, wrist, finger and toe joints.

Condyle - a smooth large round bump at the end of a long bone that forms part of a joint, for example the knee.

Congenital - a condition that is present at birth regardless of the cause, characterised by structural deformities or birth defects, congenital heart disease is the most common type of congenital disorder.

Coccyx - the tail bones at the bottom of the spinal column, comprising of three to five separate or fused coccygeal vertebrae.

Coracoid process - a bony process palpable at the front of the shoulder but attached at the back to the top of the scapula (shoulder blade). It serves as the origin of muscles and ligaments.

Deep - away from the surface of the body.

Deep vein thrombosis (DVT) - a blood clot that forms in a deep vein in your body, usually in your legs. There may be no symptoms, or it can cause leg pain and swelling.

Disc - see intervertebral disc.

Distal - a relative term comparing the position of two body parts relative to the centre of the body, so for example, the wrist is distal to the elbow.

Dorsiflexion - movement of the foot where the toes are brought closer to the shin, decreasing the angle between the dorsum (top) of the foot and the leg, for example, the foot is dorsiflexed when walking on the heels.

Dowager hump - an abnormal forward curvature or kyphosis in the upper thoracic spine due to poor posture, genetic susceptibility or disease such as osteoporosis.

Elevation - movement in a superior or upwards direction, for example, shrugging the shoulders is elevation of the scapula.

Epicondyle - a small round rough bump, at the end of a long bone, that serves as an attachment for muscles and ligaments. An epicondyle is a projection on a condyle.

Eversion - tilting the sole of the foot away from the median plane so the outside is raised.

Extension - a straightening movement, increasing the joint angle in sagittal plane, for example straightening the knee; but in joints that can move forward and backwards such as the spine and wrist, extension is backward bending or movement in a posterior direction.

External rotation - turning a limb or body part away from the midline of the body, also known as lateral rotation.

Fasciae / Fascia - fibrous connective tissue, primarily collagen, that form sheets or bands beneath the skin (superficial fascia), around and between muscles (deep fascia) and around organs (visceral fascia).

Fatigue - feeling of tiredness which may be physical or mental, normal or abnormal. Physical fatigue is the inability of a muscle to maintain tone and postural support; mental fatigue is a temporary decrease in performance resulting from prolonged periods of cognitive activity; normal fatigue can usually be alleviated by periods of rest and may be the result of prolonged working or other activity, mental stress, jet lag, boredom and lack of sleep; abnormal fatigue may be due to disease, minor illness, mineral or vitamin deficiency, blood loss and anaemia.

Fibres - have different meanings in the body depending on their location. In fasciae, tendons and ligaments fibres are proteins such as collagen and elastin, in muscles they are cells, while in nerves they are the axons that conducts electrical impulses away from the cell body.

Fibrocartilage - fibrous tissue with variable amounts of cartilage and other materials depending on its location and function; is present in menisci, articular discs, the annulus fibrosus of intervertebral discs, the glenoid and acetabular labra, discs of the symphysis pubis and temporomandibular joints. At the tendon-bone interface it is dense white fibrocartilage, whereas in the external ears and larynx it is yellow elastic fibrocartilage.

Fibrosis - the deposition of excess fibrous tissue in a soft tissue such as a muscle as a result of injury, burns, inflammation or disease.

Flexibility - an attribute of any viscoelastic tissue to lengthen or be compressed or the active or passive extensibility of a muscle.

Flexion - narrowing of a joint angle in a sagittal plane, for example bending the knee; but in joints that can move forwards and backwards such as in the spine and wrist, flexion is forward bending or movement in an anterior direction.

Force - energy exerted to change a body from a state of rest to one of motion, or changes its rate of motion, including muscle contraction and gravity.

Fracture - a broken bone that can range from a thin crack or partial fracture to a complete fracture and the bone can fracture lengthwise, crosswise, in one place or into many pieces.

Gait - walking or locomotion of the human body through the movement of limbs; the cyclic loss and recovery of balance with the least expenditure of energy; two phases of gait - stance and swing are further divided into smaller components, including heel strike and toe off.

Genes - the molecular units of heredity; blueprints containing the codes for the production of proteins, and which determine the shape, structure and function of all living things.

Genetics - the study of genes, heredity, and genetic variation in living organisms.

Gluteal muscles - gluteus maximus, gluteus medius and gluteus minimus

Golfers elbow strain - overuse or repetitive use of the flexor muscles of the forearm resulting in inflammation and pain of the tendon or tendinitis on the inside of the elbow; it is usually caused by work related activity rather than golf; also known as medial epicondylitis

Groin - crease in front of the hip, where your abdomen ends and the front of your thigh begins.

Hip joint - a ball and socket joint between the thigh bone or femur and the acetabulum of the pelvis. It supports the weight of the body during standing, walking or running.

Hyperextension - movement of a joint beyond its normal limit or range of movement.

Hypothenar eminence - a group of small muscles that form a pad at the base of the little finger on the inside of the palm and assist with movement of the little finger.

Hypertonic / hypertonicity - excessive tone or tension in a muscle resulting in firmness, shortness, stiffness and increased resistance to stretching.

Hypertrophy - increase and growth of muscle cells and muscle size usually through exercise but sometimes because of overuse.

Inferior or caudal - away from the head so for example the foot is at the inferior extremity of the body

Internal rotation - turning a limb towards the midline of the body, also called medial rotation.

Intervertebral disc - a fibrocartilagenous disc acting as a shock absorber between vertebrae, helping hold the vertebral bodies together, and facilitating movement of the spinal column.

Intervertebral disc degeneration - the loss of structural integrity within a disc resulting in thinning or bulging of the disc.

Inversion - tilting the sole of the foot towards the midline of the body so the inside of the foot is raised.

Ischial tuberosities - two bony swellings at the base of the pelvis that bear the weight of the body during sitting; also called sit bones, sitting bones or buttock bones.

Joint capsule - an envelope surrounding a synovial joint, made up of an outer fibrous layer and an inner synovial layer or membrane.

Joint degeneration - joint disease that results from the breakdown of joint cartilage; also known as osteoarthritis; symptoms include joint pain and stiffness and muscle pain.

Joint movement - the degree of movement varies according to the type of joint so most fibrous joints such as in the skull permit little or no mobility, cartilaginous joints such as in the intervertebral discs permits slight mobility, and synovial joints are freely movable.

Joint stiffness - inability or difficulty moving a joint or the partial or complete loss of range of motion; may be associated with pain, swelling and other symptoms; may be caused by injury or disease in the joint, such as osteoarthritis, or injury or inflammation in an adjacent area, such as a bursae; when a joint does not move at all it is said to be ankylosed.

Joint - where two bones connect to allow movement and provide mechanical support.

Knee joint - joint between the thigh and the leg and consists of two articulations: one between the femur and tibia, and one between the femur and patella.

Kyphosis - a normal outward convex curvature of the thoracic spine; when exaggerated it is called an increased kyphosis or hunchback; when diminished it is called a decreased kyphosis or reversed kyphosis.

Lateral - away from the midline or sagittal plane of the body.

Lateral flexion - to move the spine or head sideways, also known as sidebending.

Ligaments - fibrous connective tissue that connects bones to other bones, controlling movement and providing stability.

Ligament laxity - the loss of structural integrity in a ligament because of overstretching, injury or for genetic reasons resulting in the loss of support and stability in joints.

Ligament sprain - a joint that is forced beyond its normal range of motion causing overstretched or torn ligaments; symptoms usually include swelling and pain, and, depending on the severity of the sprain, joint hypermobility and instability, for example rolling your ankle.

Load - a force which is applied to a structure; a weight or mass that is supported or carried.

Localisation - something confined to a small area of the body, for example a sign such as redness, swelling or soft tissue mass or a symptom such as pain or numbness.

Longitudinal - running in the direction of the long axis of the body or body part.

Lordosis - a normal inward, concave curvature of the lumbar or cervical spine; when the curve is exaggerated it is called an increased lordosis or swayback, when it diminished it is called a decreased or reversed lordosis.

Lower back pain - this may occur from an injury to the sacroiliac ligaments or muscles or ligament of the lumbar spine or from spinal defects, disc or joint degeneration.

Lumbar spine - the lower five vertebrae of the spine, usually forming a posteriorly concave lordotic curve and enabling the movement of the trunk and upper body.

Lymph - a type of fluid contained within the lymphatic system of the body. Like the venous system, the lymphatic system returns lymph from the tissues to the central circulation.

Massage - the application of pressure on a soft tissue of the body. The applicator can be a body part, for example the tip or pad of a finger or thumb, palm of hand or knuckle or it can be a tool, for example a ball or tightly rolled-up towel. The pressure can be light to hard or from focal to broad. Usually done by one person on another but can be done on oneself.

Malleoli - the two bony protuberances on either side of the ankle, formed by the lower ends of the tibia and fibula.

Mandible - the jawbone holds the lower teeth in place and assists chewing.

Malocclusion - a dental problems where the top and bottom teeth do not meet properly.

Manual therapy - hands-on physical therapy to correct abnormal structural changes in tissues, restore normal function in joints and reduce symptoms such as pain, by mobilising restricted joints, relaxing tense muscles, increasing circulation and breaking up scar tissue.

Medial - towards the midline or sagittal plane of the body.

Metacarpophalangeal joint - articulation between the distal end of a metacarpal bone and the proximal end of a phalanx or finger bone of the hand.

Metatarsals - the five long bones of the forefoot that articulate with the toes.

Midfoot - the part of the foot between the hindfoot and forefoot and comprised of the navicular, cuboid and the three cuneiform bones.

Mobility - the ability to move a joint, actively or passively, through a range of motion; may also be called motion or movement.

Muscle fibres - a term used when describing muscle cells.

Muscle fibrosis - the deposition of excess fibrous tissue in a muscle as a result of injury, cramps, spasms, inflammation, postural fatigue and other types of prolonged use. A fibrous muscle is less elastic and there is a firm hard end feel when compressing or stretching it.

Muscle spasm or cramp - a sudden, involuntary contraction of a muscle or group of muscles, usually accompanied by pain.

Muscle strain - an injury to a muscle where the muscle fibres are torn as a result of overstretching, commonly known as a pulled muscle.

Muscle tension / tone - the continuous and passive contraction of a muscle, affecting its ability to contract and its resistance to stretching. Optimal muscle tension or tone helps maintain posture but too much (hypertonicity) or too little (hypotonicity) can cause problems.

Muscles - a soft tissue responsible for maintaining posture, locomotion and movement of joints, and present in some organs, such as the heart and gut. Muscle cells contain the proteins that slide over one another producing muscle contraction and generating force and motion.

Myofibril - composed of proteins, myofibrils are the basic unit of a muscle; each muscle cell or fibre contains many chains of myofibrils.

Nervous system - consists of the central nervous system containing the brain and spinal cord and the peripheral nervous system consisting of nerves. It uses electrical and chemical mechanisms to send and receive signals, enables different parts to communicate with each other, and reacts to changes both outside and inside the body.

Occiput - a bone at the base of the skull that articulates with the atlas at the top of the spine.

Osteoarthritis - a form of joint disease or degeneration where the protective cartilage that cushions the ends of bones wears down, causing swelling, pain, the development of osteophytes, or bony spurs and eventual loss of movement. It can occur as a result of major or minor trauma, infection, genetic factors, compensation and natural ageing processes.

Osteophytes - bony growth or spur associated with osteoarthritis.

Osteoporosis - loss of calcium in bones that occurs more quickly than the body can replace it, causing a loss of bone density or mass which can lead to fractures. There may be no symptoms until a broken bone occurs. The most common sites are the hip, spine, forearm and wrist.

Overuse syndrome, also known as Occupational Overuse Syndrome (OOS) or repetitive strain injury - an umbrella term for many forms of tendinitis, tenosynovitis, bursitis and tunnel syndromes, and involving repetitive movements, usually with the fingers, hands, wrists, elbows and shoulders with activities like sewing, assembly line work, playing a musical instrument or using a computer. Symptoms include pain, swelling, numbness, stiffness and weakness.

Palpation - the art and skill of feeling the tissues of the body and recognising the difference between healthy and unhealthy tissues.

Patella - the kneecap is a thick, rounded, triangular bone overlying and protecting the anterior surface of the knee joint and articulating with the femur.

Pes cavus - a high-arched and supinated foot.

Pes planus - a low-arched and pronated foot or flat foot.

Pisiform bone - the smallest of the carpal bones that form part of the wrist joint, and is situated in line with the little finger, in front of the wrist.

Plantar flexion - movement of the foot away from the shin, increasing the angle between the foot and the front of the leg, for example, the foot is plantar flexed like when walking on tiptoes.

Poor posture - an extreme posture requires lots of energy to maintain, usually a forward slouching posture where posterior spinal muscles must work hard against the force of gravity.

Posterior - the back of the body or towards the back of the body or behind something.

Posture - the position of a person's body when standing or sitting; good posture depends on bony alignment, structural integrity of ligaments and muscle, and muscle tone and power supporting the joints of the body.

Postural fatigue - the exhaustion of a muscle after prolonged contraction, especially after attempting to maintain a slouched forward posture.

Processes - a small bony projection, which can form part of a joint or serve as the attachment point for ligaments and muscles.

Pronate or pronation - the inward rotation of the forearm when the elbow is at 90 degrees flexion; also, the outward movement of the foot during walking or running.

Protraction - lateral movement of the scapula along the rib cage and away from the spine.

Proximal - a relative term comparing the position of two body parts relative to the centre of the body, so for example, the elbow is proximal to the wrist.

Range of movement - distance a joint can move, for example full flexion and full extension.

Repetitive strain injury (RSI) - symptoms such as pain, swelling, numbness and stiffness caused by repetitive movements, patterns of overuse or maintaining an awkward or bad posture for a long time. Problems commonly occur in the fingers, hands, wrists and elbows.

Retraction - the medial movement of the scapula along the rib cage and towards the spine.

Reversed kyphosis - reversal of the normal outward convex curvature of the thoracic spine, so the thoracic spine is straight or is extended inwards, sometimes called a poker back.

Reversed lordosis - reversal of the normal inward, concave curvature of the lumbar or cervical spine so these parts of the spine are flexed.

Rheumatoid arthritis - a systemic inflammatory disease causing the joints of the wrist and hands to become warm, swollen, painful and stiff. The disease may also affect other parts of the body including the lungs and heart.

Rotation - a twisting or turning motion in the spine, head and limbs.

Rotator cuff tendon tears - a tear of one or more of the tendons of the four rotator cuff muscles of the shoulder, usually the supraspinatus, as it passes below the acromion.

Rounded shoulders - a faulty posture characterized by an increase thoracic kyphosis, two protracted scapula and short pectoralis muscles.

Sacroiliac joints - two joints between the sacrum and the right and left ilium of the pelvis are supported by strong ligaments and formed by irregular interlocking elevations and depressions; they are highly variable from person to person.

Sacrum - a large triangular bone at the bottom of the spinal column and wedged between the two wing shaped iliac bones of the pelvis, formed from the fusing of five sacral vertebrae.

Scapula - commonly known as the shoulder blade, this flat triangular bone covers the upper half of the back of the rib cage.

Scar tissue / Scarring - the deposition of fibrous connective tissue mainly collagen, as a result of injury, burns, disease, surgery or anything that has caused tissue damage.

Sciatica - pain or pins and needles in the buttocks, back of the thighs, calves and feet; usually from a disc bulge or herniated disc pressing on the sciatic nerve but can be from a narrowing of the spine (spinal stenosis), defect in the vertebrae (spondylolisthesis), spasm of the piriformis muscle or spinal tumour.

Scoliosis - a sidebent curvature of the cervical, thoracic, thoracolumbar, lumbar or sacroiliac spine. There may be single, double or multiple curves. Curves are usually combined with rotation.

Shoulder - consist of three bones: the upper arm bone or humerus, the shoulder blade or scapula and the collarbone or clavicle, all connected to the trunk by four joints and supported by a series of muscles, tendons and ligaments.

Shoulder joint - a ball-and-socket joint or glenohumeral joint with the ball part at the top of the humerus bone and the socket formed by the outer edge of the scapula.

Shoulder pain - can be from muscle tension, a fracture, frozen shoulder, dislocation, rotator cuff strain or tendinitis, bursitis, osteoarthritis or can be referred from a nerve in the neck.

Sidebending - to move the spine or head sideways, also known as lateral flexion

Skin - the outer layer of the human body is made up of epidermis, dermis and hypodermis. It contains fat, connective tissue, hair follicles, sweat glands, receptors and sensory nerve endings, which provide information on pain, touch, heat, and cold. Our skin regulates our body temperature and protects us from the outside environment.

Soft tissue - tissues that connect, support or surround other structures; all tissues, including muscles, fascia, tendons and ligaments, but not bone, teeth, nails, hair, and cartilage.

Spasm - a sudden involuntary muscle contraction or cramp often accompanied by pain.

Spasticity - stiff inflexible motion, muscle excitability and incomplete range of movement, caused by a spinal cord or brain lesion.

Spine - made up of twenty-four bones called vertebrae, divided into three groups: cervical, thoracic and lumbar, plus five fused bones forming the sacrum. In between each vertebrae is an intervertebral disc that acts as a cushion.

Spinous process - a bony projection at the back of each spinal vertebra, which serves as the attachment for spinal ligaments and muscles.

Sprain - see Ligament sprain.

Stability - is concerned with the proper alignment of joints so that the bones are taking most of the stress, not the overlying tissues. Joint stability depends on the resistance offered by various tissues that surround a joint.

Sternum - commonly known as the breastbone, the sternum is a large flat bone, which articulates with the clavicle and costal cartilages of the rib cage and helps protect the heart, lungs, and major blood vessels from injury.

Subacromial bursitis - painful swelling of the bursae situated within the subacromial space of the shoulder, usually after irritation by the supraspinatus tendons passing over it.

Suboccipital spine - this consists of the occiput, which forms the base of the skull, the first two vertebrae of the spine, the atlas and axis, and the suboccipital muscles, a group of small muscles located at the top and back of the neck, deep under the base of the skull and trapezius muscle.

Superficial - near or towards the surface of the body.

Superior or cranial - toward the head end of the body.

Supinate or supination - rotating the forearm outwards

Swelling - abnormal enlargement of a part of the body, as a result of an accumulation of fluid.

Synovial fluid - viscous fluid found in the cavities of synovial joints and functioning to reduce friction between the articular cartilage of joints during movement.

Synovial joint - a joints that contains synovial fluid to aid friction-free movement.

Synovial membrane - inner membrane of synovial joints which secretes synovial fluid into the joint cavity.

Temporomandibular joint (TMJ) - a synovial joint between the mandible (jaw) and the temporal bones of the skull, which permits a sliding hinge action for speaking, eating and facial expression.

Tendinitis - also known as tendonitis, this is an acute tendon injury or irritation accompanied by inflammation, examples include Achilles tendinitis, patellar tendinitis and tennis elbow.

Tendons - tough fibrous connective tissue, mainly of collagen, that connect muscle to bone.

Tennis elbow strain - overuse or repetitive use of the extensor muscles of the forearm resulting in inflammation and pain of the tendon or tendinitis on the outside of the elbow; it is usually caused by work related activity rather than tennis; also known as lateral epicondylitis.

Tension - may be related to increased psychoemotional stress or muscle tension.

Thoracic spine - the middle twelve vertebrae of the spine, usually forming a posteriorly convex kyphotic curve and enabling the movement of the trunk, ribs and upper body.

Tension headache - the most common type of headache with symptoms that range from a diffuse, mild to moderate pain behind the eyes and across the front, sides or back of the head, a tight band and feeling of pressure around the forehead, and associated neck and shoulder muscle pain and tension.

Thenar eminence - a group of small muscles that form a pad at the base of the thumb on the outside of the palm and assist with movement of the thumb.

Thoracic outlet syndrome - a group of disorders that occur when blood vessels or nerves between the clavicle and first rib are compressed, resulting in shoulder pain and numbness in the fingers. Causes include trauma, poor posture and anatomical defects such as having an extra rib.

Tonic fibres - relating to slow-twitch postural muscles that contract slowly but can go for a long time before they fatigue; they are slow to fatigue and quick to recover.

Torticollis, spasmodic or spastic torticollis - commonly known as a wry neck this is a painful involuntarily neurological disorder causing the neck to bend to one side; it may be congenital, chronic, acquired or acute.

Transverse - situated or extending across something.

Transverse process - one of two small bony projections either side of a spinal vertebra, which serve as the attachment point for spinal ligaments and muscles.

Tubercle - a round lump projecting from a bone, sometimes an alternative name to a tuberosity.

Tuberosity - a round lump projecting from a bone, for example the humerus, tibia, ulna, radius and ischium bone of the pelvis.

Upper back pain - upper thoracic, rib and shoulder pain may be caused by whiplash injuries, overuse, strains or postural fatigue, especially when there is an increased kyphosis or scoliosis.

Vertebra - one of a series of small bones forming the spinal column, made up of a body at the front and projections for articulation and muscle attachments at the back, with a hole through the middle where the spinal cord passes.

Whiplash - a neck injury due to forceful, rapid backward and forward head movement. Symptoms include pain in the neck, shoulders, upper back and arms, neck stiffness, headaches, dizziness and tingling or numbness down the arms.

Appendix 2

Muscles involved with joint movement in the upper and lower limbs

Movement involves the prime movers, which are the main muscles that move the joint, assistants to the prime movers, stabilisers that hold a bone steady so the prime movers can work, antagonists that work against the prime mover which must relax when the prime mover contracts. Here are the prime mover and assistant muscles and the direction they act.

The Shoulder is a complex of joints working in anatomical cooperation.

Flexion	Anterior Deltoid (especially after 90°)
	Pectoralis major (clavicular portion)
	Assistants: Biceps and Coracobrachialis
Extension	Latissimus dorsi
	Teres major
	Posterior Deltoid
	Pectoralis major (sternal portion)
	Assistant: Triceps
Adduction	Pectoralis major (sternal)
	Latissimus dorsi
	Teres major
	Assistants: Posterior Deltoid, Biceps and Triceps
Abduction	First phase (0 - 90°)
	Supraspinatus then Middle Deltoid.
	Second phase (90 - 150°)
	Trapezius and Serratus anterior.
	Third phase (150 - 180°)
	Erector spinae muscles and Pectoralis minor
External Rotation	Teres minor
	Infraspinatus
	Assistant: Posterior Deltoid
Internal Rotation	Latissimus dorsi
	Teres major
	Subscapularis
	Pectoralis major
	Assistants: Coracobrachialis and Anterior Deltoid
Horizontal Flexion	Anterior Deltoid
	Pectoralis major (all fibres)
	Subscapularis
	Coracobrachialis.
	Assistant: Biceps
Horizontal Extension	Posterior and Middle Deltoid
	Latissimus dorsi
	Teres major
	Infraspinatus
	Teres minor
Scapula Elevation	Levator scapulae
	Upper Trapezius
	Rhomboids
Abduction/Protraction	Serratus Anterior
	Pectoralis Minor
Adduction/Retraction	Rhomboids
	Middle Trapezius

The Elbow includes the humeroulnar joint, humeroradial joint and proximal radioulnar joint.

Flexion	Biceps
	Brachialis
	Brachioradialis
	Assistants: Pronator teres
Extension	Triceps
	Assistant: Anconeus
Pronation	Pronator Teres
	Pronator Quadratus
Supination	Supinator
	Biceps

The Wrist and Hand include the proximal and distal carpal joints and distal radioulnar joint.

Flexion	Flexor carpi radialis
	Flexor carpi ulnaris
	Palmaris longus.
	Assistants: The finger flexor muscles
	Flexor digitorum profundus and Flexor digitorum superficialis
Extension	Extensor carpi radialis longus
	Extensor carpi radialis brevis
	Extensor carpi ulnaris
	Assistants: The finger extensor muscles
	Extensor digitorum and Extensor pollicis longus
Abduction or Radial deviation	Extensor carpi radialis longus
	Extensor carpi radialis brevis
	Assistants: Flexor carpi radialis, Abductor pollicis longus
	Extensor pollicis longus and brevis
Adduction or Ulnar deviation	Extensor carpi ulnaris
	Flexor carpi ulnaris

The Hip

Flexion	Iliopsoas
	Sartorius,
	Pectineus
	Tensor fasciae latae
	Assistants: Rectus femoris, Gracilis,
	Adductor longus and Adductor brevis
Extension	Hamstrings (Semimembranosus, Semitendinosus, Biceps femoris)
	Gluteus maximus (especially in flexion).
	Assistant: Adductor magnus (especially in flexion)
Adduction	Adductor Longus
	Adductor Brevis
	Adductor Magnus
	Gracilis
	Assistants: Pectineus, Gluteus maximus and Hamstrings
Abduction	Gluteus Medius Gluteus Minimus
	Tensor Fasciae Latae (especially in extension)
	Assistant: Gluteus maximus
External Rotation	Piriformis
	Quadratus Femoris
	Obturator Internus
	Obturator externus
	Gemellus superior
	Gemellus inferior
	Gluteus maximus

210

Internal Rotation	Gluteus medius
	Gluteus minimus
	Assistants: Tensor fasciae latae and
	Adductor magnus

The Knee

Flexion	Hamstrings
	Sartorius
	Gracilis
	Assistants: Popliteus and Gastrocnemius
Extension	Quadriceps Femoris (Vastus lateralis, medialis, intermedius and Rectus femoris)
Lateral Rotation	Biceps Femoris
	Tensor fascia lata
Medial Rotation	Popliteus
	Semimembranosus
	Semitendinosus
	Assistants: Sartorius and Gracilis

The Ankle and Foot

Plantar Flexion	Gastrocnemius
	Soleus
	Assistants: Peroneus longus and brevis, Tibialis posterior, Flexor digitorum longus and Flexor hallucis longus
	Tibialis anterior
Dorsi Flexion	Extensor digitorum longus
	Extensor hallucis longus
	Peroneus tertius

Index

www.ingramcontent.com/pod-product-compliance
Lightning Source LLC
Chambersburg PA
CBHW060957030426
42334CB00032B/3267